Springer Series on Geriatric Nursing

Mathy D. Mezey, EdD, RN, FAAN, Series Editor
New York University Division of Nursing

Advisory Board: Margaret Dimond, PhD, RN, FAAN; Steven H. Ferris, PhD; Terry Fulmer, PhD, RN, FAAN; Linda Kaeser, PhD, RN, ACSW, FAAN; Virginia Kayser-Jones, PhD, RN, FAAN; Eugenia Siegler, MD; Neville E. Strumpf, PhD, RN, FAAN; May Wykle, PhD, RN, FAAN; Mary K. Walker, PhD, RN, FAAN

Terry Fulmer, PhD, RN, FAAN, is a Professor of Nursing at New York University Division of Nursing. She is also the co-Director for The John A. Hartford Foundation Institute for the Advancement of Geriatric Nursing Practice and Director of the Consortium of New York Geriatric Education Centers. She received her bachelor's degree from Skidmore College and her master's and doctoral degrees from Boston College. Dr. Fulmer has held academic appointments at the Boston College School of Nursing, the Harvard Division of Health Policy, the Yale School of Nursing, Columbia University, and has been the Florence Seller Visiting Professor of Geriatric Nursing at Case Western Reserve University School of Nursing. She has held hospital appointments at the Beth Israel Hospital in Boston and the Yale–New Haven Hospital and currently at the Mt. Sinai—NYU health system, where she is an attending in nursing. Dr. Fulmer is a Fellow of the American Academy of Nursing, Gerontological Society of America, and the New York Academy of Medicine. She completed a Brookdale Fellowship and is a Distinguished Practitioner of the National Academies of Practice.

Marquis D. Foreman, PhD, RN, FAAN, is an Associate Professor of Medical-Surgical Nursing at the College of Nursing, University of Illinois at Chicago. Dr. Foreman earned his diploma at St. Vincent Hospital School of Nursing, Toledo, OH, his BSN from the University of Toledo, an MSN from the Medical College of Ohio at Toledo, and his PhD in nursing from the University of Illinois at Chicago. Dr. Foreman completed a postdoctoral fellowship at the University of Illinois and has focused his research on the nursing care of hospitalized elderly. Dr. Foreman is a fellow of the American Academy of Nursing and has received numerous awards for his work, including the Mary Opal Wolanin Award for Excellence in Gerontological Clinical Nursing Research, the Harriet H. Werley New Investigator Award, and the Mosby-Cameo Nursing Research Award for his work on delirium in the hospitalized elderly.

Mary F. Walker, PhD, RN, FAAN, is Dean and Professor at the School of Nursing, Seattle University.

Kristen S. Montgomery, PhD, RNC, IBCLC, is an Assistant Professor of Nursing at The University of Texas at Austin School of Nursing. She received her doctorate in nursing at the Frances Payne Bolton School of Nursing, Case Western Reserve University in Cleveland, OH. She earned her MSN from The University of Pennsylvania, in Philadelphia, and her BSN from Oakland University. Dr. Montgomery is Co-Editor of *Maternal Child Health Nursing Research Digest*, and *Internet Resources for Nurses*, both of which received *American Journal of Nursing* Book of the Year Awards.

Critical Care Nursing
of the Elderly

Second Edition

Terry T. Fulmer, PhD, RN, FAAN
Marquis D. Foreman, PhD, RN, FAAN
Mary Walker, PhD, RN, FAAN
Editors

Kristen J. Montgomery, PhD, RN, IBCLC
Assistant Editor

 Springer Publishing Company

Copyright © 2001 by Springer Publishing Company, Inc.

Springer Publishing Company, Inc.
536 Broadway
New York, NY 10012-3955

Acquisitions Editor: Sheri W. Sussman
Production Editor: Pamela Lankas
Cover design by Susan Hauley

01 02 03 04 05 / 5 4 3 2 1

Library of Congress Cataloging-in-Publication Data

Critical care nursing of the elderly / Terry Fulmer, Marquis D. Foreman, Mary Walker, editors. Kristen S. Montgomery, assistant editor. — 2nd ed.
    p. cm. — (Springer series on geriatric nursing)
    Includes bibliographical references and index.
    ISBN 0-8261-1409-1
    1. Geriatric nursing. 2. Intensive care nursing. I. Fulmer, Terry T. II. Foreman, Marquis D. III. Walker, Mary K. IV. Series.
    [DNLM: 1. Critical Care—Aged. 2. Geriatric Nursing, WY 152 C934 2001]
  RC954.C75 2001
  610.73'61—dc21   00-067022
                                                       CIP

Printed in the United States of America by Sheridan Press.

Contents

Part III: Specialized Practice in Critical Care Nursing

Part IV: Social and Policy Issues

Foreword

Today's acute care hospital has evolved into an institution that primarily serves older people and their families. Nationally, close to 40% of patients are 65 and over, and in many hospitals this percentage grows to more than half of the patients. Even the very old, including centenarians, are now commonly treated in critical care and specialty units throughout the hospital. Yet, although the notion that children have unique needs when hospitalized is readily accepted, we have been slow to acknowledge the special needs of the hospitalized elderly. Admittedly, until recently, the knowledge necessary to advise nurses and physicians as to how to best manage older patients was sparse. Now, however, and as is so evident in this volume, our knowledge base has expanded sufficiently to offer sound guidelines for professionals who care for the hospitalized elderly.

This volume serves as an important milestone in nursing for two reasons. First, as a second edition, it reaffirms that the practice of critical care geriatric nursing has come of age. The volume reflects the increasing number of nurses actively involved in geriatric care and clinical research in hospitals.

The book continues to be an important and integral volume in the Springer Series on Geriatric Nursing. As editor of this series, I hope that, in joining with Drs. Fulmer, Foreman, and Walker and the numerous other nurses working with the elderly, we can build on the growing body of knowledge in geriatric nursing and make it widely available in book form. This should improve our practice, and thus improve the health care of all older citizens and their families.

MATHY MEZEY, EdD, RN, FAAN
New York University
Division of Nursing &
The John A. Hartford Foundation Institute for Geriatric Nursing

Preface

Critical care for older adults is commonplace today, with thousands of older adults receiving such care in emergency units, coronary care units, and recovery rooms daily. As recently as 20 years ago, such care was unusual. Elderly patients were not always recommended for open-heart surgery because it was felt that they would do poorly postoperatively. It was also common to limit surgeries on elderly patients because the "cost-benefit" was suspect. These patients were not expected to do well or to live for very long, so why do the surgery? Today we know that function, not chronological age, is a better parameter for decision making regarding therapies for health problems. Today, vigorous older adults have shown us that they can do extremely well under the rigors of very complex surgeries and therapies. Intensive care units across the country are filled with older patients who might not have been there previously.

Nurses in those same settings have begun to appreciate the need for special knowledge and skills for best practices with the elderly. Although few nurses in these settings would identify with the label of "gerontological nurse," most recognize that the majority of the patients for whom they care are increasingly frail and older. Fifty percent of all inpatient, acute-care admissions in this country are for individuals over the age of 75 and account for 21% of all inpatient days. The dramatic technological advances in health care of the past 30 years have spurred an exponential increase in availability of technology for patient care, and older patients are having joint replacements, organ transplants, and cardiac-pacing implants in numbers previously unimaginable. The challenge to be met relates to appropriate *geriatric* nursing care in critical care settings.

THE EVOLUTION OF GERONTOLOGICAL NURSING

The need for gerontological nursing was documented in the context of early almshouses by Lavinia Dock, who was struck by the special needs of elders in her practice (Dock, 1948). Burnside (1988) has summarized the evolution of gerontological nursing according to two eras: 1900 to 1940 and 1940 to the present. She states that "an exhaustive search of the nursing literature for historical information about gerontological nursing revealed little" (p. 41). This may be in part because the average life expectancy in 1900 was 47 years of age and thus was a less pressing issue for the medical profession. Stone (1969) concurred that little was written in the early 1900s about gerontological nursing. There was no theory base for practice, nor any status in the specialty. It was not until 1962 at the American Nurses Association (ANA) convention that any special meeting focused on gerontological nursing. The first geriatric nursing practice group of the ANA was formed in 1966, and in 1968 nine standards were developed by the ANA Geriatric Division. In the 1970s the first gerontological nurses were certified through the ANA. Graduate-level collegiate programs for gerontological nursing became more visible following the first such program in 1966 at Duke University under the direction of Virginia Stone. Since then, federal funding has largely driven the growth and development of gerontological nursing. Medicare, Medicaid, and the Older Americans Act have had tremendous impact on the shape of health care for the elderly in this country. The 1981 Omnibus Reconciliation Act, which modified home health benefits under Medicare, created a tremendous surge in community health nursing needs in elders and the use of gerontological nurse practitioners. With this as background, there is no doubt that federal regulations and the reimbursement structures for health care drive the development and use of the specialty. In 1996, the John A. Hartford Foundation added the development of gerontological nursing leadership to its agenda with an award of $5 million to the New York University Division of Nursing for the John A. Hartford Institute for the Advancement of Geriatric Nursing Practice. That foundation, based in New York City, has an ongoing ambitious agenda for gerontological nursing development that is expected to have an enormous impact on the profession throughout the country over the next decade and will most certainly have an impact on critical care geriatric nursing.

THE EVOLUTION OF CRITICAL CARE NURSING AS A SPECIALTY

It is interesting to review gerontological nursing history in contrast with the historical development of critical care nursing. Critical care nursing evolved in the early 1960s as medical and technical advances created a need for specialized nursing services. The intensive coronary care unit dates back to 1962, and early units relied on "dedicated patient surveillance" (Kinney, Dear, Packe, & Voorman, 1981). Medical–surgical critical care units were developed in the early 1960s for the purpose of providing intense surveillance and special technology to those who required such care (e.g., patients who required hemodialysis). Today there are more than 60,000 nurses who are members of the American Association of Critical Care Nurses (AACN), the largest specialty nursing organization. The intense pace of the critical care science has always had enormous appeal, and nurses choose these areas in large numbers. Gerontological nursing, in contrast, is one of the smallest specialty areas, with far to go in terms of student recruitment, development of specialty meetings, and impact on the profession. In the past decade, our two leading journals, *The Journal of Gerontological Nursing* and *Geriatric Nursing*, have made solid strides in the quality of the manuscripts and overall circulation. However, we must go even further if we are to have a workforce prepared to care for the growing number of older adults in this country. There is a need for more nurses certified in gerontological nursing, more geriatric nurse practitioners, and more generalists who have the requisite knowledge and skills to give excellent care in all settings where there are older adults.

The Office of Technology Assessment (1987) report entitled *Life Sustaining Technologies and the Elderly* chronicled the convergence of the two specialties. In the overview chapter, it was noted that in the early 1900s there were few, if any, successful treatments for life-threatening diseases. Care was palliative in nature, and nursing was directed primarily toward providing comfort measures. The advent of antibiotics in the 1930s, hemodialysis in the late 1940s, and pacemakers in the early 1960s forever changed the life expectancy of human beings. It was not until 1920 that insulin was isolated for the treatment of diabetes. Mechanical ventilators became routine technological support for patients (Office of Technology Assessment, 1987). The 1970s and 1980s brought with them stunning technology of a "Buck Rogers" nature. Organ transplants, artificial organs, pharmacological advances, and diagnostic capabilities reshaped health care and lifespan expectations. The issues for us today are quality of life and access to affordable health care.

There has been an interesting shift in the use of hospitals as places to die. In 1937, 37% of all individuals, regardless of age, died in institutions. By 1948, the percentage had increased to 50, and in 1961, the percentage was 61. By the 1970s, more than 70% of all deaths occurred in institutions (Scitovsky, 1984). This is not true for elders as a specific age group. With increasing age, the percentage likely to die in institutions decreases; however, the rate is still an extraordinary 50% by the age of 85 years. The palliative care movement sweeping the country promises to bring about new paradigms for the dying process.

Daniel Callahan, cofounder of the Hastings Center, a special institution dedicated to the field of medical ethics, published a very controversial text entitled *Setting Limits: Medical Goals in an Aging Society* (Callahan, 1987) that is still very relevant today. That text argued that the quality of life of elderly persons is given little consideration in proportion to the amount of health care dollars that are spent to preserve life. He argued that the focus of geriatric care should be the relief of suffering, and those heroic measures that merely extend life should not be employed. Obviously, his text generated tremendous controversy, much like the activities of Dr. Jack Kevorkian, who has championed "assisted suicide." Such controversies are often framed as "dilemmas" and the questions have stayed remarkably constant since our first edition:

- Who should receive advanced technological care?
- How old is old?
- Who should pay?
- When should care stop?
- How should care be stopped?
- Who determines viability?

In the past, the question of who should receive advanced technological care was moot because there were limited technologies available, and few people lived to be "old," as we know it today. At the turn of the century only 4% of the total population lived beyond the age of 65. Today, 13% of the population is over 65, with the most rapid growth in the oldest group, those over the age of 85 years. Although chronological age gives us little information about the individual, it is the nationally accepted marker, widely used in demographic statistics and federal and state health programs. Chronological age is useful as a baseline, but it is essential to describe the biological, physiological, and cognitive functions whenever an "old" person is assessed. As elders reach the age of 85 years and older, it is more likely that chronic disease and disorders are taking their toll. This age cohort is becoming more and more apparent in critical care units and has already filled the existing 1.9 million nursing home beds in this country. Between the years 2000 and 2020 the baby boom generation will come of age and join the ranks of the elderly. At that time, the extraordinary demands placed on the health care system will require dramatic adaptation of that system. The past two decades of hospital care have focused on acute diseases and disorders. Changes in survival rates for heart disease, cancer, diabetes, and renal failure have reshaped the mortality figures. Prolonged morbidity is now the rule, and individuals who are faced with signs and symptoms of and disability from chronic disorders are requiring an increasing number of hospital days.

The question of who should pay for care is one that our society continues to wrestle with. Although we espouse equal care for all, it is clear that the cost of equal care is staggering. In the absence of increased taxes for health care and higher copayments, rationing takes place in subtle forms every day. The way in which scarce resources are allocated is another major concern for professionals and the public alike.

When and how care stops and who determines viability are questions that our court system wrestles with daily. Advanced directives and health care proxy laws have helped, but too many Americans still struggle with issues such as who should make decisions regarding termination of life supports, for what reasons, and under what conditions.

GOALS OF CARE

Goals of care for older adults are the same as for younger adults in critical care, unless special advanced directives and decisions have been made. Older adults are in the critical care area for the extra technology and vigilance these areas afford. The special capacity of nurses in these areas to provide excellent geriatric critical care lies in their ability to not only restore physiological stability but also prevent functional decline and iatrogenesis. The recent Institute of Medicine (IOM) report on negative outcomes for patients of any age who are hospitalized especially affect the elderly (Childs, 2000). The decreased capacity to maintain homeostasis under stress and the barrage of therapies can lead to falls, medication side effects, infection, incontinence, and delirium. The goal of this book is to look at critical care nursing practice for older adults through a prism, inclusive of both specialties, for the best possible outcomes for older patients. This text provides the collective thinking of experts in the field who are striving to address these questions.

TERRY T. FULMER

REFERENCES

Burnside, I. (1988). *Nursing and the aged: A self-care approach* (3rd ed.). St. Louis: C. V. Mosby.

Callahan, D. (1987). *Setting limits: Medical goals in an aging society.* New York: Simon and Schuster.

Childs, N. (2000). IOM report spurs patient safety activity on Capitol Hill. *Provider, 26* (2), 10–11.

Dock, L. (1948). *American Journal of Nursing, 48,* 680.

Kinney, M. R., Dear, C. B., Packe, D. R., & Voorman, D. M. (1981). *AACN's clinical reference for critical care nursing.* New York: McGraw-Hill.

Office of Technology Assessment. (1987). *Life sustaining technologies and the elderly* (OTA-BA-3061). Washington, DC: U.S. Government Printing Office.

Scitovsky, A. A. (1984). The high cost of dying: What do the data show? *Milbank Memorial Fund Quarterly/Health and Society, 62,* 591–608.

Stone, V. (1969). Nursing of the aged. In F. Busse & F. Pfeiffer (Eds.), *Behavior and adaptation in late life.* Boston: Little, Brown.

Contributors

Ivo L. Abraham, PhD, RN, FAAN
Principal and CEO
The Epsilon Group LLC
Charlottesville, VA

Richard W. Besdine, MD, FACP
Professor of Medicine
Director of UConn Center on
    Aging
University of Connecticut Health
    Center
School of Medicine
Farmington, CT

Kathryn Bowles, PhD, RN
University of Pennsylvania
School of Nursing
Philadelphia, PA

Roberta L. Campbell, MSN, RN
Doctoral Candidate
University of Pennsylvania
Heart Failure Study
School of Nursing
Philadelphia, PA

Eunice Choi, DNSc, RN, CS
Postdoctoral Student
The University of Iowa
College of Nursing
Iowa City, IA

Deborah Chyun, PhD, RN
Assistant Professor and Director
Adult Advanced Practice Nursing
    Program
Yale University
School of Nursing
New Haven, CT

Sabina DeGeest, PhD, RN, NFESC
Professor of Nursing & Director
Institute of Nursing Science
University of Basel
Switzerland

**Herman H. Delooz, MD, PhD,
    FCCM, FFAEM**
Professor and Chairman
Katholieke Universiteit Leuven
Department of Emergency
    Medicine
University Hospitals
Leuven, Belgium

Catherine M. Eberle, MD
University of Nebraska Medical
    Center
Section of Geriatrics
Omaha, NE

Janet Enslein, MA, RN
Doctoral Student
The University of Iowa
College of Nursing
Iowa City, IA

Donna Fick, PhD, RN, CS
Assistant Professor
Medical College of Georgia
School of Medicine
Augusta, GA

Ellen Flaherty, MSN, RN, GNP
New York University
Division of Nursing
New York, NY

Mary Beth Happ, PhD, RN
Assistant Professor
University of Pittsburgh
Pittsburgh, PA

Susan M. Heidrich, PhD, RN
Associate Professor
University of Wisconsin-Madison
School of Nursing
Madison, WI

**Martha Highfield, PhD, RN,
   AOCN**
Associate Professor
California State University,
   Northridge
Department of Health Sciences
Northridge, CA

**Karen L. Johnson, PhD, RN,
   CCRN**
Clinical Nurse Specialist
Lecturer
University of Arizona
School of Nursing/University
   Medical Center
Tucson, AZ

Steven B. Johnson, MD
Chief, Surgical Critical Care
Associate Professor of Surgery
The University of Arizona Health
   Sciences Center
General Surgery/Trauma
Department of Surgery
Tucson, AZ

Lisa Skemp Kelley, MA, RN
Doctoral Candidate
The University of Iowa
College of Nursing
Iowa City, IA

**Pamela Stinson Kidd, PhD, RN,
   ARNP**
Director
Arizona State University
College of Nursing
Temp, AZ

**Ruth M. Kleinpell, PhD, RN,
   ACNP**
Clinical Nurse I
University of Illinois at Chicago
Department of Medical Surgical
   Nursing
Nursing Services
Chicago, IL

Jane S. Leske, PhD, RN
Associate Professor
University of WI–Milwaukee
School of Nursing
Milwaukee, WI

**Kathleen M. McCauley, PhD, RN,
   FAAN**
University of Pennsylvania
School of Nursing
Philadelphia, PA

**Graham J. McDougall, PhD, RN,
   CS**
The University of Texas at Austin
School of Nursing
Austin, TX

Diane J. Mick, PhD, RN, CCNS
Assistant Professor
University of Pittsburgh
School of Nursing
Acute/Tertiary Care Department
Pittsburgh, PA

Koen Milisen, PhD, RN
Assistant Professor
Center for Health Services and
  Nursing Research
Katholieke Universiteit Leuven,
  Leuven, Belgium
and Clinical Nurse Specialist
University Hospitals Leuven,
  Leuven, Belgium

Ethel Mitty, EdD, RN
New York University
Division of Nursing
246 Greene Street
New York, NY

**Linda E. Moody, PhD, MPH,
  FAAN**
Professor
University of South Florida
College of Nursing
Tampa, FL

Mary Naylor, PhD, RN, FAAN
Associate Professor
University of Pennsylvania
School of Nursing
Philadelphia, PA

Peter Pompei, MD
Associate Professor of Medicine
Stanford University Medical Center
Medical School Office Building
Stanford, CA

Gloria C. Ramsey, BSN, RN, JD
Director, Legal and Ethical Aspects
  of Practice
New York University
Division of Nursing
New York, NY

Sally Richards, MSN, RN, APRN
Yale University
School of Nursing
New Haven, CT

**Lori B. Schumacher, MS, RN,
  GNP, CCRN**
Instructor, School of Nursing
Medical College of Georgia
Augusta, GA

**Todd Semla, MS, PharmD, BCPS,
  FCCP**
Project Coordinator
Evanston Hospital
Clinical Pharmacology Unit
Evanston, IL

**Christine Tocchi, MSN, RN, C-
  GNP**
Yale University
School of Nursing
New Haven, CT

**Toni Tripp-Reimer, PhD, RN,
  FAAN**
Professor and Associate Dean for
  Research
The University of Iowa
College of Nursing
Iowa City, IA

Meredith Wallace, PhD, RN
Assistant Professor
Southern Connecticut State
  University
Department of Nursing
New Haven, CT

Margret S. Wolf, EdD, RN
Associate Professor of Nursing
New York University
Division of Nursing
New York, NY

Standards of Practice: Gerontological and Critical Care Nursing

Mary Beth Happ

As the complexity and technological demands of critical care settings continue to grow, clinicians and quality reviewers rely on standards of care to provide guidelines on scope and responsibilities of care as well as evaluation criteria for professional performance and care outcomes. The American Nurses Association (ANA) and the American Association of Critical Care Nurses (AACN) have developed standards that are relevant to the care of critically ill elders. The ANA's *Scope and Standards of Gerontological Clinical Nursing Practice* (American Nurses Association [ANA], 1995) delineates the scope, core values, and responsibilities of gerontological nursing practice, including advanced practice roles. The *AACN Standards for Nursing Care of the Critically Ill* (Sanford & Disch, 1997) establish a set of expectations about the process by which critical care nurses provide patient care and control the critical care environment. The purpose of this chapter is to provide an overview and analysis of these standards for use in guiding care of older adults in critical care settings. Portions of the standards that are most applicable to the care of critically ill older adults are described and analyzed. This chapter will distinguish between standards of practice, practice guidelines, and practice parameters to offer recommendations about additional resources that may be helpful in guiding care of critically ill older adults.

BACKGROUND

Previous reviews concluded that the gerontological nursing standards were broadly applicable, but not specific, to critical care settings or the older adult's experience of critical illness (Herman & Massey, 1992). Conversely, critical care nursing standards were very specific to critical illness and bedside critical care nursing practice but lacked attention to the special needs of older adults or gerontological nursing principles. Herman and Massey (1992) recommended that standards of practice for older patients in critical care settings be developed. Both sets of standards have since been revised and have become more similar in form and function; however, standards of practice specific to older patients in critical care settings have not yet been developed.

DEFINITION OF TERMS

Standards of practice are value statements that include criteria that can be used to determine level of performance for a nurse, unit, or institution and reflect normative behavior from nurses (Beckman, 1987). They represent a level of requirement, excellence, or attainment that is agreed upon by members of a profession (American College of Critical Care Medicine/ Society of Critical Care Medicine [ACCM], 1995a, 1995b; American Nurses Association [ANA], 1975). Standards of practice may also describe characteristics of patient or setting that reflect professional norms (Marker, 1987). Standards of practice for nursing are a public declaration to society, consumers of nursing care, and members of the profession about what constitutes quality nursing care. Standards of practice describe the mechanisms within the setting that support nursing care (structure standards), the process and content of nursing care (process standards), or the patient outcomes that will result from the nursing care (outcome standards), or a combination of these.

It is helpful to distinguish standards of practice from clinical practice guidelines, which have gained popularity during the past decade as decision-making tools, evaluation criteria, and reimbursement parameters. A *clinical practice guideline* describes a process of patient care management and is designed to convert science-based knowledge into clinical action (Agency for Health Care Policy and Research [AHCPR], 1990). Guidelines are intended to guide practice by providing linkages among diagnoses, treatments, and outcomes and by describing best treatment options available for each patient. The Agency for Health Care Policy and Research (AHCPR) has facilitated the development, dissemination, and evaluation of clinical practice guidelines for selected high-incidence conditions, including acute pain, low back pain, cancer pain, heart failure, urinary incontinence, pressure ulcers, cataracts, depression, benign prostatic hypertrophy, and Alzheimer's disease (AHCPR, 1993; Hadorn, McCormick, & Diokno, 1992). Most of these selected conditions occur with higher frequency in the aging population. The development of clinical practice guidelines is not solely the purview of a federal agency. Specialty organizations also develop and disseminate guidelines pertinent to their special populations and areas of expertise. For example, the American College of Critical Care Medicine (ACCM) has developed "practice parameters" for systemic intravenous analgesia and sedation and for sustained neuromuscular blockade in the adult critically ill patient (ACCM, 1995b). Although not as detailed or prescriptive as clinical practice guidelines, the *practice parameters* represent expert consensus on therapeutic issues with recommendations that provide a basis for appropriate clinical judgments (ACCM, 1995a). *Practice statements* are similar to practice parameters in that expert consensus is offered in the form of a professional statement of conduct or values on a particular practice issue.

DESCRIPTION OF GERONTOLOGICAL AND CRITICAL CARE NURSING STANDARDS

Guidance for the promotion of quality nursing care for older patients in critical care settings comes primarily from two documents: *Scope and Standards of Gerontological Clinical Nursing Practice* (ANA, 1995) and *AACN Standards for Nursing Care of Critically Ill* (Sanford & Disch, 1997). These two sets of standards will be described and examined for content that is unique to critical care nursing of the elderly.

Scope and Standards of Gerontological Clinical Nursing Practice

The scope of current gerontological nursing practice described in the ANA (1995) document is intended for the members of the nursing profession, other health professionals, and consumers. This document, developed by the Executive Committee of the former ANA Council on Gerontological Nursing, emphasizes the concepts of health promotion, health maintenance, disease prevention, and self-care rather than acute or critical illness. Values explicit in this document include the belief that aging is a natural lifelong process and not synonymous with disease. The wide variability or heterogeneity of the older adult population is also acknowledged. Gerontological nursing considers the following factors that are particularly applicable to the critical care setting in the nursing care of aging persons: cumulative effect of the aging person's loss(es), frequently atypical response of the elderly to disease and its treatment, and accumulated disabling effects of multiple chronic illnesses or degenerative processes. This perspective on aging and factors related to physiological response is consistent with current studies of critical care outcomes, risk of adverse events, and aging. Research demonstrates that prehospital functional status and comorbidities are more predictive of death during critical illness than is advanced age (Chelluri, Grenvik, & Silverman, 1995; Mayer-Oakes, Oye, & Leake, 1991) and that older adults are at greater risk for adverse reactions to medication and technologies than are their younger adult counterparts (Creditor, 1993; Foreman, Theis, & Anderson, 1993; Lefevre et al., 1992; Titler, 1993).

The gerontological nursing standards outline the basic preparation (baccalaureate degree in nursing), knowledge, and skills required of all professional nurses practicing gerontological nursing. The roles, scope of practice, and educational preparation (masters degree) for advanced practice in gerontological nursing are also described.

Parameters for competent care of older adults are outlined according to the nursing process. Assessment parameters include past patterns and lifestyle, coping, and advance directives. Individualized care planning and nursing interventions, fundamental principles in the nursing care of frail elders (Happ, Williams, Strumpf, & Berger, 1996), are also emphasized in these standards. Performance standards that describe competent level of behavior in the professional nurse role include expectations for participation in quality monitoring and quality improvement activities, competency evaluation, and continuing education. The performance standards also address the gerontological nurse's role in interdisciplinary collaboration, research, resource use, and ethical decision-making or concerns.

AACN Standards for Nursing Care of the Critically Ill

The second edition of *AACN Standards for Nursing Care of the Critically Ill* (Sanford & Disch, 1997) introduces the scope of critical care nursing practice by defining critically ill patient, critical care nurse, and critical care environment. Critical care nursing is defined as the diagnosis and treatment of human responses to actual or potentially life-threatening illness. The baccalaureate degree is delineated as the basic level of educational preparation. Process and structure standards are organized according to Donabedian's (1968) quality assurance model. Future editions of the critical care standards are intended to include patient-centered outcome standards. Implementation of the standards is described in a separate section. Appendices illustrate practical application of individual standards for use on a critical care unit. This feature is particularly helpful in demonstrating the usefulness of these standards as a framework for unit policy and procedure manuals, performance expectations, or quality reviews.

The process standards broadly outline the elements of the nursing process (data collection, problem identification, care planning, implementation, and evaluation) and associated nursing actions for each step of the process. Structure standards are more specific and include unit construction, configuration, equipment, patient privacy, safety, and management of sensory stimuli (noise, light, etc.). Administrative areas addressed in the structure standards include essential policies and procedures, qualifications of nurse managers and professional nursing staff, orientation programs, and minimum requirements for staffing mix. Critical care nurse competency is also a component of the structure standards. Importantly, this section

(VIIIh) includes the requirement for additional knowledge and skills "prior to assuming responsibility for the care of patient populations for which the nurse has not been prepared" (Sanford & Disch, 1997, p. 32). Age of the patient is identified as one of the characteristics to be considered when evaluating a nurse's ability to provide care to a new population. Competency in communication skills is also a requirement. Although the standards do not provide further explication, critical care nurses should be proficient in communicating with temporarily nonvocal older adults who often experience voicelessness as terrifying, frustrating, and depersonalizing (Happ, 2000; Scarpinato, Schell, & Kagan, 2000).

Comparison

The two sets of standards are broad in terms of level of abstraction. Both sets of standards emphasize the nursing process, competency requirements, and evaluation of performance and care. The baccalaureate degree is the basic level of educational preparation across both nursing specialties. In addition, the gerontological nursing standards address the role and preparation of advanced practice nurses in caring for elderly populations. Advanced practice roles and responsibilities specific to critical care nursing of older adults have not been defined by either specialty group. The gerontological nursing and critical care nursing standards both affirm the importance of patient participation in care and decision making. The critical care nursing standards are oriented to the assessment of immediate needs and priority setting in planning care to treat life-threatening conditions, rather than the more global life pattern assessment characteristic of the gerontological nursing standards. Structure standards unique to the critical care standards encompass unit organization and are at a more concrete level of abstraction. The nurse's role in equipment procurement and in ensuring safety of patients, visitors, and other health-care team members is another area exclusive to the critical care standards. Although both sets of standards acknowledge the nurse's role in promoting peaceful death, the gerontological nursing standards specifically include the consideration of palliative care interventions when appropriate for frail older adults (section V3f) and attention to symptom management, side effects, and toxicities (sections II 4e,f). The nurse's role in ethical decision making and in identifying and resolving clinical ethical dilemmas is outlined in some detail in the gerontological nursing standards. The critical care standards address three major ethical issues: advance directives, withdrawal or withholding of life-sustaining treatment, and the patient's right to refuse treatment.

In summary, neither the critical care nursing standards nor the gerontological nursing standards "have it all," yet both sets of standards are broadly applicable to the care and nursing service of critically ill older adults. Still, no items unique to critically ill elders were identified. It seems important, then, to develop clinical practice guidelines and protocols that reflect current research on interventions, outcomes, and best practice in the nursing care of critically ill older adults to augment current standards. All standards of practice, clinical practice guidelines, and practice parameters should be judged for use in the care of older adults by their ability to incorporate age-specific and developmentally and psychosocially relevant content and criteria.

ADDITIONAL RESOURCES TO GUIDE CRITICAL CARE NURSING OF THE ELDERLY

Many clinical practice guidelines are available to guide critical care nursing of the elderly. These guidelines are based either in critical care with some special considerations for the elderly or in gerontology with a more long-term or primary care focus. Selected resources are outlined later as examples of practice guidelines that nurses may consider for guiding the care of critically ill older adults.

Thirteen research-based clinical practice protocols (or guidelines) developed by Nurses Improving Care for Health System Elders (NICHE) faculty, are contained in the Hartford Institute for Geriatric Nursing's curriculum guide entitled *Geriatric Nursing Protocols for Best Practice* (Abraham, Bottrell, Fulmer, & Mezey, 1999). The topics addressed by these protocols include physical restraints; depression, delirium, and dementia; sleep disturbances; preventing pressure ulcers; and incontinence. Some adaptations to the critical care setting are needed.

The *Practice Parameters for Systemic Intravenous Analgesia and Sedation for Adult Patients in the Intensive Care Unit* (AACM, 1995a) and the *Practice Parameters for Sustained Neuromuscular Blockade in the Adult Critically Ill Patient* (ACCM, 1995b) contain several cautionary statements regarding dosing and response in elderly patients; however, the document does not present specific dosage recommendations or reductions for older adults. Although a comprehensive review of the pharmacological literature was conducted in developing these practice parameters, relatively few studies specifically analyzed the influence of age on adverse effects, drug clearance, drug distribution, or elimination.

The American Thoracic Society's statement on *Withholding and Withdrawing Life-Sustaining Therapy* (1991) defines acceptable standards of medical practice and makes recommendations related to withholding and withdrawing life-sustaining therapy. The statement applies to the medical care of adults with or without decision-making capacity and makes no special delineations or recommendations regarding the elderly. Roles of nurses are not specifically addressed; however, the definitions and discussion of ethical principles in withholding or withdrawing life-sustaining therapy are relevant for all members of the health-care team.

SUMMARY

This chapter has presented an overview of the two major standards of practice guiding the nursing care of critically ill older adults. Although no one document encompasses the scope and practice of critical care gerontological nursing, taken together the ANA *Scope and Standards for Gerontological Clinical Nursing Practice* (1995) and the *AACN Standards for Nursing Care of the Critically Ill* (Sanford & Disch, 1997) provide a reasonable framework for assessment and intervention parameters and performance competency evaluation. Nurses should supplement these standards with implementation of relevant clinical practice guidelines (parameters or protocols) to guide the care of critically ill older adults. To be useful and relevant for the care of critically ill older adults, clinical practice guidelines must reflect current research that includes the psychosocial needs and physiological changes specific to aging persons. Implementation of clinical practice guidelines may require modifications for applicability to the critical care environment, life-threatening diagnoses, and comorbidities. Given the wide variability in aging and differences among older adults, flexibility to individualize guidelines to unique needs of particular patients is essential. Critical analysis and the development of research-based modifications to standards and practice guidelines are important components of an advanced practice nurse role.

Finally, as demographic shifts and recent critical care census studies indicate (Groeger et al., 1993), older adults will continue to represent an ever-larger proportion of patients in adult intensive care units. Nurse researchers, clinicians, and educators face a growing challenge in defining specialty practice for critical care gerontology and in developing practice level, research-based guidelines to improve the care of critically ill older adults.

REFERENCES

Abraham, I., Bottrell, M. M., Fulmer, T., & Mezey, M. (1999). *Geriatric nursing protocols for best practice.* New York: Springer Publishing Company.

Agency for Health Care Policy and Research. (1990). *Agency for Health Care Policy and Research: Program note.* Rockville, MD: U.S. Department of Health and Human Services, AHCPR.

Agency for Health Care Policy and Research. (January, 1993). *Agency for Health Care Policy and Research: A profile.* U.S. Department of Health and Human Services. Public Health Service. Rockville, MD, AHCPR pub. No. 93-0027.

American College of Critical Care Medicine/Society of Critical Care Medicine. (1995a). *Practice parameters for systemic intravenous analgesia and sedation for adult patients in the intensive care unit.* Anaheim, CA: Society of Critical Care Medicine.

American College of Critical Care Medicine/Society of Critical Care Medicine. (1995b). *Practice parameters for sustained neuromuscular blockade in the adult critically ill patient.* Anaheim, CA: Society of Critical Care Medicine.

American Nurses Association. (1975). A plan for the implementation of the standards of nursing practice: A report to the Congress for nursing practice of the American Nurses Association. *ANA Publication NP51, i–vii,* 1–46.

American Nurses Association. (1995). *Scope and standards of gerontological clinical nursing practice.* Washington, DC: American Nurses Association.

American Thoracic Society. (1991). Withholding and withdrawing life-sustaining therapy. *American Review of Respiratory Disease, 144,* 726–731.

Beckman, J. S. (1987). What is a standard of practice? *Journal of Nursing Quality Assurance, 1* (2), 1–6.

Chelluri, L., Grenvik, A., & Silverman, M. (1995). Intensive care for critically ill elderly: Mortality, costs, and quality of life. Review of the literature. *Archives of Internal Medicine, 155,* 1013–1022.

Creditor, M. C. (1993). Hazards of hospitalization of the elderly. *Annals of Internal Medicine, 118,* 219–223.

Donabedian, A. (1968). The evaluation of medical care programs. *Bulletin of the New York Academy of Medicine, 44,* 117–124.

Foreman, M. D., Theis, S. L., & Anderson, M. A. (1993). Adverse events in the hospitalized elderly. *Clinical Nursing Research, 2,* 360–370.

Groeger, J. S., Guntupali, K. K., Strosberg, M., Halpern, N., Raphaely, R., Cerra, F., & Kaye, W. (1993). Descriptive analysis of critical care units in the United States: Patient characteristics and intensive care unit utilization. *Critical Care Medicine, 21,* 279–291.

Hadorn, D. C., McCormick, K., & Diokno, A. (1992). An annotated algorithm approach to clinical guideline development. *Journal of the American Medical Association, 267,* 3311–3314.

Happ, M. B., Williams, C. C., Strumpf, N. E., & Berger, S. (1996). Individualized care for frail elders: Theory and practice. *Journal of Gerontological Nursing, 22* (3), 6–14.

Happ, M. B. (2000). Interpretation of nonvocal behavior and the meaning of voicelessness in critical care. *Social Science & Medicine, 50,* 1247–1255.

Herman, J., & Massey, J. A. (1992). Standards of practice: Gerontological nursing and critical care nursing. In T. T. Fulmer & M. K. Walker (Eds.), *Critical care nursing of the elderly.* New York: Springer Publishing Company.

Lefevre, F., Feinglass, J., Potts, S., Soglin, L., Yarnold, P., Martin, G., & Webster, J. R. (1992). Iatrogenic complications in high-risk, elderly patients. *Archives of Internal Medicine, 152,* 2074–2080.

Marker, C. G. S. (1987). What is a standard of practice? *Journal of Nursing Quality Assurance, 1* (2), 7–20.

Mayer-Oakes, S. A., Oye, R. K., & Leake, B. (1991). Predictors of mortality in older patients following medical intensive care: The importance of functional status. *Journal of the American Geriatrics Society, 39,* 862–868.

Sanford, S. J., & Disch, J. M. (1997). *American Association of Critical Care Nurses Standards for Nursing Care of the Critically Ill* (2nd ed.). Aliso Viejo, CA: American Association of Critical Care Nursing.

Scarpinato, N., Schell, E., & Kagan, S. H. (2000). Nursing rounds at the University of Pennsylvania: Kitty's dilemma. *American Journal of Nursing, 100* (3), 49–51.

Titler, M. G. (1993). Technology dependency and iatrogenic injuries. *Nursing Clinics of North America, 28,* 459–473.

PART I

Basic Clinical Issues with Elderly Populations

2

Common Geriatric Problems

Terry T. Fulmer and Marquis Foreman

Geriatric patients bear the major burden of cardiac disease and cancer in this country. It has been well documented that with each decade the prevalence of these diseases rises in the population. There is also an increase in what are known as "geriatric syndromes" with advanced age. These syndromes, including iatrogenic infections, urinary incontinence, sensory problems, eating and feeding disorders (discussed in chapter 9), falls and dizziness, pressure ulcers, sleep disorders, and depression, are all known to have an impact on the quality of life of older adults. In this chapter, we discuss most of these syndromes, with special attention to their prevalence, presentation, and likely treatment in the hospital setting.

IATROGENIC INFECTIONS

Nosocomial infections, also known as iatrogenic infections, have been studied in great detail in the nursing home setting. However, less is known about the current scope, epidemiology, and management strategies for infection in the hospitalized elderly. A recent Institute of Medicine (IOM) report (Childs, 2000) suggests that iatrogenesis is a serious and prevalent problem. In that report, the IOM stated that:

> medical errors kill some 44,000 people in U.S. hospitals each year. Another study puts the number much higher, at 98,000. Even using the lower estimate, more people die from medical mistakes each year than from highway accidents, breast cancer, or AIDS. Moreover, while errors may be more easily detected in hospitals, they afflict every health care setting: day-surgery and outpatient clinics, retail pharmacies, nursing homes, as well as home care. Deaths from medication errors that take place both in and out of hospitals—more than 7,000 annually—exceed those from workplace injuries. (Childs, 2000, p. 10)

Although these data are not specific to the elderly, older patients account for the majority of hospital days and are more vulnerable to iatrogenic sequelae, given their decreased reserve. Common infections include urinary tract infections (UTIs), respiratory infections, and tissue infections. In the acute care setting, UTIs may be induced by nonsterile techniques with urinary catheter placement and can cause serious *E-coli* infections in the elderly. Indwelling urinary catheters are another major source of infection during hospitalization (Franson, Duthie, Cooper, Van Oudenhoven, & Hoffman, 1986). In the critical care area, the nonsterile technique may be used in an emergent situation, for example, during a cardiac arrest, when dramatic measures are needed to restore a patient's heartbeat. Therefore, less care may be taken for sterile technique, for example, during urinary catheter placement. Although no one argues that such events occur, it is extremely important for critical care nurses to anticipate UTIs in the elderly when a catheter has been placed temporarily. Clinical observation of the urine for any change in smell, appearance, or odor is the first-line assessment, followed by urine cultures to rule out UTIs in this group. Elderly individuals may be asymptomatic for UTIs until the advanced stages, when there may be evidence of septic shock. Judicious attention to any symptoms of UTI, not just the presence of fever, should be a routine critical care nursing practice with the elderly.

URINARY INCONTINENCE

Urinary incontinence is another common geriatric syndrome that increases in prevalence with each decade and further increases by setting. It is estimated that hospitalized elderly may have an increase in prevalence of urinary incontinence of up to 50%. Although normal changes of the aging urinary system (Table 2.1) may play a part, the genesis of urinary incontinence in the hospital is felt to have several sources. These sources include mechanical barriers to the use of the toilet (i.e., restraints, bedrails, and uncertainty regarding locations of the bathroom), indwelling devices that reduce mobility, and episodes of delirium that may be triggered by medication. In the latter case, it may be a delirium reaction to medication that triggers an incontinence episode. Furthermore, medications that are usually therapeutic (e.g., furosemide) may cause an iatrogenic episode of incontinence when the older person is not prepared for the drug effect and the sudden need to void is not anticipated. Whether the reason for urinary incontinence is external (the environmental milieu) or internal to the patient or physiological and pathophysiological responses to therapies or disease, it is an unpleasant and uncomfortable geriatric syndrome that warrants careful attention. In the past, it would be usual for an intensive care unit nurse to insert a urinary catheter in any patient who was incontinent. This was felt to be an appropriate practice given the need to pay careful attention to fluid balance. It was also thought to be for the patient's

TABLE 2.1 Urinary Function in Older Adults

Age-related changes	Negative functional consequences	Risk factors
Degenerative changes in cerebral cortex	Decline in efficiency of homeostatic mechanisms	Genitourinary disease (e.g., prostatic hyperplasia)
Decreased number of nephrons	Delayed excretion of water-soluble medications	Systemic disease (e.g., cerebrovascular accident, dementia, dehydration)
Decreased renal blood flow	Diminished bladder capacity	
Decreased glomerular filtration rate	Nocturia	Medications (e.g., diuretics, anticholinergics)
Hypertrophy of muscles in the urinary tract	Urinary urgency and frequency	Any factor that interferes with socially appropriate urinary elimination (e.g., impaired mobility)
Relaxation of pelvic floor muscles	Chronic residual urine	
Contractions during bladder filling		
Decreased bladder capacity		Environmental barriers
		Unfamiliar environments
		Indwelling catheters

From *Nursing care of older adults: Theory and practice*, 3rd ed., by C. A. Miller, 1999, Philadelphia: Lippincott, p. 273.

comfort. It is now known that the insertion of an indwelling catheter is likely to cause infection and is not comfortable, and it is not the treatment of choice. These common causes of transient urinary incontinence have been carefully described in the Agency for Health Care Policy and Research (AHCPR) guidelines for urinary incontinence (Agency for Health Care Policy and Research [AHCPR], 1992) and are noted in Table 2.2.

The types of urinary incontinence are listed in Table 2.3. A major category of urinary incontinence in the hospital is urge incontinence. This occurs when an individual has a sudden urge to void and cannot get to the bathroom in time. Urge incontinence may happen when an individual is seated on an over-the-seat toileting commode device that is not properly in place when the patient sits (T. Wells, personal communication, 1999). The physiological urge to void once the learned patterns of sitting on a commode are in place frequently triggers this response. Again, careful attention to cues in the environment, which may initiate an urge response, is important.

Stress incontinence takes place when an individual sneezes or coughs or in other ways increases intra-abdominal pressure, which then causes pressure on the bladder and causes a person to void. In this instance, a regular

TABLE 2.2   Common Causes of Transient Urinary Incontinence

Potential causes	Comment
Delirium (confusional state)	In the delirious patient, incontinence is usually an associated symptom that will abate with proper diagnosis and treatment of the underlying cause of confusion.
Infection (symptomatic urinary tract infection)	Dysuria and urgency from symptomatic infection my defeat the older person's ability to reach the toilet in time. Asymptomatic infection, although more common than symptomatic infection, is rarely a cause of incontinence.
Atrophic urethritis or vaginitis	Atrophic urethritis or vaginitis may present as dysuria, dyspareunia, burning or urination, urgency, agitation (in demented patients), and occasionally incontinence. Both disorders are readily treated by conjugated estrogen administered either orally (0.3–1.25 mg/d) or locally (2 g or fraction/d).
Pharmaceuticals Sedative hypnotics	Benzodiazepines, especially long-acting agents such as flurazepam and diazepam, may accumulate in elderly patients and cause confusion and secondary incontinence. Alcohol, frequently used as a sedative, can cloud the sensorium, impair mobility, and induce a diuresis, resulting in incontinence.
Diuretics	A brisk diuresis induced by loop diuretics can overwhelm bladder capacity and lead to polyuria, frequency, and urgency, thereby precipitating incontinence in a frail older person. The loop diuretics include furosemide, ethacrynic acid, and bumetanide.

Anticholinergic agents
    Antihistamines
    Antidepressants
    Antipsychotics
    Disopnamide
    Opiates
    Antispasmodics (dicyclomine and Donnatal)
	Nonprescription (over-the-counter) agents with anticholinergic properties are taken commonly by older patients for insomnia, coryza, pruritus, and vertigo, and many prescription medications also have anticholinergic properties. Anticholinergic side effects include urinary retention with associ-

TABLE 2.2 *(continued)*

Potential causes	Comment
Antiparkinsonian agents (trihexyphenidyl and benztropine mesylate)	ated urinary frequency and overflow incontinence. Besides anticholinergic actions, antipsychotics such as thioridazine and haloperidol may cause sedation, rigidity, and immobility.
Alpha-adrenergic agents Sympathomimetics (decongestants) Sympatholytics (e.g., prazosin, terazosin, and doxazosin)	Sphincter tone in proximal urethra can be decreased by alpha antagonists and increased by alpha agonists. An older woman whose urethra is shortened and weakened with age, may develop stress incontinence when taking an alpha antagonist for hypertension. An older man with prostate enlargement may develop acute urinary retention and overflow incontinence when taking multicomponent "cold" capsules that contain alpha agonists and anticholinergic agents, especially if a nasal decongestant and a nonprescription hypnotic antihistamine are added.
Calcium channel blockers	Calcium channel blockers can reduce smooth muscle contractility in the bladder and occasionally can cause urinary retention and overflow incontinence.
Psychological problems	Severe depression may occasionally be associated with incontinence but is probably less frequently a cause in older patients.
Excessive urine production	Excess intake; endocrine conditions that cloud the sensorium and induce a diuresis (e.g., hypercalcemia, hyperglycemia, and diabetes insipidus); and expanded volume states, such as congestive heart failure, lower extremity venous insufficiency, drug-induced ankle edema (e.g., nifedipine, indomethacin), and low albumin states, cause polyuria and can lead to incontinence.
Restricted mobility	Limited mobility is an aggravating or precipitating cause of incontinence that can frequently be corrected or im-

(continued)

TABLE 2.2   (continued)

Potential causes	Comment
	proved by treating the underlying condition (e.g., arthritis, poor eyesight, Parkinson's disease, or orthostatic hypotension). A urinal or bedside commode and scheduled toileting often help resolve the incontinence that results from hospitalization and its environmental barriers (e.g., bed rails, restraints, and poor lighting).
Stool impaction	Patients with stool impaction present with either urge or overflow incontinence and may have fecal incontinence as well. Disimpaction restores continence.

From Urinary incontinence in adults. In *Clinical practice guidelines* by the Agency for Health Care Policy and Research, 1992, Rockville, MD: U.S. Department of Health and Human Services, Public Health Service, pp. 7–9.

toileting schedule of every 2 hours is the appropriate approach to keep the bladder empty and avoid distention.

Neurogenic incontinence comes about when patients have a spinal cord injury that leaves them incapable of controlling their bladder impulses. In this case, the nurse should understand from the patient the way he or she usually controls urinary incontinence and urinary patterns at home. Every effort should be made to maintain the bladder program during hospitalization. Failure to do so may needlessly disrupt a bladder program that has taken months to establish.

SENSORY PROBLEMS

Sensory problems in the critical care setting are to be anticipated given the unusual array of machines that emit noises and lights. Such sensory stimuli can create an environment in which the patient feels overwhelmed. Philbin and Ballweg (1994) have reported increasing concern that environmental stimuli in the neonatal intensive care unit (NICU) may be detrimental to the preterm infants hospitalized there. In that study, chicks were incubated, hatched, and reared in either a quiet or NICU-sound environment. Habituation was measured by the length of time that chicks delayed their ongoing peeping on hearing a white noise stimulus. NICU-sound–reared 4-day-old chicks failed to habituate, showing as much responsiveness at the end of repeated stimulation as at the beginning. This demonstration

TABLE 2.3 Urinary Incontinence: Manifestations and Underlying Mechanisms

Type	Manifestations	Underlying mechanisms
Transient	Acute onset but may be ignored for a long time; associated with identifiable causes	Delirium, infections, pathological conditions, fecal impaction, limited mobility, medications (see Table 2.2)
Stress	Sudden leakage of small amounts of urine as a result of an activity that increases abdominal pressure (e.g., coughing, lifting, laughing, sneezing, or exercising)	Medications, obesity, estrogen deficiency, weakness of the pelvic floor muscles, effects of postradiation of post–prostrate surgery, urethral sphincter weakness
Urge	Inability to hold urine long enough to get to the toilet despite the perception of the urge to void (cognitive impairments can impair this perception)	Medications, stroke, dementia, parkinsonism, urinary tract infection, detrusor overactivity or instability
Overflow	Leakage of small amounts of urine, periodically or continually, without the urge to void or without being able to pass large amounts	Medications, fecal impaction, enlarged prostate, diabetic neuropathy, severe pelvic prolapse
Functional	Intermittent or consistent total incontinence in a person with an intact urinary tract but with other functional impairments	Medications, mobility limitations or cognitive impairments in combination with external factors (e.g., caregiver inattention, restraints, environmental barriers)

From *Nursing care of older adults: Theory and practice,* 3rd ed. by C. A. Miller, 1999, Philadelphia, PA: Lippincott, p. 272.

showed that atypical sound exposure alone can alter a fundamental aspect of neurosensory competence in an otherwise healthy neonate (Philbin & Ballweg, 1994). Such studies need to be replicated in the elderly in order to detect physiological parameters that may be affected by ICU noise.

PRESSURE ULCERS

Pressure ulcers are one of the leading causes of morbidity and mortality in the elderly. In the critical care environment, they can develop in hours and take years to heal. Evidence suggests that the development of a stage II or greater pressure ulcer in the hospital increases hospital costs and length of stay significantly (Allman, Goode, Burst, Bartolucci, & Thomas, 1999; Resources in Wound Care, 1999). Pressure ulcers are ready sources of infection in the elderly and are also known to cause pain and discomfort for those who are unfortunate to develop a pressure ulcer in the hospital setting. AHCPR guidelines (1994) have documented appropriate approaches to assessing pressure against the skin, and the scales, such as the Braden Scale (Bergstrom, Braden, & Boynton, 1995) (Table 2.4), have done much to help nurses understand appropriate ways to assess pressure in the hospital environment.

Once an older person develops a pressure ulcer, the array of therapeutic interventions available is overwhelming to the practicing nurse, and there is still much confusion as to how therapeutic intervention should be chosen and evaluated. In one summary, 20 pages were required to list all of the products (more than 1000) available to use for pressure ulcers (Resources in Wound Care, 1999). Interventions for managing pressure ulcers are listed in Figure 2.1.

SLEEP DISORDERS

Sleep is a mechanism for restoring the body and its function and for maintenance of energy and health (Spenceley, 1993). It has a renewing and replenishing effect, both physically and emotionally. Consequently, sleep is a necessity for survival (Carskadon & Dement, 1994). When sleep is disrupted, physical, emotional, and behavioral disturbances arise. With severe sleep disruption, physiological instability may occur. Common sleep disturbances are associated with poorer outcomes of care, for example, delayed healing, protracted recuperation, transient states of cognitive impairment, and physiological instability. Sleep disturbances also are associated with a decreased ability to function and to perform daily activities and therefore frequently result in institutionalization. Thus, for patients to recuperate from critical illness, sleep is an essential component of care.

Sleep is a complex combination of physiological and behavioral processes and has been defined as "a reversible behavioral state of perceptual disengagement from and unresponsiveness to, the environment" (Carskadon & Dement, 1994, p. 16). Within the sleep cycle, there are two states: Rapid eye movement (REM) (or desynchronized) sleep and nonrapid eye movement (NREM) (or synchronized) sleep (Carskadon & Dement, 1994). The sleep cycle usually progresses from stage 1 NREM sleep to stages 2, 3, and 4 and then to REM sleep (Table 2.5). REM sleep typically occurs after a change from stage 3 or 4 NREM to stage 2 NREM sleep and continues to alternate between REM and NREM stages in 70- to 120-minute cycles. Typically there are 4–6 cycles per night. According to Carskadon and Dement (1994), in the first third of a typical night, stages 3 and 4 NREM sleep predominate, whereas in the last third, stage 2 NREM and REM sleep predominate and stage 4 NREM sleep may be absent. Deprivation of REM sleep is associated

TABLE 2.4   The Braden Scale

Clients name			Evaluator's name		Date of assessment
Sensory Perception Ability to respond meaningfully to pressure-related discomfort	1. **Completely limited** Unresponsive (does not moan, flinch, or grasp) to painful stimuli because of diminished level of consciousness or sedation OR limited ability to feel pain over most of body surface	2. **Very limited** Responds only to painful stimuli; cannot communicate discomfort except by moaning or restlessness OR has a sensory impairment that limits the ability to feel pain or discomfort over 1/2 of the body	3. **Slightly limited** Responds to verbal commands but cannot always communicate discomfort or need to be turned OR has some sensory impairment that limits ability to feel pain or discomfort in 1 or 2 extremities	4. **No impairment** Responds to verbal commands; has no sensory deficit that would limit ability to feel or voice pain or discomfort
Moisture Degree to which skin is exposed to moisture	1. **Completely moist** Skin is kept moist almost constantly by perspiration, urine; dampness is detected every time the client is moved or turned	2. **Moist** Skin is often but not always moist; linen must be changed at least once a shift	3. **Occasionally moist** Skin is occasionally moist, requiring an extra linen change approximately once a day	4. **Rarely moist** Skin is usually dry; linen requires changing only at routine intervals

(continued)

TABLE 2.4 *(continued)*

Clients name _____ Evaluator's name _____ Date of assessment _____

Activity Degree of physical activity	1. **Bedfast** Confined to bed	2. **Chairfast** Ability to walk severely limited or nonexistent; cannot bear own weight and must be assisted into chair or wheelchair	3. **Walks occasionally** Walks occasionally during the day but for very short distances, with or without assistance; spends the majority of each shift in bed or chair	4. **Walks frequently** Walks outside the room at least twice a day and inside the room at least once every 2 hours during waking hours
Mobility Ability to change or control body position	1. **Completely immobile** Does not make even slight changes in body or extremity position without assistance	2. **Very limited** Makes occasional slight changes in body or extremity position but unable to make frequent or significant changes independently	3. **Slightly limited** Makes frequent though slight changes in body or extremity position independently	4. **No limitations** Makes major and frequent changes in position without assistance

TABLE 2.4 (*continued*)

Clients name		Evaluator's name		Date of assessment
Nutrition Usual food intake pattern	**1. Very poor** Never eats a complete meal; rarely eats more than 1 serving of any food offered; eats 2 servings or less of protein (meat or dairy products) per day; takes fluids poorly; does not take a liquid dietary supplement OR Is NPO or maintained on clear liquids or IV for more than 5 days	**2. Probably inadequate** Rarely eats a complete meal and generally eats only about 1/2 of any food offered; protein intake includes only 3 servings of meat or dairy products per day; occasionally will take a dietary supplement OR Receives less than optimal amount of liquid diet or tube feeding	**3. Adequate** Eats over half of most meals; eats a total of 4 servings of protein (meat, dairy products) each day; occasionally will refuse a meal but will usually take a supplement if offered OR Is receiving tube feeding or total parenteral nutrition, which probably meets most nutritional needs	**4. Excellent** Eats most of every meal; never refuses a meal; usually eats a total of 4 or more servings of meat and dairy products; occasionally eats between meals; does not require supplementation

(*continued*)

TABLE 2.4 *(continued)*

Clients name		Evaluator's name	Date of assessment
Friction and shear	**1. Problem** Requires moderate to maximum assistance in moving; complete lifting without sliding against sheets is impossible; frequently slides down in bed or chair, requiring frequent repositioning with maximum of assistance; spasticity, contractures, or agitation leads to almost constant friction	**2. Potential problem** Moves feebly or requires minimum assistance; during a move, skin probably slides to some extent against sheets, chair, restraints or other devices; maintains relatively good position in chair or bed most of the time but occasionally slides down	**3. No apparent problem** Moves in bed and in chair independently and has sufficient muscle strength to lift up completely during move; maintains good position in bed or chair at all times

Total score

(Source: Barbara Braden and Nancy Bergstrom. Copyright, 1998.)

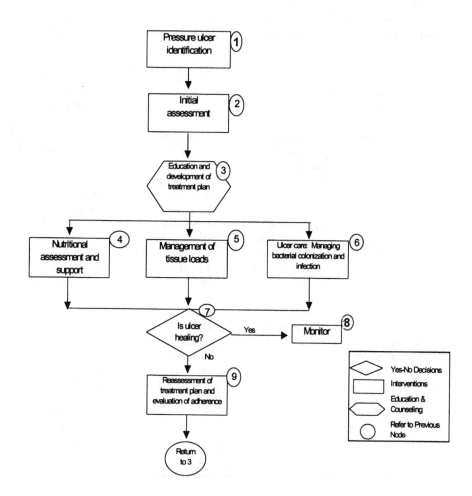

FIGURE 2.1   Management of pressure ulcers: Overview.

From Treatment of pressure ulcers. In *Clinical Practice Guidelines #15* by the Agency for Health Care Policy and Research, 1994, Rockville, MD: U.S. Department of Health and Human Services, Public Health Service, p. 22.

with anxiety, irritability, and inability to concentrate and, if severe enough, disturbed behavior (Carskadon & Dement, 1994; Gottlieb, 1990).

Changes in sleep occur with aging, as is the case for other human mechanisms (Prinz, Vitiello, Raskind, & Thorpy, 1990). The changes in sleep that are observed with aging are

TABLE 2.5   Stages of Sleep

Stage of sleep	Description	Duration	Observable behaviors
Non–rapid eye movement (NREM) sleep		75–80% total sleep time	Characterized by a minimum of mental activity in a movable body
Stage 1 NREM	Transitional stage between waking and sleep	1–7 minutes; 2–5% total sleep time	Person relaxed but easily aroused
Stage 2 NREM		10–25 minutes; 45–55% of total sleep time	Person more relaxed but remains arousable
Stage 3 NREM and Stage 4 NREM	Deep sleep stages; responsible for essential restorative aspect of sleep	Start about 20 minutes after Stage 1; 10–20% of total sleep time	Person is very relaxed; pulse rate is slower; body temperature is lower; stronger stimuli needed for arousal
Rapid eye movement (REM) sleep	Considered essential for well-being;	Starts 60–90 minutes into the sleep cycle; accounts for 20–25% total sleep time	Characterized by an abundance of mental activity and is associated with dreaming; muscle atonia; blood pressure, pulse, and respiration increase and fluctuate

- decrease in actual sleep time
- increase in total sleep time (i.e., more time in bed but less of it asleep)
- increase in sleep latency (i.e., more time required to fall asleep)
- increase in the number of awakenings each night
- REM sleep more interrupted
- increase in stage 1 sleep
- stages 3 and 4 sleep less deep
- decreased sleep efficiency
- more easily disturbed by environmental factors
- more frequent comments about poor quality of sleep
- increase in daytime sleepiness and napping

Overall, these changes lead to sleep that is lighter, shorter, and interrupted. These changes are for the most part minor, still allowing sleep to perform its restorative function. Recent evidence indicates that these changes observed in sleep are more likely to be the result of chronic health problems and their treatment than of aging (Bliwise, 1994). However, the elderly are predisposed to poor sleep as a result of heightened autonomic activity and an increased susceptibility to external arousal (Beck-Little & Weinrich, 1998). In addition to these "normal" changes in sleep that accompany aging, there are disturbances in the sleep–wake cycle that are not normal. These alterations in sleep require prompt and appropriate assessment and intervention because they are associated with increased morbidity, mortality, and a reduction in quality of life (Gottlieb, 1990; Prinz et al., 1990; Spenceley, 1993). Alterations in the sleep–wake cycle have been classified into four major categories: (a) dyssomnias, (b) parasomnias, (c) sleep disorders associated with medical or psychiatric disorders, and (d) proposed sleep disorders (Thorpy, 1994). Only sleep disorders associated with medical or psychiatric disorders will be described here. For a more detailed discussion of other sleep disorders, please refer to and Foreman, Wykle, and the NICHE Faculty (1999) and to Thorpy (1994).

Sleep disorders associated with medical and psychiatric conditions are those disturbances in sleep and wakefulness associated with a large number of health problems and their treatment. This category is further subdivided into three groups: those sleep disorders associated with mental, neurological, and medical disorders. These disturbances in sleep, referred to by some as secondary sleep problems, are frequent concomitants of hospitalization for critical illness in older patients and are easily remedied by a variety of nursing strategies outlined in this chapter (for a more detailed discussion see Foreman et al., 1999). Despite the negative consequences of sleep disturbances outlined earlier, the sleep of critically ill patients generally is not carefully assessed by nurses. Interventions are predominately pharmacologically based and more likely to exacerbate the sleep disturbance they were intended to solve (Table 2.6). The practice protocol outlined in Table 2.7 provides parameters for the assessment of sleep and nursing strategies for the prevention and management of sleep.

Pharmacologically based interventions should be used as a temporary means and last resort for treating sleep disorders. These parameters have been selected on the basis of their relevance to critical care nursing; a more comprehensive listing of nursing strategies is outlined in Foreman et al. (1999).

The etiologies of sleep disturbances in the elder patient population include the critical illness and its treatment, characteristics of the intensive care unit (ICU) environment, characteristics of the older individual, and changes in daily routines associated with the critical illness. As a result, an assessment of sleep and sleep disturbances should encompass the parameters of (a) usual sleep and wake patterns, (b) bedtime routines and rituals, (c) diet and drug use (not to overlook over-the-counter medications), (d) environmental factors, (e) physiological factors, and (f) illness factors.

TABLE 2.6   Medications and Sleep Disturbances

Drug type	Specific drug	Effect on sleep
Central nervous system depressants		
Barbiturates	Phenobarbital Nembutal Seconal	Suppress REM sleep
Opiate narcotic analgesics	Morphine	Decrease REM activity Increase number of arousals Increase stage I sleep
	Demerol	Suppress REM sleep
Benzodiazepines	Ativan Valium Halcion Serax	Increase stage IV sleep Alter REM sleep Reverse normal sleep patterns
Antipsychotics	Mellaril Haldol Thorazine Navane	Delay onset of sleep Interfere with REM sleep
Monoamine oxidase inhibitors	Marplen Nardel Parnate	Improve sleep in depressed persons
Central nervous system stimulants		
General	Theophylline Caffeine Amphetamine	Decrease total sleep time Increase arousals Delay onset of sleep Interfere with REM sleep
Catecholamines	Dopamine	Increase wakefulness
Autonomic agents	Nasal sprays Cough syrups with dextromethorphan Sudafed	Cause daytime sleepiness
Antihypertensives	Methyldopa Reserpine Atenolol Nifedipine	Cause drowsiness
Miscellaneous drugs		
Diuretics	Lasix	Nighttime awakenings caused by nocturia
Steriods	Hydrocortisone	Interfere with sleep

Adapted from Sleep disturbances in the elderly by M. Foreman, M. Wykle, & NICHE Faculty, 1999. In I. Abraham, M. M. Bottrell, T. Fulmer, & M. Mezey (Eds.), *Geriatric nursing protocols for best practice*. New York: Springer Publishing Company, pp. 8–21.

TABLE 2.7 Nursing Strategies for Sleep Disturbances in Critically Ill Elders

Promote physiological stability

    Administer medications (as prescribed) to promote breathing prior to sleep time

    Complete any health care treatments about 1 hour prior to sleep time

Maintain normal sleep pattern

    Schedule nighttime treatment and care activities to provide uninterrupted periods of sleep of at least 2–3 hours

    Balance daytime rest and activity

Avoid/minimize drugs that negatively influence sleep

    Pharmacological treatment of sleep disturbances is treatment of last resort; therefore, if a sleep-promoting medication is required, use the lowest effective dose of a drug with a short half-life for the least amount of time

    Discontinue or adjust the dose or dosing schedule of any/all offending medication (see Table 2.6).

    Select a dosing schedule of other medications to promote sleep, e.g., give diuretics at least 4 hours prior to bedtime

Promote comfort

    Minimize pain by using scheduled analgesics

    Promote sleep using back massage, progressive relaxation, or guided imagery

    Reposition patient for comfort

Create an optimal environment for sleep

    Keep noise to an absolute minimum

    Set room temperature according to patient preference

    Use night light as desired but keep ambient lighting low

    Provide soft music or white sound to mask the noise of the unit activities

    Use remote equipment alarms at nurses' station

Specific areas of questioning are found in Table 2.7. Information elicited should include objective data as well as subjective appraisals of the quality of sleep. Questions of family or significant others also may provide insight into usual patterns and certain aspects of sleep.

The sleep assessment is focused to elicit information relative to indicators, or defining characteristics, of sleep disturbance that include verbal comments by the individual of not sleeping well, of not feeling rested, of being tired, of being awakened earlier than usual, or of having interrupted sleep. Changes in behavior or performance, or both, also should be observed. For example, the individual may be irritable, restless, lethargic, listless, or apathetic. Additionally, the individual may be observed to have difficulty concentrating, an increased reaction time, a greater sensitivity to pain, and diminished daytime alertness. If ambulatory, this individual may be prone to accidents and falls.

Nursing strategies suggested for promoting sleep in the critically ill elderly were selected upon two basic principles. First, for the strategy to be effective, it must be individualized, considering the specific characteristics of the patient and the nature of the sleep disturbance, as determined by the sleep assessment (Vitello, 1996). Second, pharmacological treatment, for example, prescription and administration of sedatives or hypnotics, should be considered an intervention of last resort. Additionally, when pharmacological treatment is considered appropriate, only a short-acting, low-dose medication with a wide margin of safety is recommended on a temporary basis (Vitello, 1996). Nonpharmacological strategies are emphasized.

Sleep disturbances can be a serious detriment to the recovery process from critical illness for the frail elder. Careful attention and documentation with thoughtful intervention can make an important difference in speeding the recovery time of these vulnerable individuals. We direct the reader to chapter 5 for detailed coverage of confusion and delirium and to chapter 10 for a discussion on falls.

REFERENCES

Agency for Health Care Policy and Research. (1992). Urinary Incontinence in Adults. In *Clinical Practice Guidelines* (pp. 7–9). Rockville, MD: U.S. Department of Health and Human Services, Public Health Service.

Agency for Health Care Policy and Research. (1994). Treatment of Pressure Ulcers. In *Clinical practice guidelines* (Vol. 15, p. 22). Rockville, MD: U.S. Department of Health and Human Services, Public Health Service.

Allman, R., Goode, P., Burst, N., Bartolucci, A., & Thomas, D. (1999). Pressure ulcers, hospital complications and disease severity: Impact on hospital costs and lengths of stay. *Advances in Wound Care, 12* (1), 22–30.

Beck-Little, R., & Weinrich, S. P. (1998). Assessment and management of sleep disorders in the elderly. *Journal of Gerontologic Nursing, 24* (4), 21–29.

Bergstrom, N., Braden, B., & Boynton, P. (1995). Using research based assessment scales in clinical practice. *Nursing Clinics of North America, 30,* 539–551.

Bliwise, D. L. (1994). Normal aging. In M. H. Kryger, T. Roth, & W. C. Dement (Eds.), *Principles and practice of sleep medicine* (2nd ed., pp. 26–39). Philadelphia: W. B. Saunders.

Carskadon, M. A., & Dement, W. C. (1994). Normal human sleep: An overview. In M. H. Kryger, T. Roth, & W. C. Dement (Eds.), *Principles and practice of sleep* (2nd ed., pp. 16–25). Philadelphia: W. B. Saunders.

Childs, N. (2000). IOM report spurs patient safety activity on Capitol Hill. *Provider, 26* (2), 10–11.

Foreman, M., Wykle, M., & the NICHE Faculty. (1999). Sleep disturbances in elderly patients. In I. Abraham, M. M. Bottrell, T. Fulmer, & M. Mezey (Eds.), *Geriatric nursing protocols for best practice* (pp. 13–25). New York: Springer Publishing Company.

Franson, T. R., Duthie, E. H. Jr., Cooper, J. E., Van Oudenhoven, G., & Hoffmann, R. G. (1986). Prevalence survey of infections and their predisposing factors at a hospital-based nursing home care unit. *Journal of the American Geriatric Society, 34,* 95–100.

Gottlieb, G. L. (1990). Sleep disorders and their management. *American Journal of Medicine, 88* (suppl. 3A), 29–33.

Philbin, M., & Ballweg, D. (1994). The effect of an intensive care unit sound environment on the development of habituation in healthy avian neonates. *Developmental Psychobiology, 27* (1), 11–21.

Prinz, P. N., Vitiello, M. V., Raskind, M. A., & Thorpy, M. J. (1990). Geriatrics: Sleep disorders and aging. *New England Journal of Medicine, 323* (8), 520–526.

Resources in Wound Care: 1999 Directory, Products by Categories, Manufacturers, A–Z . . . and much more. (1999). *Advances in Wound Care, 12* (4), 1–223.

Spenceley, S. M. (1993). Sleep inquiry: A look with fresh eyes. *Image—The Journal of Nursing Scholarship, 25* (3), 249–256.

The National Academies. *Preventing Death and Injury from Medical Errors Requires Dramatic, System-wide Changes: November 29, 1999, Press Release.* http:www.nationalacademies.org.news, 12/6/99: Washington, DC.

Thorpy, M. J. (1994). Classification of sleep disorders. In M. H. Kryger, T. Roth, & W. C. Dement (Eds.), *Principles and practice of sleep medicine* (2nd ed., pp. 426–436). Philadelphia: W. B. Saunders.

Vitello, M. V. (1996). Sleep disorders and aging. *Current Opinion in Psychiatry, 9,* 284–289.

3

Becoming Frail: Failure to Thrive

Graham J. McDougall, Jr.

The term "frailty" may be used to describe older adults who are dependent on others for one or more activities of daily living and in whom there is a precarious balance between the assets for maintaining health and the deficits that threaten it (McDougall & Balyer, 1998). Frailty is often described in purely physical terms, the mental and psychological aspects omitted. The goal of this chapter is to appraise the evolution of critical care and geriatric nursing, with an emphasis on frailty.

FRAILTY AND VULNERABILITY IN THE ELDERLY

Pressley and Patrick (1999) found that functional status is an important predictor of developing frailty in community-dwelling populations. Walston and Fried (1999) associate frailty with advanced age and validated a phenotype of frailty. Women are twice as likely to develop the syndrome as men. Predictors of frailty are inactivity and weight loss, and men may be protected because of higher levels of muscle mass, testosterone, and growth hormones (Chin et al., 1999).

Frail older adults are often dependent on others for one or more activities of daily living. Strawbridge, Shema, Balfour, Higby, and Kaplan (1998) examined risk factors associated with frailty, conceptualized as having problems or difficulties in two or more functional domains: physical, nutritive, cognitive, and sensory. In the sample of 574 adults from California between the ages of 65 and 102 years of age, one fourth scored as frail; there were no gender differences. The strongest predictors of frailty were drinking, cigarette smoking, physical inactivity, depression, social isolation, fair or poor perceived health, and chronic conditions. However, in another study of 516 older adults from Berlin with a mean age of 85 years, Smith and Baltes (1998) found that women had a 1.6 higher risk than men had for developing physical frailty that ultimately affected their psychological functioning. The results of studies indicate a beginning knowledge development in understanding the influence of gender, functional ability, and activity in predicting the development of frailty.

Mental Frailty

The physical manifestations of frailty are often emphasized, and the mental and psychological aspects of this phenomenon are omitted. However, older adults with psychiatric illness as well as major physical illness are considered to have mental frailty. Mental abilities may be linked to a compromised memory or vulnerability in the cognitive domain and to anxiety and depression in the emotional and affective domains. Compromised thinking and insecurity about mental ability are symptoms of mental frailty. Depression has a negative influence on memory performance, and it often causes anxiety and forgetfulness and may lead to a decrease in intellectual ability. Mentally frail elderly often have a low opinion of the state of their memories and a faltering confidence in their cognitive abilities. This is particularly devastating when a critically ill older adult is recovering from an illness.

Nursing has a poor representation in this category of clinical practice, with few published studies. Delirium is a contributor to mental frailty in hospitalized elderly. Inouye, Rushing, Foreman, Palmer, and Pompei (1998) found that even though the associations between delirium and death and delirium and length of stay were not significant, delirium predicted nursing home placement, functional decline, and death at hospital discharge or at 3-month follow up. At hospital discharge, nursing home placement occurred in 60 (9%) of the 692 patients evaluated; the odds ratio for delirium was 3. This finding indicates that if delirium was present at hospital admission, there is a three times higher risk of being discharged to a nursing home. The findings of two studies of mental frailty are provided for contrasts and illustration, one in the community and the other in a nursing home (Inouye et al., 1998).

As one loses confidence in memory, anxiety increases and sense of self-efficacy regarding using memory in everyday contexts and memory-demanding situations erodes. In a study of elders living in their own homes (McDougall, Strauss, Holston, & Martin, 1999), one cohort of 218 older adults from the midwest, 96 blacks (24 men, 72 women) and 122 whites (45 men, 77 women) age 70 and older, were drawn from a random telephone sample to participate. A three-stage telephone screening procedure was initiated. At the third telephone call, and after consent was given, the Short Portable Mental Status Questionnaire was administered; those with more than two errors were not interviewed further. The mean age of subjects was 77.75 years, and Mini Mental State Exam scores were in the nonimpaired range $M = 27.45$, $SD = 2.29$. There were no racial differences on variables of memory performance measured with the Rivermead Behavioral Memory (RBM), memory self-efficacy with the Memory Self-Efficacy Questionnaire (MSEQ), memory anxiety with the Metamemory In Adulthood (MIA) questionnaire, and depression with the Center for Epidemiological Studies in Depression (CES-D) scale. The correlations ($n = 218$) of individual measures with memory performance varied from 0.03 to 0.45. The correlations between memory performance and memory self-efficacy ($r = 0.31$, $p < 0.05$) and memory anxiety ($r = -0.16$, $p < 0.05$) were significant. The correlations between memory performance and depression ($r = -0.14$, $p < 0.05$) were significant. Persons with higher depression and anxiety scores performed more poorly on memory. The correlations between metamemory variables and memory performance ranged from 0.03 to 0.23. The correlations between memory performance and metamemory change ($r = 0.23$, $p < .05$), capacity ($r = 0.13$, $p < 0.05$), external strategy ($r = 0.15$, $p < 0.05$), and total strategy ($r = 0.15$, $p < 0.05$) were significant. Persons with higher memory performance had greater capacity, were more stable (decline), and used greater numbers of external strategies and total memory strategies.

Based on a median split, subjects were divided into high (> 3.143) and low (< 3.143) memory anxiety. Those in the high-anxiety group scored significantly lower on memory self-efficacy ($M = 26.12$, $SD = 15.80$, whereas those in the low-anxiety group scored significantly higher ($p < .05$) on memory self-efficacy ($M = 34.39$, $SD = 18.66$). In the first regression model age explained 11% of the variance in memory performance. In the second model the addition of memory self-efficacy contributed an additional 6%. In the third model age and the interaction term memory efficacy, X anxiety contributed a total R_2 of 15% of the variance. Clearly, anxiety and confidence about one's cognitive ability can influence actual memory performance. Even though these individuals were living independently, their confidence and cognitive ability were compromised.

This lack of confidence or mental frailty in memory ability may include a generalized negative self-concept, a false perception that everyone else has a better memory, a lack of control over strategic behaviors, and an unrealistic fear of developing Alzheimer's disease. Individuals with this type of vulnerability may purchase expensive medications or dietary supplements in an effort to improve their memory or avoid social interactions that make demands on their faltering cognitive ability.

In older adults living in nursing homes, mental frailty is devastating to cognitive function and quality of life. McDougall (1998) evaluated memory awareness in 106 nursing home residents. Forty-three percent of the sample were depressed, and 46% were cognitively impaired. Depression negatively influenced perceptions of memory capacity (less) and change (decline). The sample was divided into high ($n = 64$) and low ($n = 42$) locus of control groups. *Locus* is the individual's perceived personal control over remembering abilities; a higher score indicates a greater internal locus, a lower score indicates less control. Those individuals in the high control group used more internal and external memory strategies to help their memories; those in the low control group used significantly fewer strategies to remember. In addition, individuals in the low control group had lived in the nursing home significantly longer than had those in the high group (4.56 versus 4.11 years). Those individuals who lived the longest in a nursing home were less likely to use internal and external memory strategies to improve their everyday memory. This same principle could be extrapolated to elderly in critical care units.

ATTITUDES TOWARD THE ELDERLY

Research on attitudes and beliefs of nurses and physicians toward the elderly offers insight into the care received and the resources used by critically ill older adults. Although Wolanin's (1977) seminal research on health-care providers' attitudes was conducted in a nursing home, it has broad application. She studied labeling by nurses and doctors of older patients as confused. Each attributed different characteristics to the residents in Wolanin's (1977) study. Nurses classified the residents as socially inaccessible; physicians classified them as cognitively inaccessible. Cilberto, Levin, and Arluke (1981) studied nurses' ($n = 186$) clinical decision-making process that permits the systematic labeling of patients as senile. When compared to a younger person, older patients with identical neuropsychiatric symptoms were given the diagnosis of organic brain syndrome with a concomitant poor prognosis for recovery. The treatment was of a palliative, rather than interventive, nature. Armstrong-Esther and Brown (1986) found that nurses had significantly less psychosocial interaction with confused patients.

During the 1970s nephrology nurses, social workers, physicians, and ethicists were writing about critical care and older adults. Although only 4 publications appear in the database during this time period, issues were debated. Each discipline expressed concerns regarding the decision making associated with issues of death with dignity and the reactions of patients, family, and staff to the illness. When moving forward to the decade of the 1980s, there were 16 publications appearing in the database. Almost equal numbers of nursing and medical references were available. The topics were not divergent but related to the concerns of the disciplines. For example, nurses were examining decision making, do-not-resuscitate orders, endotracheal procedures, sleep, and the critical care environment. Physicians were examining nursing home care, resuscitation, aggressiveness of the therapy delivered, quality-of-life ethics, and tracheotomy versus intubation. Clearly, the technology was a concern.

During the 1990s the number of citations increased to 54. Ethical concerns related to advance directives and end-of-life care were rigorously debated, and mechanical ventilation was a continuing concern for these patients. Families of the patients and the spiritual concerns of patients were being addressed. What is evident is the international research being generated in China and Europe. In summary, during the 1990s at least 25 of the 54 citations were nursing references. Other interdisciplinary journals may in fact represent nursing authors; however, this is not evident from the citation.

CRITICALLY ILL ELDERLY SURVIVORS AND HOME-BASED CARE

In 1987, Zaren and Hedstrand examined quality of life in 717 individuals 1 year after their admission to an intensive care unit. Of those adults 65 years of age and older, 90% were living independently at the time of the study. Mahul et al. (1991) followed 216 adults 70 years of age and older discharged from intensive care units. At 1 year, 103 patients had survived the illness, and in 72% of the survivors, functional ability permitted their continued independent living. Konopad, Noseworthy, Johnston, Shustack, and Grace (1995) followed 504 patients, 55 years of age and older, for 1 year after they were hospitalized in intensive care. They found that at 1 year post discharge, 89% of the study participants had returned to their homes, and health status increased in the very old. With greater numbers of older adults surviving critical illnesses, not only is survival a concern, but the quality of their lives becomes even more important when reconstructing their lives from before the illness.

With the discharges from acute care hospitalization occurring sooner, investigators became interested in the cost effectiveness of home care. Nurses have been providing care in the homes but not always documenting and testing their interventions systematically. Weinberger, Smith, Katz, and Moore (1988) provided discharge information to outpatient nurses, and a clinical trial with 1001 patients was implemented. They found that even though high-risk patients in the intervention group had greater outpatient costs, their inpatient costs were significantly lower than those for the high-risk patients in the control group. Their findings significantly reduced the costs associated with hospital readmissions. Prigerson (1991) found that geriatric patients preferred care by home health hospices. Patients with diagnoses of heart failure who are being weaned from mechanical ventilation are being treated at home, and many studies have documented home-based care as a treatment of choice. The studies are usually multidisciplinary research efforts (Evans & Hendricks, 1993; Kornowski et al., 1995; Scheinhorn, Chao, Stearn-Hassenpflug, LaBree, & Heltsley, 1997).

Heart Disease

Nursing has had a significant impact on home-based care for older adults discharged with heart failure. Heart failure is now treated in the home by advanced practice and critical care nurses. Sherman (1995) documented that nurses were providing in-home dobutamine infusions to patients with heart failure. Naylor et al. (1994), in a rigorous clinical trial, tested a discharge planning protocol implemented by clinical nurse specialists and specifically designed for the elderly. Her team found the greatest impact in delaying or preventing rehospitalization to occur in the first 6 weeks post discharge. Naylor et al. (1999) replicated the original study with more intensive follow-up at 2, 6, 12, and 24 weeks for at-risk hospitalized elders. The team found that the control group was readmitted and had multiple readmissions, twice as often as the intervention group. However, there was a $.6 million savings to Medicare in the intervention group. In a secondary analysis of 202 patients with cardiac illness (angina, cardiac valve replacement, coronary artery bypass graft surgery, heart failure, and myocardial infarction), Naylor and McCauley (1999) found no differences in functional status between the experimental and control groups. Other investigators have replicated these studies in Australia and the United States and found similar positive outcomes (Kornowski et al., 1995; Rich et al., 1995; Stewart, Pearson, Luke, & Horowitz, 1998). Clearly, nurse scientists have begun a process of documenting interventions and outcomes related to the critically ill elder.

Weaning from Mechanical Ventilation

The incidence of mechanical ventilation and weaning from this technology is increasing (Douglas et al., 1997). Gracey et al. (1992) found that of the 62 patients admitted to a unit for those who were chronically ventilator dependent, 8 were discharged to home after rehabilitation. A trend in the care of these patients is to transfer to a regional weaning center before discharge. Scheinhorn et al. (1997) studied 1123 ventilator-dependent patients transferred to a weaning center and found no change in patient outcomes or in median time to wean. However, a 14% increase in those patients discharged to home occurred over the 8-year study period. Even though mortality was unchanged, the authors found that the patients being transferred to the weaning center had greater severity of illness on arrival. Douglas et al. (1997) found 33% of their sample ($n = 57$) of intensive care unit (ICU) patients were living at home 6 months after discharge. However, none of these individuals returned home without assistance. These patients seem to be sicker on arrival to weaning centers, and, in spite of this level of acuity their prognosis is positive.

Psychiatric Home Care

The incidence of psychiatric illness in the elderly continues to be a major public health crisis. The prevalence of anxiety disorders, major depression, and bipolar disorders has not gone away. If an older adult with a psychiatric diagnosis is discharged from a psychiatric facility, then he or she is considered critically ill. For these patients to return home, there must be someone to provide both the physical and the mental aspects of care in the home. Under Medicare Part B home-care guidelines, home health agencies are reimbursed for skilled nursing visits provided by master's prepared psychiatric nurses with specialized experience and education for treating older adults. The referral is made by the physician, or other health-care provider to the home health agency, and the postdischarge plan of care is given to the agency. After the advanced practice nurse provides an initial skilled home visit and before the in-home psychotherapy commences, the plan of care must be documented on the Health Care Financing Review Form 486. This plan must identify specific goals that can be reached in a 60-day period. If the individual client or patient regresses or is rehospitalized, the 60-day period may be extended with the approval and collaboration of the psychiatrist. An example of a nurse-directed study is provided here for illustration.

McDougall, Blixen, and Suen (1997) and Blixen, McDougall, and Suen (1997) examined the outcomes of life-review therapy provided by an advanced practice geropsychiatric nurse to older adults discharged from psychiatric hospitals to homebound status. Eighty elders (26 males and 54 females) over 65 years of age were seen at home for an average of 13 life review psychotherapy sessions. Depression was the primary psychiatric diagnosis in the life review group ($n = 80$). The treatment was reimbursed under Medicare Part B. Content analysis methods, both latent and manifest, were used to analyze the data and identify themes. There was a significant decrease ($p < .0001$) in the disempowerment themes ($M_1 = 11.66$; $M_2 = 8.75$) during the therapy; however, there was no change in the empowerment themes. The individuals who had access to this nursing intervention clearly benefited from the treatment.

In the entire study sample ($N = 101$), more than one third (37.6%) had a substance abuse disorder in addition to the psychiatric disorder. Of this dual diagnosis group, 71% abused alcohol and 29% abused both alcohol and other substances. This group was mentally frail; significantly more elders in the dual diagnosis group (17.7%) than in the group with only a mental disorder diagnosis (3.3%) made a suicide attempt prior to admission to the hospital. In a national sample of adults ($N = 18,352$), Grant and Hasin (1999) found major depression and alcohol dependence to be risk factors of suicidal ideation. In a study of dual diagnosis in adult men who were veterans, unipolar and bipolar disorders with concurrent alcohol use disorder were associated with increased risk for suicidality (Waller, Lyons, & Costantini-Ferrando, 1999).

The hospital admission patterns of 176 elderly, age 60 years or older, with alcohol disorders were investigated from retrospective chart audits. Twenty-nine percent of the admissions were to psychiatric services and 71%

went to medicine or surgery. In contrast, patients between the ages of 20 and 59 were overwhelmingly (78%) admitted to a psychiatric service. The findings may not apply to the United States because the study was completed in Manchester in the United Kingdom (Mulinga, 1999). Critical care nurses will most likely continue to care for older adults with alcohol and other substance abuse disorders in hospital settings.

FAILURE TO THRIVE

In 1976, Messert, Kurlanzik, and Thorning described a syndrome in adults that they called "failure to thrive" (FTT). Their analogy compared this adult neurological syndrome to a similar syndrome seen in children. At that time, their hypothesis was clinically based, and they believed that the pathology was the result of a random aggregate of lesions rather than the result of a verifiable discrete hypothalamic deficit. Their conclusions were based on observations from patients exhibiting a variety of central nervous system diseases that seemed to follow an unusual course and resulted in weight loss. Temperature variations, intractable decubitus ulcerations, and decreased consciousness were the primary manifestations of the disease process.

Berkman, Foster, and Campion (1989) linked the FTT syndrome to frail elderly. They studied the charts of 82 elderly patients who were unresponsive to health-care interventions. In 1990, Palmer described FTT as a gradual decline of an elderly patient in both physical and cognitive function. Dr. Palmer expanded on the definition to include the original symptom of weight loss and included social withdrawal that occurs without an explanation. He determined that dementia, depression, delirium, drug reactions, and some chronic diseases were a part of the syndrome. The original conceptualization of FTT was in 1976; the Institute of Medicine (IOM) comprehensively reported on the phenomenon in 1991. The IOM report (1991) determined that FTT is a syndrome of nutritional abnormalities with many etiologies: starvation, undiagnosed disease, and a unique process associated with aging. In addition to malnutrition, FTT is associated with immune activation, physiological stress response, involutional changes in anabolic hormones, and the chronic-acute phase response.

Although there are dozens of articles describing the phenomenon, interventions have not been developed to reverse this process (Carr-Lopez & Phillips, 1996; Egbert, 1996; Gordon, 1997; Hildebrand, Joos, & Lee, 1997; Katz, Beaston-Wimmer, Parmelee, Friedman, & Lawton, 1993; Markson, 1997; Roubenoff & Harris, 1997; Verdery, 1997a, 1997b). Nursing began to describe the syndrome in 1992 (Newbern, 1992), and nursing authors are at the descriptive stage, evaluating the clinical manifestations of the phenomenon (Groom, 1993; Jamison, 1997; Kimball, & Williams-Burgess, 1995; Newbern & Krowchuk, 1994; Osato, Takano Stone, Phillips, & Winne, 1993).

Recently, clinicians have hypothesized that depression and dementia may lead to FTT in older adults (Katz & DiFillippo, 1997). Schreiber and Lerer (1997) believe that FTT is an extreme form of clinical depression and that treating the depression has intrinsic clinical value. Regardless of the etiology of this syndrome, the next step is to develop and test interventions to reverse the course of this syndrome.

REFERENCES

Armstrong-Esther, C. A., & Browne, K. D. (1986). The influence of elderly patients' mental impairment on nurse-patient interaction. *Journal of Advanced Nursing, 11,* 379–387.

Berkman, B., Foster, L. W., & Campion, E. (1989). Failure to thrive: Paradigm for the frail elder. *Gerontologist, 29,* 654–659.

Blixen, C. E., McDougall, G. J., & Suen L. J. (1997). Dual diagnosis in elders discharged from a psychiatric hospital. *International Journal of Geriatric Psychiatry, 12,* 307–313.

Carr-Lopez, S. M., & Phillips, S. L. (1996). The role of medications in geriatric failure to thrive. *Drugs & Aging, 9,* 221–225.

Chin, A., Paw, M. J., Dekker, J. M., Feskens, E. J., Schouten, E. G., & Kromhout, D. (1999). How to select a frail elderly population? A comparison of three working definitions. *Journal of Clinical Epidemiology, 52,* 1015–1021.

Cilberto, D. J., Levin, J., & Arluke, A. (1981). Nurses' diagnostic stereotyping of the elderly. *Research on Aging, 3,* 299–310.

Douglas, S. L., Daly, B. J., Brennan, P. F., Harris, S., Nochomovitz, M., & Dyer, M. A. (1997). Outcomes of long-term ventilator patients: A descriptive study. *American Journal of Critical Care, 6,* 99–105.

Egbert, A. M. (1996). The dwindles: Failure to thrive in older patients. *Nutrition Reviews, 54* (1 Pt 2), S25–S30.

Evans, R. L., & Hendricks, R. D. (1993). Evaluating hospital discharge planning: A randomized clinical trial. *Medical Care, 31,* 358–370.

Gordon, M. (1997). Failure to thrive in older adults. *Annals of Internal Medicine, 126,* 669.

Gracey, D. R., Viggiano, R. W., Naessens, J. M., Hubmayr, R. D., Silverstein, M. D., & Koenig, G. E. (1992). Outcomes of patients admitted to a chronic ventilator-dependent unit in an acute-care hospital. *Mayo Clinic Proceedings, 67,* 131–136.

Grant, B. F., & Hasin, D. S. (1999). Suicidal ideation among the United States drinking population: Results from the national longitudinal alcohol epidemiologic survey. *Journal of Alcohol Studies, 60,* 422–429.

Groom, D. D. (1993). Elder care. A diagnostic model for failure to thrive. *Journal of Gerontological Nursing, 19* (6), 12–16.

Hildebrand, J. K., Joos, S. K., & Lee, M. A. (1997). Use of the diagnosis "failure to thrive" in older veterans. *Journal of the American Geriatrics Society, 45,* 1113–1117.

Inouye, S. K., Rushing, J. T., Foreman, M. D., Palmer, R. M., & Pompei, P. (1998). Does delirium contribute to poor hospital outcomes? A three-site epidemiologic study. *Journal of General Internal Medicine, 13,* 234–242.

Institute of Medicine. (1991). *Extending life, enhancing life. A national research agenda on aging.* Washington, DC: National Academy Press.

Jamison, M. S. (1997). Failure to thrive in older adults. *Journal of Gerontological Nursing, 23* (2), 8–13.

Katz, I. R., Beaston-Wimmer, P., Parmelee, P., Friedman, E., & Lawton, M. P. (1993). Failure to thrive in the elderly: Exploration of the concept and delineation of psychiatric components. *Journal of Geriatric Psychiatry & Neurology, 6,* 161–169.

Katz, I. R., & DiFilippo, S. (1997). Neuropsychiatric aspects of failure to thrive in late life. *Clinics in Geriatric Medicine, 13,* 623–638.

Kimball, M. J., & Williams-Burgess, C. (1995). Failure to thrive: The silent epidemic of the elderly. *Archives of Psychiatric Nursing, 9,* 99–105.

Konopad, E., Noseworthy, T. W., Johnston, R., Shustack, A., & Grace, M. (1995). Quality of life measures before and one year after admission to an intensive care unit. *Critical Care Medicine, 23* (10), 1653–1659.

Kornowski, R., Zeeli, D., Averbuch, M., Finkelstein, A., Schwartz, D., Moshkovitz, M., Weinreb, B., Hershkovitz, R., Eyal, D., Miller, M., et al. (1995). Intensive home-care surveillance prevents hospitalization and improves morbidity rates among elderly patients with severe congestive heart failure. *American Heart Journal, 129,* 762–766.

Mahul, P., Perrot, D., Tempelhoff, G., Gaussorgues, P., Jospe, R., Ducreux, J. C., Dumont, A., Motin, J., Auboyer, C., & Robert, D. (1991). Short- and long-term prognosis, functional outcome following ICU for elderly. *Intensive Care Medicine, 17* (1), 7–10.

Markson, E. W. (1997). Functional, social, and psychological disability as causes of loss of weight and independence in older community-living people. *Clinics in Geriatric Medicine, 13,* 639–652.

McDougall, G. J. (1998). Memory awareness in nursing home residents. *Gerontology, 44,* 281–287.

McDougall, G. J., & Balyer, J. (1998). Decreasing mental frailty in at-risk elders. *Geriatric Nursing, 19,* 220–224.

McDougall, G. J., Blixen, C. E., & Suen, L. J. (1997). The process and outcome of life review psychotherapy with depressed homebound older adults. *Nursing Research, 46,* 277–283.

McDougall, G. J., Strauss, M. E., Holston, E., & Martin, M. (1999, November). Memory self-efficacy and memory anxiety as predictors of memory performance in at-risk elderly. In S. Kwon (Chair), *Memory and cognition: Theoretical and methodological approaches to sel-ratings, control beliefs, and self-efficacy.* Symposium conducted at the meeting of the Gerontological Society of America, San Francisco, CA.

Messert, B., Kurlanzik, A. E., & Thorning, D. R. (1976). Adult "failure-to-thrive" syndrome. *Journal of Nervous & Mental Disease, 162,* 401–409.

Mulinga, J. D. (1999). Elderly people with alcohol-related problems: Where do they go? *International Journal of Geriatric Psychiatry, 14,* 564–566.

Naylor, M., Brooten, D., Jones, R., Lavizzo-Mourey, R., Mezey, M., & Pauly, M. (1994). Comprehensive discharge planning for the hospitalized elderly. A randomized clinical trial. *Annals of Internal Medicine, 120,* 999–1006.

Naylor, M. D., Brooten, D., Campbell, R., Jacobsen, B. S., Mezey, M. D., Pauly, M. V., & Schwartz, J. S. (1999). Comprehensive discharge planning and home follow-up of hospitalized elders: A randomized clinical trial. *Journal of the American Medical Association, 281,* 613–620.

Naylor, M. D., & McCauley, K. M. (1999). The effects of a discharge planning and home follow-up intervention on elders hospitalized with common medical and surgical cardiac conditions. *Journal of Cardiovascular Nursing, 14* (1), 44–54.

Newbern, V. B. (1992). Failure to thrive: A growing concern in the elderly. *Journal of Gerontological Nursing, 18* (8), 21–25.

Newbern, V. B., & Krowchuk, H. V. (1994). Failure to thrive in elderly people: A conceptual analysis. *Journal of Advanced Nursing, 19,* 840–849.

Osato, E. E., Takano Stone, J., Phillips, S. L., & Winne, D. M. (1993). Clinical manifestations. Failure to thrive in the elderly. *Journal of Gerontological Nursing, 19* (8), 28–34.

Palmer, R. M. (1990). "Failure to thrive" in the elderly: Diagnosis and management. *Geriatrics, 45* (9), 47–50, 53–55.

Pressley, J. C., & Patrick, C. H. (1999). Frailty bias in comorbidity risk adjustments of community-dwelling elderly populations. *Journal of Clinical Epidemiology, 52,* 753–760.

Prigerson, H. G. (1991). Determinants of hospice utilization among terminally ill geriatric patients. *Home Health Care Services Quarterly, 12* (4), 81–112.

Rich, M. W., Beckham, V., Wittenberg, C., Leven, C. L., Freedland, K. E., & Carney, R. M. (1995). A multidisciplinary intervention to prevent the readmission of elderly patients with congestive heart failure. *New England Journal of Medicine, 333,* 1190–1195.

Roubenoff, R., & Harris, T. B. (1997). Failure to thrive, sacropenia and functional decline in the elderly. *Clinics in Geriatric Medicine, 13,* 613–622.

Scheinhorn, D. J., Chao, D. C., Stearn-Hassenpflug, M., LaBree, L. D., & Heltsley, D. J. (1997). Post-ICU mechanical ventilation: Treatment of 1,123 patients at a regional weaning center. *Chest, 111,* 1654–1659.

Schreiber, S., & Lerer, B. (1997). "Failure to thrive" in elderly depressed patients: A new concept or a different name for an old problem?. *Israel Journal of Psychiatry & Related Sciences, 34,* 108–114.

Sherman, A. (1995). Critical care management of the heart failure patient in the home. *Critical Care Nursing Quarterly, 18* (1), 77–87.

Smith, J., & Baltes, M. M. (1998). The role of gender in very old age: Profiles of functioning and everyday life patterns. *Psychology & Aging, 13,* 676–695.

Stewart, S., Pearson, S., Luke, C. G., & Horowitz, J. D. (1998). Effects of home-based intervention on unplanned readmissions and out-of-hospital deaths. *Journal of the American Geriatrics Society, 46,* 174–180.

Strawbridge, W. J., Shema, S. J., Balfour, J. L., Higby, H. R., & Kaplan, G. A. (1998). Antecedents of frailty over three decades in an older cohort. *Journal of Gerontology. Series B, Psychological Sciences & Social Sciences, 53* (1), S9–16.

Verdery, R. B. (1997a). Failure to thrive in old age: Follow-up on a workshop. *Journal of Gerontology, 52A,* M333–M336.

Verdery, R. B. (1997b). Clinical evaluation of failure to thrive in older people. *Clinics in Geriatric Medicine, 13,* 769–778.

Waller, S. J., Lyons, J. S., & Costantini-Ferrando, M. F. (1999). Impact of comorbid affective and alcohol use disorders on suicidal ideation and attempts. *Journal of Clinical Psychology, 55,* 585–595.

Walston, J., & Fried, L. P. (1999). Frailty and the older man. *Medical Clinics of North America, 83,* 1173–1194.

Weinberger, M., Smith, D. M., Katz, B. P., & Moore, P. S. (1988). The cost-effectiveness of intensive postdischarge care. A randomized trial. *Medical Care, 26,* 1092–1102.

Wolanin, M. O. (1977). Confusion study: Use of grounded theory as methodology. *Communicating Nursing Research, 8,* 68–75.

Zaren, B., & Hedstrand, U. (1987). Quality of life among long-term survivors of intensive care. *Critical Care Medicine, 15,* 743–747.

4

Delirium

Koen Milisen, Sabina De Geest, Ivo L. Abraham, and Herman H. Delooz

Delirium is a condition primarily characterized by a disturbance of consciousness, attention, cognition, and perception, but it can also affect sleep, psychomotor activity, and emotions (American Psychiatric Association [APA], 1999). In general, the syndrome occurs in 14 to 56% of older hospitalized patients (Inouye, 1998) and is the most common form of psychopathology in this patient population (Britton & Russel, 1998). The marked variability in the epidemiology of delirium results from the differences in study populations, diagnostic criteria, and case-finding and research techniques (Milisen, Foreman, Godderis, Abraham, & Broos, 1998). The emergency department (ED) is the entry point to inpatient wards for most of elderly patients, and the prevalence rates of delirium in this setting are therefore expected to be high (Rousseau, 1999). Limited evidence suggests that prevalence rates for alterations in mental status in elderly ED patients range between 33.5 and 39.9% (Gerson, Counsell, Fontanarosa, & Smucker, 1994; Naughton, Moran, Kadah, Heman-Ackah, & Longano, 1995) of which 10 to 24% present a delirium (Lewis, Miller, Morley, Nork, & Lasater, 1995; Naughton et al., 1995).

Compared to nondelirious elderly, delirious patients experience a higher in-hospital functional decline, more postoperative complications, longer and costlier hospitalizations, and an increased risk for residential care placement (Cole & Primeau, 1993; Francis & Kapoor, 1992; Inouye, Rusing, Foreman, Palmer, & Pompei, 1998; Jacobson, 1997; Naughton et al., 1995). Moreover, hospital mortality rates are higher in delirious patients, ranging from 10% to 65% (Inouye et al., 1998), further emphasizing the danger of this syndrome. Although factors such as severity of illness and comorbidity, pre-existing dementia, or advanced age may contribute to this poor prognosis, delirium itself has been demonstrated to independently contribute to poor outcomes of hospital care (Inouye et al., 1998; O'Keefe & Lavan, 1997).

Unfortunately, the diagnosis of delirium is frequently missed in elderly patients admitted to the ED (Lewis et al., 1995). Early recognition and correct diagnosis of the syndrome are essential to prevent or treat delirium effectively because delirium is mainly a reversible condition. The ED is therefore a strategic place for risk identification or detection of delirium and for referral to appropriate services for further evaluation and treatment (Gerson et al., 1994; Rousseau, 1999). The purpose of this chapter is to present an in-depth discussion of issues of delirium relevant for ED nurses in order to optimize early recognition of this syndrome in elderly patients.

WHAT IS DELIRIUM?

Delirium is characterized by a disturbance of mental functioning that may take days (sometimes weeks) to resolve and sometimes only results in partial recovery (Levkoff et al., 1992). The core features of delirium refer to acute onset and fluctuation of symptoms and impairment in consciousness and cognition or perception (APA, 1994, 1999).

Delirium typically begins suddenly, and in the prodromal stage unusual restlessness is common. The patient may report confused thinking, difficulty with concentration, difficulty in judging the passing of time, or just feeling mixed up (Milisen et al., 1998). Since a patient's baseline cognitive functioning is not known when he or she is admitted to the ED, it is difficult to establish the acuity of onset of delirium. In order to acquire this information, it is necessary to find a reliable informant, such as a family member or previous caregiver, who is familiar with the patient's functioning before admission (Inouye, 1998). Additionally, the course and severity of the symptoms of delirium may vary among individuals and within an individual across time (Milisen et al., 1998). Lucid intervals and delirious episodes may alternate and can be misleading in diagnosing the syndrome (Inouye, 1998).

Delirium is also characterized by a disturbance in consciousness that is manifested by a reduced clarity of awareness of the environment. The ability to focus, sustain, or shift attention is impaired (APA, 1994, 1999). The level of vigilance may vary in intensity and fluctuate over time. A patient may alternate between serious apathetic behavior and increased irritability or hypersensitivity to external stimuli (Francis, 1992; Godderis, Van de Ven, & Wils, 1992). This means, that when a patient is drowsy or lethargic, a clinician must raise the volume of his or her voice or physically stimulate the patient to get his or her attention. It is difficult to involve the patient in the care process to let him or her perform resolute actions, such as activities of daily living (ADL) (Brännström, Gustafson, Norberg, & Winblad, 1989; Francis, 1992). A patient may also be less concentrated and unable to generate or sustain attention to external stimuli and may appear easily distracted by irrelevant stimuli (Milisen et al., 1998). The patient is unable to engage adequately in a conversation or to answer specific questions (Godderis et al., 1992) because he or she easily loses the thread of what has been said.

Delirium is also associated with a change in cognitive functioning that may include disorganized thinking and memory and visuoconstructional impairment and disorientation (APA, 1994, 1999; Inouye, 1998). Disorganized thinking (rambling, illogical or incoherent) is usually a manifestation of underlying cognitive or perceptual disturbances (hallucinations, illusions, misinterpretations) and altered level of consciousness (lethargy, with reduced clarity of awareness of the environment) (Inouye, 1998).

Memory disturbances are a consequence of the previously mentioned attention and concentration deficits that lead to the inability to register recent information (Milisen et al., 1998). Disorientation to time and place is common in delirious patients, and in the worst cases may extend to disorientation to other persons; however, disorientation to self is rare (APA, 1999; Godderis et al., 1992). Although the latter two symptoms are not cardinal features, they are frequently associated with delirium, together with disturbances in sleep–wake cycle (e.g., daytime sleepiness, nighttime agitation, reversal of the cycle); emotional lability, such as fear, anxiety, depression, anger and apathy; and psychomotor agitation or retardation, the so-called "hyperactive," "hypoactive," and mixed variant of both forms (APA, 1999; Inouye, 1998; Milisen et al., 1998).

The hypoactive form (decreased psychomotor activity) is the most common form of delirium in older persons but is difficult to recognize and is associated with a poorer overall prognosis (Inouye, 1998). This quiet state of withdrawal, apathy, and clouded inattention differs from the drowsiness seen in persons dozing or sleeping, in that these latter subjects can be quickly aroused to (and remain at) normal consciousness by mild stimuli. In contrast, the hypoactive delirium necessitates strong physical or verbal stimuli (e.g., vigorous shaking or shouting) to arouse the patient, and, despite these stimuli, arousal is incomplete and transient at best (Milisen et al., 1998). The hyperactive form of delirium (increased psychomotor activity) is rarely missed and is characterized by agitation, verbal and physical aggression, and hallucinations (Inouye, 1998; Milisen et al., 1998).

RISK FACTORS FOR INCIDENCE

Risk factors for developing new-onset delirium include advanced age (Schor, Levkoff, & Lewis, 1992; Williams et al., 1985; Williams-Russo, Urquhart, Sharrock, & Charlson, 1992), pre-existing cognitive impairment such as dementia and depression (Fisher & Flowerdew, 1995; Inouye, Viscoli, Horwitz, Hurst, & Tinetti, 1993; Marcantonio et al., 1994; Pompei et al., 1994; Schor et al., 1992; Williams et al., 1985), severe and multiple underlying illnesses (Inouye et al., 1993; Pompei et al., 1994), substance and alcohol use (Marcantonio et al., 1994; Williams-Russo et al., 1992; Pompei et al., 1994), dehydration (Inouye et al., 1993), and functional (poor mobility) and sensory (vision and hearing) impairment (Inouye et al., 1993; Williams et al., 1985). Older patients presenting in the ED with any of these conditions, should be "flagged" as at high risk for developing delirium in the ED or during their further stay in the hospital.

Together with these risk factors, the stressful experience (psychological and physiological) characteristic for a sudden admission to a critical care environment makes older patients even more vulnerable for development of delirium. As suggested by a multifactorial model for delirium (Inouye & Charpentier, 1996) that represents the complex interrelationship between a vulnerable patient with pertinent predisposing factors and noxious insults or precipitating factors, a highly vulnerable patient (e.g., a hip fracture patient, 80 years old, cardiological comorbidity, and vision impairment) may develop delirium with even relatively benign precipitating factors, such as a single dose of analgesics or use of urinary catheters.

Finally, it is important to note that almost any physiological derangement can cause delirium in a susceptible person. Special interest should be given to older patients admitted for medical conditions such as fluid and electrolyte imbalance, infection, drug toxicity and withdrawal, metabolic disturbances, intracranial processes, and low-perfusion states (Naughton et al., 1995). Moreover, acute cognitive impairment may present in ways that often obscure these causes of illness (Wofford, Loehr, & Schwartz, 1996).

DIFFERENTIATING DELIRIUM FROM DEMENTIA AND DEPRESSION

According to Lewis et al. (1995), underdetection of delirium results from a lack of recognition of the disorder and the failure to recognize signs and symptoms associated with delirium. The need for differentiation of delirium from dementia and depression difficulties is common because many of their features overlap (Table 4.1). As a result, delirium is often misdiagnosed as one of the latter two conditions. Moreover, patients with dementia and depression may present with delirium that is superimposed on their pre-existing cognitive impairment.

As mentioned previously, the symptoms for delirium develop suddenly, are often transient, and vary in intensity. One of the core features of delirium is a disturbance in attention. In contrast, dementia has an insidious onset and a chronic, progressive course (Milisen et al., 1998). Cognitive disturbances, such as memory impairment, are common to both delirium and dementia; however, the patient with dementia usually is alert and does not have the disturbance of consciousness or arousal that is characteristic of delirium (APA, 1999; Inouye, 1998).

TABLE 4.1 Differential Diagnosis of Delirium, Dementia, and Depression

Feature	Delirium	Dementia	Depression
Onset	Acute	Insidious	Acute
Course	Fluctuating, lucid periods in a day	Relatively stable	Relatively stable
Duration	Days to weeks	Months to years	Weeks to months
Consciousness	Reduced	Clear	Clear
Attention	Impaired	Normal, except severe cases	May be disordered
Hallucinations	Usually visual or visual and auditory	Often absent	Predominantly auditory
Delusions	Fleeting, poorly systematized	Often absent	Sustained, systematized
Orientation	Usually impaired, at least for a time	Often impaired	May be impaired
Memory	Immediate and recent memory impaired, remote memory intact	Immediate memory intact, recent memory impaired more than remote memory	May be selectively impaired
Psychomotor	Increased, reduced or shifting unpredictably	Often normal	Varies from retardation to hyperactivity (in agitated depression)
Speech	Often incoherent, slow or rapid	May have difficulty finding words, perseveration	Normal, slow or rapid
Thinking	Disorganized or incoherent	Impoverished and vague	Impoverished, retarded
Physical illness or drug toxicity	One or both are present	Often absent, especially in Alzheimer's disease	Usually absent, but debatable

From "Delirium in the elderly patient," by Z. J. Lipowski, 1989, *New England Journal of Medicine, 320*, p. 578–581. Copyright 1989 by Massachusetts Medical Society. Reprinted with permission of the author.

Differentiation between delirium and depression is even more difficult in the elderly with hypoactive features of delirium (slow speech, apathy, reduced psychomotor activity, fatigue) because these symptoms are similar to those for depression. Depression, however, differs from delirium because impairments in attention and cognition are not pronounced and onset is more gradual. Moreover, perceptual disturbances are uncommon in depression, and the patient is alert. Thinking in depressed persons tends to be intact, although patients may verbalize hopelessness or helplessness (Milisen et al., 1998).

The differential diagnosis among delirium, dementia, and depression is enhanced by the constellation of findings, the rapidity of their onset, and the associated medical and environmental risk factors.

IMPORTANT ISSUES FOR SCREENING AND DETECTING DELIRIUM

Systematic monitoring of mental status of all elderly patients, and especially of those who are at risk for delirium (see earlier), is of major importance at the time of admission and during the hospital stay at the ED. Integration of input from everyone involved in the care process is imperative to improve detection and diagnosis of delirium (Zou, Cole, Primeau, McCusker, Bellavance, & Laplante, 1998). Nurses are best positioned strategically to play a central role in the detection of delirium. Despite the limited time frame in which patients remain in critical care, nurses have the most frequent and ongoing contact with the patient compared with physicians and are therefore more able to detect the minor fluctuations in cognitive functioning (Milisen et al., 1998).

Systematic monitoring of cognitive function can be realized by use of standardized, "observed-rated" instruments that incorporate observations over a certain period of time. This approach is preferred over the use of "performance-based" screening instruments, which may be administered only once at a certain point in time (e.g., formal testing by using the Mini-Mental State Examination [MMSE] [Folstein, Folstein, & McHugh, 1975]) and increase the chance of not detecting a transient syndrome like delirium (Pompei, Foreman, Cassel, Alessi, & Cox, 1995). The usefulness of these performance-based measures can be questioned further because they pose significant response and administration burdens on patients and nurses (Neelon, Champagne, Carlson, & Funk, 1996). Moreover, the interpretation of the resulting score is not always clear and can be misleading because the severity of the cognitive impairment, the level of formal education, fatigue, and the characteristics of the testing environment adversely influence performance on mental status testing (Tombaugh & McIntyre, 1992). Nurses prefer instruments that can be completed based on the observation of behavior and that can be used in the course of usual practice, repetitively and without respondent burden, rather than instruments that necessitate formal testing (Williams, 1991).

The selection of an instrument for cognitive assessment will also be guided by the purpose of the measurement; in other words, screening, monitoring, or diagnosis (Foreman, Fletcher, Mion, Simon, & NICHE Faculty, 1996). Screening is needed for determining the presence of an impairment of cognitive functioning, rather than knowing whether the impairment is, for example, delirium, dementia, or depression. Conversely, diagnostic methods are used to identify the exact nature and cause of the impairment. Monitoring is used to determine cognitive status or severity of cognitive dysfunctioning over time and can be useful in documenting an individual's response to treatment (Foreman et al., 1996).

THE NEECHAM CONFUSION SCALE AS AN INSTRUMENT FOR SCREENING AND MONITORING MENTAL FUNCTIONING

The Neecham Confusion Scale (Neelon et al., 1996) can be regarded as the best screening instrument for delirium in clinical practice. (An example of this instrument and more specific guidelines for use in clinical practice can be found in Letkan-Rutledge [1997].) The Neecham Confusion Scale consists of nine components organized into three subscales, allowing the detection not only of changes in mental status but also of changes and different patterns of physiological and behavioral manifestations over short time frames (Neelon et al., 1996). Subscale 1 (Processing) (0 to 14 points) focuses on the primary components of cognition: attention/alertness, verbal and motor command of information, and memory and orientation. Subscale 2 (Behavior) (0 to 10 points) measures behavioral manifestations associated with more physical performance functions: appearance/posture control, sensorimotor performance, and verbal manifestations accompanying or heralding delirium-like syndromes. Subscale 3 (Physiologic Control) (0 to 6 points) consists of physiological control and stability, including vital functions, oxygenation, and continence. These last three components in subscale 3 are an attempt to link the cognitive and behavioral symptoms of delirium with alteration in various physiological parameters to facilitate the identification of the underlying etiology(ies) (Neelon et al., 1996; Williams, 1991).

The use of this instrument is feasible during routine nursing assessments and real-world patient-nurse interactions. The Neecham Confusion Scale causes a minimal response burden for patients. Completion of the instrument after clinical assessment by nurses takes only 5 to 10 minutes and can thus be done at the same time nurses write their clinical report. The Neecham Confusion Scale comprises items that are not associated with learning effect, and testing can therefore be repeated at frequent intervals to monitor for changes in the patient's mental status during a possible further hospital stay.

The Neecham total score is calculated by adding the scores for the three subscales and ranges from 0 (minimal responsiveness) to 30 (normal function). The following cut-off points are suggested for clinical practice: 0 to 19 indicates moderate to severe confusion; 20 to 24 indicates mild or early development of confusion; and scores greater than 24 indicate normal cognitive functioning or no confusion (Lekan-Rutledge, 1997). The scores for subjects with severe chronic cognitive impairment may differ from the above ranges (with or without superimposed delirium). Recent research indicates that there is need for further differentiation between the different syndromes (e.g., delirium versus dementia versus depression) through clinical assessment because the Neecham shows low positive predictive value for diagnosing delirium when using the aforementioned cut-off points (Milisen, 1999). Additionally, identifying delirium superimposed on dementia may be better addressed by examining changes in scores over time rather than comparing single scores with threshold values developed for individuals without pre-existing cognitive impairment (Pompei et al., 1995).

Based on these findings, the Neecham Confusion Scale is a good instrument for screening and rating or monitoring of cognitive dysfunctioning but not for the diagnosis of delirium.

THE CONFUSION ASSESSMENT METHOD AS A METHOD TO DIFFERENTIATE DELIRIUM FROM DEMENTIA AND DEPRESSION

Delirium must be considered when recent changes in an older patient's level of mental and behavioral functioning are observed. It is imperative to collect baseline data on the patient's mental history before admission. Elderly patients, especially those who are already confused upon admission, are not able to provide a clear clinical history. Relatives or previous caregivers accompanying the patient should be asked for baseline cognitive data. This can be achieved by describing the patient's behavior on a typical day concerning his or her interaction style with other people; responsiveness to stimuli; and memory, orientation, and perceptual patterns. Further, the ability to engage in basic activities of daily living (feeding, grooming, toileting oneself) may be the most sensitive indicator of cognitive status and is an excellent baseline measure that can be observed over time (Dellasega, 1998). Special interest should be given to onset (e.g., was the onset sudden or insidious), duration (when did the changes first become apparent, how long did it last) and course (has the patient's condition been constant or variable) of abnormal behavior of the patient.

More specifically, these issues refer to the first feature of the Confusion Assessment Method (CAM) (Table 4.2), a diagnostic algorithm proven to be an efficient and effective method to detect delirium in the elderly by nonpsychiatric-trained clinicians (Inouye et al., 1990). Although some formal evaluation (e.g., interview) of the patient is needed to test the patient's attention (feature 2, Table 4.2), specific questions in this regard may be kept to a minimum (e.g., days of the week backwards, count backwards from 20, and a five-item forward digit-span), as shown by Lewis et al. (1995). Thinking and level of consciousness and alertness (features 3 and 4, Table 4.2) can be easily observed during the routine care process.

TABLE 4.2   The Confusion Assessment Method: Diagnostic Algorithm

Feature 1.   Acute onset and fluctuating course
This feature is usually obtained from a family member or nurse and is shown by positive responses to the following questions: Is there evidence of an acute change in mental status from the patient's baseline? Did the (abnormal) behavior fluctuate during the day, that is, tend to come and go or increase and decrease in intensity?

Feature 2.   Inattention
This feature is shown by a positive response to the following question: Did the patient have difficulty focusing attention, for example, being easily distractible, or having difficulty keeping track of what was being said?

Feature 3.   Disorganized thinking
This feature is shown by a positive response to the following question: Was the patient's thinking disorganized or incoherent, such as rambling or irrelevant conversation, unclear or illogical flow of ideas, or unpredictable switching from subject to subject?

Feature 4.   Altered level of consciousness
This feature is shown by any answer other than "alert" to the following question: Overall, how would you rate this patient's level of consciousness? (alert [normal], vigilant [hyperalert], lethargic [drowsy, easily aroused], stupor [difficult to arouse], or coma [unarousable])

From "Clarifying confusion: The confusion assessment method," by S. K. Inouye, C. H. van Dyck, C. A. Alessi, S. Balkin, A. P. Siegal, & R. I. Horwitz, 1990, *Annals of Internal Medicine, 119*, p. ___. Copyright XXXX by __. Reprinted with permission of the author.

To classify a patient as delirious, the first two and at least one of the other two criteria must be fulfilled (Inouye et al., 1990). However, because a patient mostly stays for a limited period of critical care and a relative is not always available for additional baseline information, it is often very difficult to assess criterion 1 or 2 of the CAM. A distinct category of probable delirium is therefore added (Lewis et al., 1995), in which evidence for either acute change in or fluctuation of mental status (but not both) is required. This allows increased sensitivity for detection of all possible delirium cases.

CONCLUSIONS

Geriatric patients are at high risk for developing delirium while admitted for critical care. Delirium is associated with an increased risk for morbidity and mortality. The syndrome often remains unrecognized or is misdiagnosed as dementia or depression. Nurses are best positioned to monitor the fluctuations in elderly patients' cognitive status because of their intensive contact with the patient. Nurses' observations should be communicated to other health-care workers in order to enhance correct diagnosis of delirium. A thorough, reliable, and systematic clinical assessment of delirium in elderly patients is crucial. Several standardized instruments are available for this purpose. Attention should be given to the differentiation among delirium, dementia, and depression in order to optimize effective management of these patients.

REFERENCES

American Psychiatric Association. (1994). *Diagnostic and statistical manual of mental disorders* (4th ed.). Washington, DC: American Psychiatric Press.
American Psychiatric Association. (1999). Practice guideline for the treatment of patients with delirium. *American Journal of Psychiatry, 156* (Suppl.), 5.
Brännström, B., Gustafson, Y., Norberg, A., & Winblad, B. (1989). Problems of basic nursing care in acutely confused and non-confused hip-fracture patients. *Scandinavian Journal of Caring Sciences, 3,* 27–34.
Britton, A. M., & Russell, R. (1998). Multidisciplinary team interventions in the management of delirium in patients with chronic cognitive impairment: A review of the evidence of effectiveness. *Cochrane Library, 4,* 1–12.
Cole, M. G., & Primeau, F. J. (1993). Prognosis of delirium in elderly hospital patients. *Canadian Medical Association Journal, 149,* 41–46.
Dellasega, C. (1998). Assessment of cognition in the elderly: Pieces of the complex puzzle. *Nursing Clinics of North America, 33,* 395–405.
Fisher, B. W., & Flowerdew, G. (1995). A simple model for predicting postoperative delirium in older patients undergoing elective orthopedic surgery. *Journal of the American Geriatrics Society, 43,* 175–178.
Folstein, M. F., Folstein, S. E., & McHugh, P. R. (1975). "Mini-Mental State": A practical method for grading the cognitive state of patients for the clinician. *Journal of Psychiatry and Research, 12,* 189–198.
Foreman, M. D., Fletcher, K., Mion, L. C., Simon, L., & NICHE Faculty. (1996). Assessing cognitive functioning. *Geriatric Nursing, 17,* 228–233.
Francis, J. (1992). Delirium in older patients. *Journal of the American Geriatrics Society, 40,* 829–838.
Francis, J., & Kapoor, W. N. (1992). Prognosis after hospital discharge of older medical patients with delirium. *Journal of the American Geriatrics Society, 40,* 601–606.
Gerson, L. W., Counsell, S. R., Fontanarosa, P. B., & Smucker, W. D. (1994). Case finding for cognitive impairment in elderly emergency department patients. *Annals of Emergency Medicine, 23,* 813–817.
Godderis, J., Van de Ven, L., & Wils, V. (1992). Delier. In J. Godderis, L. Van de Ven, & V. Wils (Eds.), *Handboek Geriatrische Psychiatrie* (pp. 129–161). Leuven/ Apeldoorn Béligium, Garant.
Inouye, S. K. (1998). Delirium in hospitalized older patients. *Clinics in Geriatric Medicine, 14,* 745–764.
Inouye, S. K., & Charpentier, P. A. (1996). Precipitating factors for delirium in hospitalized elderly persons: Predictive model and interrelationship with baseline vulnerability. *Journal of the American Medical Association, 275,* 852–857.
Inouye, S. K., Rusing, J. T., Foreman, M. D., Palmer, R., & Pompei, P. (1998). Does delirium contribute to poor hospital outcomes? A three-site epidemiologic study. *Journal of General Internal Medicine, 13,* 234–242.

Inouye, S. K., van Dyck, C. H., Alessi, C. A., Balkin, S., Siegal, A. P., & Horwitz, R. I. (1990). Clarifying confusion: The confusion assessment method. *Annals of Internal Medicine, 119,* 474–481.

Inouye, S. K., Viscoli, C. M., Horwitz, R. I., Hurst, L. D., & Tinetti, M. E. (1993). A predictive model for delirium in hospitalized elderly medical patients based on admission characteristics. *Annals of Internal Medicine, 119,* 474–481.

Jacobson, S. A. (1997). Delirium in the elderly. *The Psychiatric Clinics of North America, 20,* 91–110.

Lekan-Rutledge, D. (1997). Functional assessment. In M. A. Matteson, E. S. McConnel, & A. D. Linton (Eds.), *Gerontological nursing: Concepts and practice* (2nd ed., pp. 90–94). Philadelphia: W. B. Saunders.

Levkoff, S. E., Evans, D. A., Liptzin, B., Cleary, P. D., Lipsitz, L. A., Wetle, T. T., Reilly, C. H., Pilgrim, D. M., Schor, J., & Rowe, J. (1992). Delirium: The occurrence and persistence of symptoms among elderly hospitalized patients. *Archives of International Medicine, 152,* 334–340.

Lewis, L. M., Miller, D. K., Morley, J. E., Nork, M. J., & Lasater, L. C. (1995). Unrecognized delirium in ED geriatric patients. *American Journal of Emergency Medicine, 13,* 142–145.

Marcantonio, E. R., Goldman, L., Mangione, C. M., Ludwig, L. E., Muraca, B., Haslauer, C. M., Donaldson, M. C., Whittemore, A. D., Sugarbaker, D. J., Poss, R., Haas, S., Cook, E. F., Orav, E. J., & Lee T. H. (1994). A clinical prediction rule for delirium after elective noncardiac surgery. *Journal of the American Medical Association, 271,* 134–139.

Milisen, K. (1999). *An intervention study for delirium in elderly fracture patients.* Unpublished Doctoral Thesis, Katholicke Universiteit Leuven, Leuven, Belgium.

Milisen, K., Foreman, M. D., Godderis, J., Abraham, I., & Broos, P. L. O. (1998). Delirium in the elderly: Nursing assessment and management. *Nursing Clinics of North America, 33,* 417–439.

Naughton, B. J., Moran, M. B., Kadah, H., Heman-Ackah, Y., & Longano, J. (1995). Delirium and other cognitive impairment in older adults in an emergency department. *Annals of Emergency Medicine, 25,* 751–755.

Neelon, V. J., Champagne, M. T., Carlson, J. R., & Funk, S. G. (1996). The Neecham Confusion Scale: Construction, validation, and clinical testing. *Nursing Research, 45,* 324–330.

O'Keefe, S. O., & Lavan, J. (1997). The prognostic significance of delirium in older hospital patients. *Journal of the American Geriatrics Society, 45,* 174–178.

Pompei, P., Foreman, M. D., Cassel, C. K., Alessi, C., & Cox, D. (1995). Detecting delirium among hospitalized older patients. *Archives of Internal Medicine, 155,* 301–307.

Pompei, P., Foreman, M. D., Rudberg, M. A., Inouye, S. K., Braund, V., & Cassel, C. K. (1994). Delirium in hospitalized elderly persons: Outcomes and predictors. *Journal of the American Geriatrics Society, 42,* 809–815.

Rousseau, F. (1999). Delirium detection among emergency and hospitalized older patients. Paper presented at the Ninth Congress of the International Psychogeriatric Association, Vancouver, Canada.

Schor, J. D., Levkoff, S., & Lewis, A. (1992). Risk factors for delirium in hospitalized elderly. *Journal of the American Medical Association, 267,* 827–831.

Tombaugh, T. N., & McIntyre, N. J. (1992). The Mini-Mental State Examination: A comprehensive review. *Journal of the American Geriatrics Society, 40,* 922–935.

Williams, M. A. (1991). Delirium/acute confusional states: Evaluation devices in nursing. *International Psychogeriatrics, 3,* 301–308.

Williams, M. A., Campbell, E. B., Raynor, W. J., Musholt, M. A., Mlynarczyk, S. M., & Crane L. F. (1985). Predictors of acute confusional states in hospitalized elderly patients. *Research in Nursing and Health, 8,* 31–40.

Williams-Russo, P., Urquhart, B. L., Sharrock, N. E., & Charlson, M. E. (1992). Post-operative delirium: Predictors and prognosis in elderly orthopedic patients. *Journal of the American Geriatrics Society, 40,* 759–767.

Wofford, J. L., Loehr, L. R., & Schwartz, E. (1996). Acute cognitive impairment in elderly ED patients: Etiologies and outcomes. *American Journal of Emergency Medicine, 14,* 649–653.

Zou, Y., Cole, M. G., Primeau, F. J., McCusker, J., Bellavance, F., & Laplante, J. (1998). Detection and diagnosis of delirium in the elderly: Psychiatrist diagnosis, confusion assessment method, or consensus diagnosis? *International Psychogeriatrics, 10,* 303–308.

5

Comorbidity: Assessment and Impact

Peter Pompei

In the care of older persons in intensive care units, our primary attention is commonly focused on the acute condition for which the patient was admitted. We recognize, however, that individual patient characteristics such as illness severity, physical and cognitive functional abilities, and the presence of other chronic medical problems will influence the patient's treatment and recovery. Although advanced chronological age often serves as a reasonable surrogate measure of these influential patient characteristics, it is important to remember the diversity of health and disease among older persons. In a large study of complications associated with anesthesia done in France, the rate of complications, although rising with advancing age, was largely dependent on the number of associated diseases per person (Tinet, 1986). Among patients 75 years of age and older, those with three or more associated diseases had a complication rate 10-fold greater than those with no associated diseases. This observation supports the hypothesis that physiological reserve and ability to regain homeostasis are affected partly by changes associated with aging but more importantly by the deleterious consequences of accumulating disease among older persons.

Clinicians commonly consider patient-specific factors other than the presenting problem during their initial assessment of hospitalized patients. It has been shown that physicians were comfortable rating comorbidity as none, mild, moderate, or severe within 24 hours of admission in a cohort of 604 patients admitted to a New York hospital and that these informal estimates were predictive of 1-year mortality rates (Pompei, Charlson, Ales, MacKenzie, & Norton, 1991). Although clinical judgment is appealing because of its simplicity, this method of measuring comorbidity can be influenced by the experience, knowledge, and intuition of the rater, and more objective and quantitative methods would be useful for prognostic stratification. One of the early contributions to the classification of comorbidity was prompted by the need to account for the possible influence of other conditions when evaluating vascular complications among patients with diabetes mellitus (Kaplan & Feinstein, 1974). A cohort of patients with adult-onset diabetes mellitus was followed prospectively for 5 years or until death. Medical problems other than diabetes were classified and graded according to explicit criteria. Each problem was classified as either "cogent" or expected to impair long-term survival or "noncogent." The cogent problems were divided into vascular or nonvascular, and their severity was rated as none, moderate, or severe. There was a clear gradient of mortality based on severity of comorbidity measured by this method: the 5-year mortality rate was 7% for patients with no cogent comorbidity, 33% for patients with moderate comorbidity, and 69% for patients with severe comorbidity. This study demonstrated the importance of classifying and quantitating the burden of comorbidity when evaluating the outcomes of patients with a serious condition such as diabetes mellitus.

As we examine commonly used current methods for assessing and measuring comorbidity in older persons, several areas of controversy should be kept in mind. Exactly what constitutes a comorbid condition and how these conditions are assessed regarding their severity and stability are still debated. The concept of "frailty" is used in the geriatric literature, and distinguishing frailty from the accumulated burden of comorbidity is not always clear. Many different patient outcomes such as mortality (short and longer term), duration of hospitalization, and complication rates could be related to having multiple coexisting medical problems. When a measure of comorbidity is developed to predict one of these outcomes, it may or may not perform well in predicting other seemingly related outcomes. Also, for some conditions, selected types of comorbid conditions may be more "cogent" than other types. For example, among patients undergoing pneumonectomy, the extent and severity of underlying lung disease may be more important in predicting survival than the presence or absence of diabetes mellitus. When selecting a measure of comorbidity it is important to consider the intended use of the measure and clinical characteristics of the patients being assessed. Selected measures of comorbidity and examples of their use will be reviewed in the next sections.

TARGETING ONE CONDITION AS A MEASURE OF COMORBIDITY

In some clinical situations, the presence or absence of a selected seminal condition can be used to stratify patients according to their risk for a specified outcome. Comorbid conditions such as certain cancers and congestive heart failure are associated with a mortality risk that will influence outcomes of patients being treated for many other conditions. In a recent study of 1-year mortality after hip fracture among older persons, the investigators chose the presence of cancer, other than skin cancer, as the important measure of comorbidity that would influence survival (Aharonoff, Koval, Shovron, & Zuckerman, 1997). Among older patients with a hip fracture, those with cancer had a higher 1-year mortality rate than those patients without had. Sometimes the association of a comorbid condition with an outcome such as mortality is more surprising. In a prospective cohort study of more than 500 older persons hospitalized for a medical illness, the presence of depressive symptoms was associated with an increased risk of death within 3 years (Covinsky, 1999). These examples support using the presence or absence of selected comorbid states as potential confounding variables when measuring the outcome of longer-term survival.

It has also been shown that the presence of a low serum albumin level can be an indicator of a higher risk for mortality. Although an abnormal laboratory measurement is not often what clinicians consider a comorbid condition, hypoalbuminemia can be considered a marker of malnutrition or organ dysfunction resulting from comorbidity. In a study of more than 15,000 patients older than age 40 admitted to a Boston hospital between 1984 and 1988, patients with low serum albumin were found to be have an increased risk of in-hospital mortality, longer hospital stays, and more frequent readmissions (Herrmann, Safran, Levkoff, & Minaker, 1992). Two reports from a study of more than 200,000 patients treated at Department of Veterans Affairs Medical Centers confirm the importance of a low serum albumin in predicting poor surgical outcomes. Among about 54,000 cases of major noncardiac surgery, a low serum albumin level was the strongest predictor of morbidity and 30-day mortality when compared with 61 other preoperative patient risk variables (Gibbs et al., 1999). In the specific subset of patients undergoing proctectomy for rectal cancer, presurgical hypoalbuminemia was again associated with an increased 30-day mortality rate (Longo et al., 1998). Low serum albumin is considered a nonspecific marker both because of its association with a variety of disease states and because it is considered by some to be a consequence of normal aging. Based on substantial empirical evidence, despite the many causes of hypoalbuminemia, the presence of this condition has been shown to be related to important patient outcomes such as mortality, morbidity, and prolonged hospitalizations. For this reason, serum albumin can be considered a measure of comorbidity useful to stratify patients according to their risk for selected untoward outcomes.

COUNTING DIAGNOSES TO ESTIMATE COMORBIDITY

Another strategy to assess burden of comorbidity involves counting the number of medical conditions or diagnoses a patient has. The source and accuracy of the information will clearly influence the usefulness of this approach. Most commonly, information is abstracted from the medical record, which will vary in its completeness. Also, because some medical conditions or diagnoses, for example, seborrhea or incontinence, may have little relevance to a patient outcome such as in-hospital mortality, efforts are made to count only "important" comorbid conditions. When predictors of 30-day mortality were sought among 92 patients undergoing pneumonectomy, the comorbid conditions judged worthy of counting were a significant medical history of the following: cardiac disease, diabetes, hypertension, respiratory disease, pulmonary cancer, peripheral vascular disease, liver disease, renal insufficiency, and inflammatory bowel disease (Swartz et al., 1997). Patients with one or more of these conditions were found to have an increased risk of 30-day morality after pneumonectomy. Similarly, in a study of about 100 patients undergoing total knee arthroplasty, comorbidity was assessed by determining how many of the following conditions patients had: hypertension, diabetes mellitus, coronary artery disease, atherosclerotic heart disease, peripheral vascular disease, chronic renal failure, and asthma (Wasielewski, Weed, Prezioso, Nicholson, & Puri, 1998). Patients with four or more of these comorbid conditions were found to have longer hospital stays and a worse functional status at 3 months compared with those with less than four of the conditions. These results indicate that a simple count of selected diagnoses can help identify patients at increased risk for outcomes such as survival, functional recovery, and duration of hospitalization.

Somewhat more complicated counting schemes have been designed to be more comprehensive than selecting from a short list of nonspecific and sometimes overlapping conditions. The National Cancer Institute and the Surveillance, Epidemiology, and End Results tumor registry have a systems-oriented list of comorbid conditions. In this scheme, conditions that involve the same body system are not counted twice, but each condition that is considered distinct from others is awarded 1 point. For example, a patient with arthritis and incontinence would be assigned 2 points, as would a patient with asthma and angina. However, a patient with angina and congestive heart failure would only be assigned 1 point because both conditions are heart related. Trained chart abstractors are responsible for assigning the comorbidity scores. Using this system in a study of about 1600 patients with colon carcinoma, investigators have found that the number of comorbid conditions predicted early mortality, even after taking disease stage into consideration (Yancik et al., 1998). A similar method of classification takes advantage of a mechanism for consolidating the more than 400 diagnosis related groups (DRGs) into 23 major diagnostic categories. Sixteen of the categories correspond to major body systems, and the remaining represent conditions that may involve multiple body systems, such as sepsis or major trauma. Clinical diagnoses can be consolidated into these major diagnostic categories and the number of different involved categories can be summed. This strategy avoids counting related conditions more than once. For instance, a patient with hypertension, angina, and aortic valvular stenosis has three diagnoses, but only one major diagnostic category is involved. When comorbidity was assessed using this system in a cohort of about 400 older persons admitted to the medical service of a Chicago hospital, it was found to be an important predictor of delirium (Pompei et al., 1994). Delirium, in turn, has been shown to be significantly related to both an increased risk of in-hospital mortality and a prolonged duration of hospitalization (Pompei et al., 1994). Various methods for counting comorbid conditions are useful in determining the risk for such important patient outcomes as survival and length of hospital stay among older persons.

INDICES OF COMORBIDITY

For some, a significant limitation of counting diagnoses as a means of quantifying comorbidity relates to the clinical importance of some of the conditions being counted. If the goal is to assess a person's ability to regain or maintain homeostasis, an assessment of the degree of organ impairment seems warranted. Clinicians often make implicit judgments regarding overall organ function that are reasonably accurate. Making these judgments explicit and quantitative is another method to assess comorbidity. This strategy was adopted by those who developed the Cumulative Illness Rating Scale (CIRS), a brief tool used to estimate prognosis and evaluate the impact of patient characteristics on the effect of treatments (Linn, Linn, & Gurel, 1996). To use this scale, physicians are asked to rate the involvement of 13 separate organ systems on a scale from none to extremely severe, as shown in Table 5.1. The total score is the sum of the values assigned to each of the 13 organ systems. Although the authors report excellent interrater reliability, as with any instrument that involves clinical judgment, this should be reconsidered at each clinical site where the scale might be applied. This method for quantifying comorbidity has been used to predict survival and length of hospital stay in patients with spinal cord injuries (Rochon et al., 1996). In addition, it has been used in an observational study of older patients with spinal stenosis to assess whether baseline patient characteristics might explain results from different treatment approaches (Katz et al., 1997). Researchers coordinated a multicenter study involving 272 patients with spinal stenosis who underwent a lumbar laminectomy. A principle finding was improved pain relief among those patients who had a simultaneous noninstrumented arthrodesis compared with patients with no arthrodesis or with an instrumented arthrodesis. The degree of comorbidity in the three groups was similar and did not explain the differences in patient outcomes. The CIRS index of comorbidity has been shown to be useful as a measure of case mix and to predict survival and duration of hospitalization in selected patient populations.

TABLE 5.1   The Cumulative Illness Rating Scale*

Cardiovascular-respiratory system
   1. _____ Cardiac
   2. _____ Vascular
   3. _____ Respiratory
   4. _____ EENT (eyes, ears, nose, throat)

Gastrointestinal system
   5. _____ Upper GI
   6. _____ Lower GI
   7. _____ Hepatic

Genitourinary system
   8. _____ Renal
   9. _____ Other GU

Musculoskeletal-integumentary system
   10. _____ Muscles, bone, skin

Neuropsychiatric system
   11. _____ Neurologic
   12. _____ Psychiatric

General system
   13. _____ Endocrine-metabolic

---

*Each of the following 13 systems are rated on a 5-point scale where 0 = none, 1 = mild, 2 = moderate, 3 = severe, 4 = extremely severe. The ratings are summed to determine the final score.

From "Cumulative Illness Rating Scale," by B. S. Linn, M. W. Linn, and L. Gurel, 1996, *Journal of the American Geriatrics Society, 16,* pp. 622–626. Reprinted with permission of the authors.

A commonly used index to measure comorbidity is one now known as the Charlson index (Charlson, Pompei, Ales, & Mackenzie, 1987). This is an empirically derived prognostic taxonomy of comorbid conditions relevant to short-term survival. It was derived from a cohort of about 600 patients admitted to the medical service of New York Hospital during a 1-month period in 1984. All recorded comorbid conditions were organized into a list of those that were cogent from the point of view of short-term prognosis. Based on the 1-year mortality of the patients enrolled, a weighted index of the selected comorbid conditions was derived based on the number and seriousness of the diseases. The specific conditions considered and their associated weights are shown in Table 5.2. Since it was initially developed, others have enhanced the usefulness of the index by adapting it for use with administrative databases using ICD-9-CM codes (Deyo, Cherkin, & Ciol, 1992; Romano, Roos, & Jollis, 1993). When the index was first developed, it was applied to a cohort of 685 women with breast cancer and proved useful in stratifying patients according to their risk of mortality at 10 years (Charlson et al., 1987). Since then it has been used in many clinical

TABLE 5.2   The Charlson Weighted Index of Comorbidity
Weights are assigned for each condition the patient has, and the sum of the weights is the score.

Condition	Weight
Myocardial infarction	1
Congestive heart failure	1
Peripheral vascular disease	1
Cerebrovascular disease	1
Dementia	1
Chronic pulmonary disease	1
Connective tissue disease	1
Ulcer disease	1
Mild liver disease	1
Diabetes	1
Hemiplegia	2
Moderate or severe renal disease	2
Diabetes with end-organ damage	2
Any tumor	2
Leukemia	2
Lymphoma	2
Moderate or severe liver disease	3
Metastatic solid tumor	4
AIDS	4

From "A New Method of Classifying Prognostic Comorbidity in Longitudinal Studies: Development and Validation," by M. E. Charlson, P. Pompei, K. L. Ales, and C. R. Mackenzie, 1987, *Journal of Chronic Disease, 40,* pp. 373–383. Reprinted with permission of the authors.

studies. The index has been shown to be useful in predicting 5-year mortality among older men undergoing prostatectomy for benign prostatic hypertrophy (Krousel-Wood, Abdah, & Re, 1996) and 18-month mortality among patients treated for a spinal cord injury (Rochon et al., 1996). Among 201 patients admitted to an intensive care unit, the method of quantifying comorbidity developed by Charlson was useful at stratifying the patients according to their risk of in-hospital death (Poses, McClish, Smith, Bekes, & Scott, 1996). In a study of more than 21,000 cases of open cholecystectomy among older persons, both 30- and 90-day mortality were associated with comorbidity measured using the Charlson index (Escarce, Shea, Chen, Qian, & Schwartz, 1995). This method of classifying comorbid conditions has proved extremely useful in categorizing patients according to their risk of mortality for a variety of different clinical conditions. When compared with other methods such as counting diagnoses and the CIRS, it has performed well (Rochon et al., 1996; Krousel-Wood et al., 1996), and it has served as the template for developing a questionnaire that could avoid the need for medical record review when measuring comorbidity (Katz, Chang, Sangha, Fossel, & Bates, 1996).

ASSESSING COMORBIDITY: PROMISES AND PITFALLS

Clinicians commonly make informal judgments about patient-specific characteristics such as severity of illness, stability, functional status, and burden of comorbid illness. These assessments, in combination with their knowledge of specific disease states afflicting patients, have proved useful to them in estimating clinical outcomes including prognosis. The concept that comorbidity, or interacting illnesses, has an important role in patient outcomes is especially relevant among older persons. The combination of age-related decline in physiological function and the accumulation of chronic illness with advancing age can significantly impair homeostatic mechanisms essential for healing and recovery. The challenge of documenting the contribution of comorbid illness to impaired homeostasis has been taken up by several investigators. As described in this chapter, several different measures of comorbidity have been shown to be helpful at predicting patient outcomes, from simply identifying the presence of a particular condition to counting diagnoses, to more elaborate methods of counting and assigning a degree of importance to coexisting illness. These varied methods of defining comorbidity have contributed to improved assessments of patient outcomes such as acute and longer-term mortality, morbidity or complications, and duration of hospitalization. Some studies have demonstrated that measuring comorbidity offers prognostic information beyond other similarly important clinical constructs such as severity of illness, case mix, and functional status (Corti, Guralnik, Salive, & Sorkin, 1994; Zenilman, Bender, Magnuson, & Smith, 1996).

With the advances in measurement strategies and the convincing impact of comorbidity on important patient outcomes, several limitations of our current assessment tools should be mentioned. The fact that there are several different approaches to quantifying comorbidity is evidence that they all have benefits and limitations so that no one strategy has become universally accepted. Measures of comorbidity that include clinical judgment will continue to be limited by the variability of that assessment based on the experience of the clinician, the availability of information, and the stability of the condition. Measures that rely on documentation in the medical record or the use of administrative data will be limited by incomplete documentation and a bias against coding comorbid conditions among patients who die (White, 1996). There is evidence that improved estimates of prognosis result from using a combination of clinical judgment and data abstraction tools or by combining comorbidity measures with measures of severity and case mix (Vaca, 1994; Corti et al., 1994). In addition to comorbidity and severity, especially among older persons, functional status can have an important and independent impact on patient outcomes (Zenilman et al., 1996). Assessing the burden of comorbidity in older hospitalized patients can be important in predicting critical clinical outcomes. Improved taxonomies and metrics for comorbidity and other important patient-specific characteristics are needed for both clinical care and research.

REFERENCES

Aharonoff, G. B., Koval, K. J., Shovron, M. L., & Zuckerman, J. D. (1997). Hip fractures in the elderly: Predictors of one year mortality. *Journal of Orthopaedic Trauma, 11*, 162–165.

Charlson, M. E., Pompei, P., Ales, K. L., & Mackenzie, C. R. (1987). A new method of classifying prognostic comorbidity in longitudinal studies: Development and validation. *Journal of Chronic Disease, 40*, 373–383.

Corti, M. C., Guralnik, J. M., Salive, M. E., & Sorkin, J. D. (1994). Serum albumin level and physical disability as predictors of mortality in older persons. *JAMA, 272*, 1036–1042.

Covinsky, K. E. (1999). Depressive symptoms and 3-year mortality in older hospitalized medical patients. *Annals of Internal Medicine, 130*, 563–569.

Deyo, R. A., Cherkin, D. C., & Ciol, M. A. (1992). Adapting a clinical comorbidity index for use with ICD-9-CM administrative databases. *Journal of Clinical Epidemiology, 45*, 613–619.

Escarce, J. J., Shea, J. A., Chen, W., Qian, Z., & Schwartz, J. S. (1995). Outcomes of open cholecystectomy in the elderly: A longitudinal analysis of 21,000 cases in the prelaparoscopic era. *Surgery, 117*, 156–164.

Gibbs, J., Cull, W., Henderson, W. G., Daley, J., Hur, K., & Khuri, S. F. (1999). Preoperative serum albumin level as a predictor of operative mortality: Results from the National VA surgical risk study. *Archives of Surgery, 134*, 36–42.

Herrmann, F. R., Safran, C., Levkoff, S. E., & Minaker, K. L. (1992). Serum albumin level on admission as a predictor of death, length of stay, and readmission. *Archives of Internal Medicine, 152*, 125–130.

Kaplan, M. H., & Feinstein, A. R. (1974). The importance of classifying initial comorbidity in evaluating the outcome of diabetes mellitus. *Journal of Chronic Disease, 27*, 387–404.

Katz, J. N., Chang, L. C., Sangha, O., Fossel, A. H., & Bates, D. W. (1996). Can comorbidity be measured by questionnaire rather than medical record review? *Medical Care, 34*, 73–84.

Katz, J. N., Lipson, S. J., Lew, R. A., Grobler, L. J., Weinstein, J. N., Brick, G. W., Fossel, A. H., & Liang, M. H. (1997). Lumbar laminectomy alone or with instrumented or noninstumented arthrodesis in degenerative lumbar spinal stenosis: Patient selection, costs, and surgical outcomes. *Spine, 22*, 1123–1131.

Krousel-Wood, M. A., Abdah, A., & Re, R. (1996). Comparing comorbid-illness indices assessing outcome variation: The case of prostatectomy. *Journal of General Internal Medicine, 11*, 32–38.

Linn, B. S., Linn, M. W., & Gurel, L. (1996). Cumulative illness rating scale. *Journal of the American Geriatrics Society, 16*, 622–626.

Longo, W. E., Virgo, K. S., Johnson, F. E., Wade, T. P., Vernava, A. M., Phelan, M. A., Henderson, W. G., Daley, J., & Khuri, S. F. (1998). Outcome after proctectomy for rectal-cancer in department-of-Veterans-Affairs hospitals: A report from the national surgical quality improvement program. *Annals of Surgery, 228,* 64–70.

Pompei, P., Charlson, M. E., Ales, K., MacKenzie, C. R., & Norton, M. (1991). Relating patient characteristics at the time of admission to outcomes of hospitalization. *Journal of Clinical Epidemiology, 44,* 1063–1069.

Pompei, P., Foreman, M., Rudberg, M. A., Inouye, S. K., Braund, V., & Cassel, C. K. (1994). Delirium in hospitalized older persons: Outcomes and predictors. *Journal of the American Geriatric Society, 42,* 809–815.

Poses, R. M., McClish, D. K., Smith, W. R., Bekes, C., & Scott, W. E. (1996). Prediction of survival of critically ill patients by admission comorbidity. *Journal of Clinical Epidemiology, 49,* 743–747.

Rochon, P. A., Katz, J. N., Morrow, L. A., McGlinchey-Berroth, R., Ahlquist, M. M., Sarkarati, M., & Minaker, K. L. (1996). Comorbid illness is associated with survival and length of hospital stay in patient with chronic disability: A prospective comparison of three comorbidity indices. *Medical Care, 34,* 1093–1101.

Romano, P. S., Roos, L. L., & Jollis, J. J. (1993). Further evidence concerning the use of a clinical comorbidity index with ICD-9-CM administrative data. *Journal of Clinical Epidemiology, 46,* 1085–1090.

Swartz, D. E., Lachapelle, K., Sampalis, J., Mulder, D. S., Chiu, R. C.-J., & Wilson, J. (1997). Perioperative mortality after pneumonectomy: Analysis of risk factors and review of the literature. *Canadian Journal of Surgery, 40,* 437–444.

Tinet, L. (1986). Complications associated with anesthesia. *Canadian Anesthetists Society Journal, 33* (3), 336–344.

Vaca, K. J. (1994). Cardiac surgery in the octogenarian: Nursing implications. *Heart and Lung, 23* (5), 413–422.

Wasielewski, R. C., Weed, H., Prezioso, C., Nicholson, C., & Puri, R. D. (1998). Patient comorbidity: Relationship to outcomes of total knee arthoplasty. *Clinical Orthopaedics and Related Research, 356,* 85–92.

White, S. R. (1996). Secondary diagnoses as predictive factors for survival or mortality in Medicare patients with acute pneumonia. *American Journal of Medical Quality, 11* (4), 186–192.

Yancik, R., Wesley, M. N., Ries, L. A. G., Havlik, R. J., Long, S., Edwards, B. K., & Yates, J. W. (1998). Comorbidity and age as predictors of risk for early mortality of male and female colon cancer patients. *Cancer, 82,* 2113–2134.

Zenilman, M. E., Bender, J. S., Magnuson, T. H., & Smith, G. W. (1996). General surgical care in the nursing-home patient: Results of a dedicated geriatric surgery consult service. *Journal of the American College of Surgeons, 183* (4), 361–370.

6

Pain

Meredith Wallace and Ellen Flaherty

Pain is one of the most pervasive yet undertreated problems among older adults. Complaints of pain vary, but it is estimated that about half of all community-dwelling older adults and about two thirds of nursing home residents experience problems with pain. In 1994, the Iowa 65+ Rural Health Study, which was sponsored by the United States National Institute on Aging, sponsored a significant epidemiological study of the elderly. An analysis of pain in the elderly was conducted using data obtained in this project (Mobily, Herr, Clark, & Wallace, 1994). The study included all noninstitutionalized persons 65 years and older living in two rural midwestern counties ($N = 4592$). The sample size for the pain analysis component was 64.3% ($n = 3097$) of the entire target population. The results demonstrated that 86% ($n = 2477$) of this rural elderly population reported pain of some type in the past year. Fifty-nine percent ($n = 1827$) reported multiple pain complaints. A significant relationship between pain and age was reported.

Pain results in depression, decreased socialization, sleep disturbances, impaired ambulation, and increased health care use and costs (American Geriatrics Society Panel [AGS], 1998). For nurses, pain assessment and management are paramount in providing nursing care to older adults and preventing these sequelae of pain. However, the detection and management of pain is complex and must include routine pain assessment, diagnosis, the careful use of analgesic drugs, and the use of nonpharmacological approaches such as physical therapy interventions and nontraditional approaches.

One barrier to providing effective pain management to older adults is lack of knowledge. An investigation into nurses' knowledge and experience with pain and elderly patients was conducted by Closs (1996). Data for this study were obtained through a mailed questionnaire that was completed by 208 hospital nurses. Results from this questionnaire demonstrated an awareness of the prevalence of chronic pain and its negative consequences, along with knowledge of assessing pain. However, Closs (1996) reported concerns that one third of the nurses believed pain and discomfort are unavoidable consequences of aging, which may lead to the neglect of potentially treatable pain. In another study, a sample of 78 Oncology Nursing Society (ONS) members and community hospital nurses responded to a questionnaire developed to evaluate nursing pain assessment and management. The results of this investigation led the author to recommend that nursing research, education, and practice should include teaching nurses to assess quality of life and coping skills related to the pain experience, how to interpret family information, and how to teach patients to use pain management strategies (Dalton, 1989). This research clearly illustrates the need for nurses caring for critically ill older adults to understand the current information on pain assessment and management in order to plan and provide the most efficient pain treatment.

This chapter begins with an overview of the concept of pain. The experience of pain in the elderly population is reviewed and explored. The clinical assessment of pain in cognitively impaired and normal cognitively functioning older adults is presented along with commonly used pain assessment instruments. Diagnosis of pain and the use of both pharmacological and nonpharmacological pain management strategies are reviewed. The chapter concludes with implications for future nursing research and practice.

THE CONCEPT OF PAIN

The study of pain has historical roots dating back to the 1600s, when Descartes developed the concept of the pain pathway (Melzack & Wall, 1982). Descartes describes this specificity theory by comparing it to the bell ringing mechanism in a church. He believed a distinct system exists that communicates a signal from the bottom of the tower (the skin) to the belfry (the brain). Specificity theory evolved and was taught in medical schools as fact until the 19th century, when physiology emerged as a science (Melzack & Wall, 1982).

The gate control theory of pain was developed in the mid-1960s, which incorporated the physiological theories of pain and also accounted for the psychological process on pain perception and response (Melzack & Wall, 1982). Turk and Melzack (1992) were the first to introduce pain as a multidimensional concept that integrated motivational-affective and cognitive-evaluative components with sensory-physiological ones. The gate control theory addressed the complicated system of physiological transmission of pain through fibers in the spinal cord to the brain, involving the ventrobasal and intralaminar thalamus, somatosensory cortex, and the limbic system. This theory also states that influencing factors such as cognitive information related to past experience, probability of outcome of response, and motivational tendency affect the complex pattern that characterizes pain (Melzack & Wall, 1982).

THE EXPERIENCE OF PAIN IN THE ELDERLY

In 1962, Schludermann and Zubeck conducted an experimental study involving 171 male subjects divided into four groups ages 12–29, 30–45, 45–59, and 60–83 years. Each group was administered the Hardy, Wolff, Goodell dolorimeter to elicit and measure pain response in five areas. Subjects were asked to stop the watch at the first perception of pain. The results of the study revealed that pain sensitivity declines with age. Three years later (Collins & Stone, 1965), an experimental, correlational study of 18 male schizophrenic patients age 32–82 from one hospital was conducted. Subjects were asked to report pain sensitivity and intensity when a stimulator was placed on the dorsal surface of one hand, three times on each occasion. The study was repeated once a week for 5 weeks. The authors concluded that there is no relationship between age and pain intensity (Collins & Stone, 1965). Research attempts to clarify these conflicting findings were conducted in 1976 and 1977 when Harkins and Chapman conducted experimental studies of pain sensitivity by stimulating subjects' teeth with electrodes. Response to pain was measured by pressing 1 of 6 response buttons ranging from no sensation to moderate pain. The findings of this study suggest that older individuals were significantly less willing to report painful shocks than was the younger population.

Inducing pain in subjects is clearly not an acceptable method of studying the relationship of pain and aging. Therefore, these types of studies have not been repeated. However, further descriptive and quasi-experimental studies have revealed both collaborative and conflicting findings. Farrell, Gibson, and Helme (1996) in reporting on the clinical presentation of pain in elders state that several attributes of aging may affect the clinical presentation of pain in older people.

Physiologically, the mechanisms that communicate pain impulses to the brain are presumably subjected to age-related changes in function and may affect presentation. Physiological studies on the pain response of older adults have been conducted in an attempt to determine the presence and cause of altered pain perception with aging. In an experimental study (Levasseur, Gibson, & Helme, 1990) of 25 subjects with a mean age of 70.8 years, subjects were divided into three groups according to their origin of pain: chronic lower lumbar pain, postherpetic neuralgia, and pain of nonorganic origin (psychiatric foundation). Capsaicin ointment was applied to two sites, and pain was measured with two instruments at baseline. After application of the ointment, flare responses were measured using a doppler flowmeter. The results indicated that alteration in the function of capsaicin-sensitive sensory fibers is a possible a cause of decreased subjective reports of pain in older adults and should be regarded as a clinical possibility, warranting further research (Levasseur, Gibson, & Helme, 1990).

In another experimental study of 15 subjects ages 20–40 and 15 healthy subjects over the age of 65, nerve block efficacy was monitored during preblock, block, and postblock while measuring cold, warm, mechanical threshold, and simple reaction time. Qualitative reports of the pain experience were also recorded. The results determined that older adults rely primarily on C-fibre input when reporting pain, which should caution clinicians that pain presentation, diagnosis, and subsequent treatment could be potentially compromised (Chakour, Gibson, Bradbeer, & Helme, 1996). Because of the barriers in studying pain among older adults, understanding the pain sensitivity of these individuals remains a complicated problem.

VARIABLES INFLUENCING THE RESPONSE TO PAIN

Pain has been shown to extend beyond physical dimensions, underscoring the need for effective pain assessment. The effect of other variables influencing the experience of pain among older adults is the subject of much research. The influence of cognitive status on the reports of pain was the subject of a study by Parmalee, Smith, and Katz (1993). The study used a cross-sectional, correlational method with 750 nursing home and congregate housing residents. Self-reports of pain intensity and complaints were correlated with medical reports of cognitive status and functional ability at one period of time. The researchers concluded that decreased reports of pain should be suspected in cognitively impaired elderly. In another study (Porter et al., 1996), similar findings evolved using a quasi-experimental design with 51 cognitively intact community-dwelling adults 65 or over and 44 community- or nursing home–dwelling adults age 65 or over with dementia. Subjects were assessed for cognitive status by clinical exam. Responses to the pain were measured by heart rate, amplitude of sinus arrythmia, videotaped facial expressions, and self-report of pain and anxiety before, during, and after venipuncture. The data again revealed that cognitive status in elderly individuals influences physiological reactivity, self-reported perception of anxiety and pain, and facial expression in response to a mildly painful event and emphasizes the difficulty clinicians confront when attempting to diagnose or effectively manage the pain of cognitively impaired older adults (Porter et al., 1996).

The influence of depression on the experience of pain among older adults has been illustrated in several studies. Sixty-three chronic pain patients, age 25–76 were assessed for pain and depression using diaries, medication intake, and other interviews and questionnaires. The results showed that depression and pain are highly related in women and that when one is present, the other should be suspected. Impaired activity is highly related to depression in older men and should be viewed as potential symptom of the disease (Haley, Turner, & Romano, 1985). In another study of the relationship between pain and depression, Herr and Mobily (1992) surveyed 69 subjects age 64–90 who had experienced back pain for at least 3 months. The results again indicated a relationship between pain and depression. Turk, Okifuji, and Scharff (1995) found similar results when they conducted a correlational descriptive study of 100 chronic pain patients who were selected from 1800 patients referred from physician practices. Patients were divided into two groups, age 69 and younger and age 70 and older and were compared on the variables of demographics, depression, adaptation, coping, and control of pain and function. The results showed that depression and pain severity mediate each other, and one should be suspected when the other is present. The researchers suggested that those nursing the elderly with pain complaints can enhance assessment and intervention by increasing their understanding of the relationship between depression and pain. Therefore, treatment of depression should be incorporated into a total pain management program when necessary (Magni, Schifano, & DeLeo, 1985).

Anxiety and pain were found to be highly correlated in a descriptive correlational study of 479 residents age 61–99 of a multilevel nursing care facility (Casten, Parmelee, Kleban, Powell, Lawton, & Katz, 1995). Subjects were assessed using the *Diagnostic and Statistical Manual of Mental Disorders, third edition revised* (*DSM-III-R*; ADA, 1987) criteria for anxiety and depression and the profile of mood states and pain and depression instruments. The researchers suggested that depression should also be suspected in pain patients but may be demonstrated as anxiety. The findings suggested that anxiety and depression may be used as predictors of pain.

The International Association for the Study of Pain appointed a task force in 1993 to study pain in the elderly. Recognizing age-related changes, this report stressed the need for an approach to pain in the elderly that was different from that for younger populations. The task force surveyed research that demonstrated high prevalence rates of pain in the elderly, necessitating additional research that will ultimately lead to further education and improved practice. Factors, including the physiological changes of aging, sensory deficits, cognitive impairment, and underreporting affect all aspects of this complex phenomena. Psychological factors, including the belief that pain is a normal function of aging, also inhibit reporting and treatment (Farrell et al., 1996). An individualistic approach to pain in older adults, with a focus on the potential influence of these variables on the perception of pain, will result in the most effective assessment and management.

PAIN ASSESSMENT

Assessment of pain for older adults is an essential part of pain management. When nurses do not ask about specific pain symptoms or pain effects, older clients are placed at risk for unidentified, misdiagnosed, and undertreated pain (Greipp, 1992). Pain management is most effective when pain assessment results in the identification of the underlying cause of pain. In addition, it is necessary to distinguish acute pain from chronic pain in order to plan care accordingly. Because there are no objective biological markers of pain, the patient's self-report is the most effective method for gathering information regarding pain. The National Consensus Panel suggestions for comprehensive pain assessment are located in Figure 6.1.

Assessment in Cognitively Impaired Older Adults

Ferrell, Ferrell, and Rivera (1995) concluded that cognitive impairment is a substantial barrier to objective pain assessment, stating "these patients were not comatose or incapable of feeling pain. They were able to make most of their needs known in a qualitative but not always quantitative way" (Ferrell et al., 1995, p. 597). The barriers in objective pain assessment among cognitively impaired older adults was illustrated in a descriptive study of 46 residents, age 73–95, of two medical units in one hospital. Subjects were assessed on admission for pain, cognitive impairment, and functional status using several instruments. The researchers concluded that current standards of practice that rely on patient self-report of discomfort are not an adequate means of assessment with confused older adults. When working with acutely confused elderly patients, nurses need to anticipate the likelihood of discomfort as they assist with activities of daily living and intervene appropriately (Miller et al., 1996).

Alternatives to objective pain assessment in cognitively impaired older adults were evaluated in further studies conducted to develop and validate the Discomfort Scale—Dementia or the Alzheimer's type (DS-DAT) pain assessment tool for use in those with Alzheimer's disease. The first qualitative study, describe by Hurley, Volicer, Hanrahan, Houde, and Volicer (1992), developed the tool content by interviewing 45 nurses. The second study, noted by Hurley et al., attempted to validate the tool and reduce the number of items by using nurse-observers of 68 residents of nine long-term care units of one VA hospital. The third study tested the validity of the developed tool on 82 older subjects at baseline and then monthly over a 6-month period. The study resulted in the conclusion that the nine-item DS-DAT tool is an appropriate instrument for assessing pain in Alzheimer's patients (Hurley et al., 1992).

Pain Assessment Instruments

There are many standardized tools for objectively assessing pain in older adults. However, these instruments are not always used by the nursing staff.

GERIATRIC PAIN ASSESSMENT

Date:_____   Medical Record Number_____

Patient's Name_____

Problem List: Medications:

_____   _____
_____   _____
_____   _____
_____   _____

Pain Description:

Pattern: Constant   Intermittant   Pain Intensity:
Duration:_____   0 1   2   3   4   5   6   7   8   9 10
Location:_____   None   Moderate   Severe
Character:
Lancinating Burning   Stinging   Worst Pain in Last 24 hours:
Radiating   Shooting   Tingling   0 1   2   3   4   5   6   7   8   9 10
                                        None   Moderate   Severe
Other Descriptors:
                                        Mood:_____
_____
                                        Depression Screening Score: _____
_____
                                        Gait and Balance Score: _____
Exacerbating Factors: Impaired Activities:

_____   _____
_____   _____

Relieving Factors: Sleep Quality: _____
_____   Bowel Habits: _____
_____   _____

Other Assessments or Comments: _____
_____
_____

Most Likely Cause of Pain:_____

Plans: _____
_____
_____
_____

FIGURE 6.1 Example of a medical record form that can be used to summarize pain assessment in older persons.

In researching pain assessment tools for the elderly, Herr and Mobily stated that "although pain is a multidimensional concept, subjective intensity is probably the component most often measured in both clinical practice and in treatment-outcome research" (1993, p. 39). When nurses' ratings for pain were compared with those of their patients, Weiner, Ladd, Pieper, and Keefe (1995) found that patient's ratings were routinely higher. These findings underscore the need to use an objective pain assessment instrument for initial and ongoing pain assessment.

The most frequently used measure of pain assessment is a numeric rating scale in which the client is asked to choose a position on a scale of 1 to 10, with 1 being very little pain and 10 being the worst pain imaginable. However, Weiner et al. (1995) reports that the scale is difficult for some older adults because of its abstract design. Furthermore, the scale has not been found to be reliable in a cognitively impaired population (Ferrell, Ferrell, & Rivera, 1995).

Because of numerous factors, including sensory deficits and cognitive impairments, simple questions and tools that can be easily used are the most effective with an older population. Visual Analogue Scales (VAS) provide such a measure. The VAS is a straight horizontal 100-mm line anchored with "no pain" on the left and "worst possible pain" or "pain as bad as it could possibly be" on the right, and patients are told to indicate where on the scale would represent their pain. Another type of pain intensity scale is a faces scale that depicts facial expressions on a scale of 0–6, with 0 = smile and 6 = crying grimace. These two scales are featured in Figure 6.2. Studies that have compared simple pain intensity measures have demonstrated reliability and validity using varying forms of visual analogue scales in an elderly population. Herr and Mobily (1993) report a failure rate of 7.1% with the VAS when used among older adults and a poor test–retest reliability.

The McGill Pain Questionnaire (MPQ; Melzack, 1975) is a widely used instrument consisting of 78 words categorized into 20 groups, a body drawing, and a Present Pain Intensity (PPI) subscale consisting of a six-point ordinal scale. In some cases the PPI is used effectively apart from the entire MPQ among older adults. Several researchers found the tool to be effective in both cognitively intact and cognitively impaired older adults (Ferrell et al., 1995; Mosier, Nusser-Gurlach, Manz, & Bergstrom, 1998; Raway, 1994; Weiner et al., 1995). However, Herr and Mobily (1993) found that older adults with visual and hearing impairments had difficulty understanding this tool and became tired during the assessment. The Verbal Descriptor Scale is a variation of the PPI with simple language used to describe pain. Herr and Mobily (1993) found this subscale to be have a low failure rate and a high correlation with other pain measures. Ethnic, cultural, and spiritual factors play an important role in patient's perception and response to pain. Variations exist among cultures that must be explored with the patient and family. A descriptive, correlational study of 411 Mexican-Ameri-

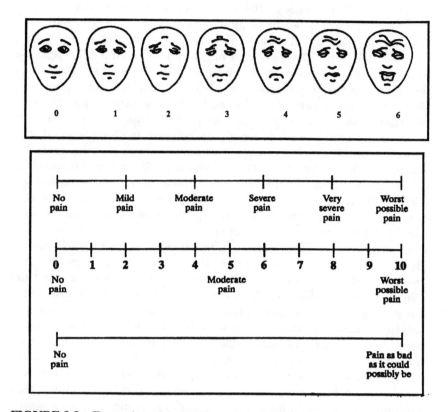

FIGURE 6.2   Examples of pain intensity scales for use with older persons. A faces scale and visual analogue scales.

Reprinted from *Pain, 41,* pp. 139–150, 1990, with permission from Elsevier Science.

can and non-Hispanic white subjects age 65–74 using the MPQ and several other pain questionnaires revealed that the MPQ is a valid tool for pain assessment in an older, community-based, multicultural sample (Escalante, Lichtenstein, White, Rios, & Hazuda, 1995).

The Pain Experience Measure (PEM) was originally developed by Ferrell, Wisdom, and Wenzl (1989) while studying cancer pain and was modified slightly to become the Pain Experience Interview (PEI). The PEI consists of 31 questions in mostly a yes/no format. In a study of 20 older adults in a veteran's care facility, the PEI demonstrated internal consistency of 0.85 (Cronbach's alpha) and test-retest reliability of 0.87 (Ferrell et al., 1995). A study comparing the PEI with the PPI showed a significant correlation between the two instruments (Ferrell, Ferrell, & Osterweil, 1990).

A descriptive study of 1193 subjects age 67–99 used the SF-36 health survey comparatively with two osteoarthritis indices, 2–7 years post knee replacement. The results of this study support the inclusion of both a generic and a disease-specific health-related quality of life (HRQOL) measure to assess patient pain outcomes fully (Bombardier et al., 1995). In a correlational study of 39 cognitively intact subjects more than 65 years old with back pain, subjects were administered both self-report and observational instruments to assess pain, pain behavior, and disability. X-rays were also taken of lumbosacral spine. Again, the data revealed that pain behavior observation, especially during activities of daily living (ADLs), is a more sensitive and valid way of assessing pain behavior in older adults than is self-report of pain (Weiner, Pieper, McConnell, Martinez, & Keefe, 1996).

Lewis, Lewis, and Cumming (1995) conducted three studies to assess the reliability and validity of the Prompting Intensity of Pain Electronic Recorder (PIPER). The first study asked 40 subjects age 51–83 to rate recent pain using both the VAS and the PIPER. The second study used the same sample and instruments to assess current pain. The final study concerned 26 subjects aged 31–83 and used five instruments, including the VAS and PIPER, to assess for long-term use of the PIPER. The findings indicated that frequent measures of pain should be taken to fully understand the pain experience of patients. The PIPER is a valid and reliable instrument that is easily used by the elderly, both by itself and with other instruments.

Accurate pain assessment is necessary to achieve effective pain management; therefore, it is essential to determine the most appropriate method of assessment for each client. Herr and Mobily (1993) in their correlational study of 49 community-dwelling subjects age 65–93 with chronic leg pain, found that no single measure of pain is good for all older adults. They recommended determining an elderly client's preference for pain measurement tool prior to choosing one tool over the other. A consensus panel of the agency for Health Care Policy and Research (U.S. Department of Health and Human Services [DHHS], 1992) recommends that pain assessment instruments be chosen with regard to age and physical, emotional, and cognitive condition, as well as available time and knowledge of the nurse administering the instrument.

DIAGNOSIS OF PAIN

Following the assessment of pain, diagnosis of pain is a necessary step for appropriate intervention to be implemented. The North American Nursing Diagnosis Association (NANDA) provides defining characteristics of pain that may be used in conjunction with assessment findings to form a diagnosis. Chang (1995) conducted assessments of 120 patients, age 50–96 with chronic pain and found that the assessments correlated with current defining characteristics of the nursing diagnosis of pain using a standard computer assessment tool administered by both nurses and a clinical nurse specialist (CNS). Chang concluded that the defining characteristics of the nursing diagnosis of pain provide an accurate and consistent clinical picture of the patient.

PAIN MANAGEMENT

Pharmacological Pain Management

Pain is often treated with pharmacotherapeutics. However, managing pain in the elderly through the use of pharmacological interventions is complicated by adverse reactions and analgesic sensitivity. Popp and Portenoy (1996) report that safe, effective use of analgesic drugs in the elderly requires in-depth knowledge of age-related changes in pharmacokinetics and pharmacodynamics. A decline in the therapeutic index of most drugs among older adults further complicates treatment because often little time exists between favorable effects and adverse drug effects. The old adage "start low and go slow" (AGS, 1998) is an appropriate rule for administration of pain medications in older adults.

Because of assessment and other barriers, administration of pharmacological treatment of pain is not always provided. A retrospective, descriptive study of 80 cardiac surgery patients was conducted. The subjects were divided into two groups of those age 65 and older and those younger than 65. The results showed that younger adults received more analgesia than older adults did. These findings may suggest an increased suffering among the elderly population that should be avoided (Lay, Puntillo, Miaskowski, & Wallhagen, 1996).

The complexity of pain management in older adults frequently requires the use of collaborative pain medications. These medications may include antidepressants, anticonvulsants, and anxiolytics. These medications are summarized in Table 6.1. For the most effective pain management, medications should be given on a regular basis, with extra doses added during treatment and activities likely to result in pain (AGS, 1998). The delivery of pain medication in older adults presents several options. However, little research is available to support the use of one method over another in the older adult population. The options for administration of pain medication include by mouth (PO), intravenous (IV) (bolus, continuous drip of patient-controlled analgesia [PCA]); intramuscularly (IM), and subcutaneous (SQ). The physiological changes of the aging body as well as the medication distribution should be considered when deciding on a route of administration.

The use of pain medication among the elderly presents significant challenges to clinicians. In a descriptive study of 3097 subjects age 65 and older, as part of the Iowa 65+ rural health study, subjects were interviewed regarding analgesic drug use. Although some multiple analgesic use ap-

TABLE 6.1   Nonopioid Drugs for Analgesia

Drug	Starting dose (po)	Specific indications	Pharmaco-logic changes	Precautions and recom-mendations
Corticoste-roids (pred-nisone)	2.5–5.0 mg daily	Inflammatory disease	Increased risk of hypergly-cemia, os-teopenia, and Cush-ing pheno-menon	Avoid high dose for long-term use
Antidepres-sants (ami-triptyline, desipra-mine, doxe-pin, imipra-mine, nor-triptyline)	10 mg HS	Neuropathic pain, sleep disturbance	Increased sen-sitivity to side effects, especially anticholiner-gic effects	Monitor care-fully for anti-cholinergic adverse ef-fects; desi-pramine may be as ef-fective as amitripty-line with fewer side ef-fects; start at lowest available dose, 10 mg, and ti-trate HS dose up-ward by 10 mg every 3–5 days
Anticonvul-sants				
Clonazapam	0.25–0.5 mg	Neuropathic pain		
Carbamazep-ine (Tegra-tol)	100 mg	Only for lanci-nating pain, e.g., trigemi-nal neu-ralgia	Can cause som-nolence, ataxia, dizzi-ness, leuko-penia, thrombocy-topenia, and rarely aplastic an-emia	Start at 100 mg qd, in-crease slowly bid, 200 mg qd, then bid; check LFTs, CBC, RF at baseline; CBC at 2 then 8 weeks

TABLE 6.1 *(continued)*

Drug	Starting dose (po)	Specific indications	Pharmaco- logic changes	Precautions and recom- mendations
Gabapentin (Neurontin)	100 mg	Neuropathic pain	May prove to have less se- rious side ef- fects than carbama- zepine	Start with low dose (100 mg) and ti- trate up slowly to ef- fect; neuro- pathic doses not yet es- tablished; ti- trate to tid dosing; monitor for idiosyncratic side effects, e.g., ankle swelling, ataxia; dose range for ef- ficacy anec- dotally reported 100–800 mg tid
Anti- arrhythmics Mexiletine (Mexitil)	150 mg	Neuropathic pain	Side effects such as tremor, diz- ziness, un- steadiness, paresthesias are com- mon; rarely hepatic damage and blood dys- crasias occur	Avoid use in patients with pre-ex- isting heart disease; start with low dose and ti- trate slowly; recommend initial and follow-up ECGs; ti- trate to tid- qid dosing

(continued)

TABLE 6.1   *(continued)*

Drug	Starting dose (po)	Specific indications	Pharmaco-logic changes	Precautions and recom-mendations
Local Anesthetics (intravenous) Lidocaine	3–5 mg/kg infused every 15–30 minutes	Diagnostic test	Delirium commom	May be useful predictor of response to mexiletine or other oral local anesthetics for neuropathic pain; diagnostic test only in a monitored environment where seizure, delirium, airway control, and hemodynamic alterations can be managed
Other agents Baclofen	5 mg	Neuropathic pain, muscle spasms	Probable increased sensitivity and decreased clearance	Monitor for weakness, urinary dysfunction; avoid abrupt discontinuation due to CNS irritability

CBC = complete blood cell count; CNS = central nervous system; ECG = electrocardiogram; HS = hour of sleep or at bedtime; LFT = liver function tests; RF = renal function.

From American Geriatrics Society. (1998). Clinical practice guidelines. The management of chronic pain in older persons. *Journal of the American Geriatrics Society, 46,* 643–644.

pears to be motivated by significant pain, polypharmacy does not result in additional pain relief and places the elderly individual at increased risk of many potential adverse effects and should be discouraged (Chrischilles, Lemke, Wallace, & Drube, 1990).

Nonsteroidal Anti-Inflammatory Drugs for Pain

Nonopiod pain management among older adults has received much interest in the literature yet is not without complications. A list of these medications, dosages, pharmacological changes, and precautions and recommendations are listed in Table 6.2. However, such medications should be used discriminately in the elderly population because of the risk of side effects. Skander and Ryan (1988) report a descriptive study of two groups of patients, age 65–74 and 75+, visualized during endoscopy to assess for the presence of ulcers. Results were correlated with a history of nonsteroidal antiinflammatory drug (NSAID) use for the 6 weeks preceding the procedure, and they revealed that NSAIDs contribute to ulceration and mask pain that leads to ulcer diagnosis.

In addition to the gastrointestinal side effects, hospitalized elderly patients are at risk for developing indomethacin-related renal dysfunction. Addition of misoprostol can minimize renal impairment and decrease gastrointestinal bleeding without affecting pain control (Nesher, Sonnenblick, & Dwolatzky, 1995). In a quasi-experimental study of 42 subjects over the age of 65, subjects were randomly assigned to receive either indomethacin or indomethacin plus misoprostal. Response to treatment was assessed using the VAS for pain and plasma evaluation of renal function. The authors found that misoprostol can minimize renal impairment without effecting pain control (Nesher et al., 1995).

The addition of misoprostol, histamine$_2$-receptor antagonists, proton pump inhibitors, and antacids has been supported as an adjunct to NSAIDs in the elderly. However, these medications are not entirely effective in alleviating the risk of side effects with NSAID use (AGS, 1998). Protective medications are not without effects, and the harm must be weighed against the potential benefit. NSAIDs should be used with caution in older adults and may be replaced by acetaminophen when appropriate because of the high risk of renal and gastrointestinal side effects in the older population.

Opioid Treatment of Pain

The use of opiod medication to manage pain has become a popular and effective method for older adults. Examples of some commonly used opioids, their oral equivalent, starting dosage, aging effects, and precautions and recommendations are listed in Table 6.3. Ferrell, Wisdom, Wenzl, and Brown (1989) conducted a quasi-experimental, repeated-measures study of 83 subjects randomly assigned to receive either morphine sulfate contin

TABLE 6.2   Acetaminophen and Nonsteroidal Antiinflammatory Drugs*†

Drug	Maximum dosage	Pharmacologic changes	Precautions and recommendations
Acetamino-phen‡§ (Tylenol)	4000 mg/24 h (q 4–6 h dosing)	Hepatotoxic above maximum dose	Avoid exceeding maximum recommended dose
Aspirin‡§	4000 mg/24 h (q 4–6 h dosing)	Gastric bleeding; abnormal platelet function	Avoid high doses for prolonged periods of time
Ibuprofen‡ (Motrin, Advil, Nuprin, etc.)	2400 mg/24 h (q 6–8 h dosing)	Gastric, renal, and abnormal platelet function may be dose-dependent; constipation, confusion, and headaches may be more common in older patients	Avoid high doses for prolonged periods of time
Naproxen‡§ (Naprosyn)	1000 mg/24 h (q 8–12 h dosing)	Similar toxicity to ibuprofen	Avoid high doses for prolonged periods of time
Choline magnesium trisalicylate‡ˡ (Trilisate)	5500 mg/24 h (q 8–12 h dosing)	Prolonged half-life of 8–12 h; similar toxicity to ibuprofen; classic salicylate toxicity may develop at high dose	Tests for salicylate levels may be necessary occasionally to avoid toxicity

*Limited number of representative examples only for demonstrative purposes. Comprehensive lists of other classes of NSAIDs and a multitude of brand names can be located elsewhere. There is no evidence of increased efficacy or decreased adverse effects (other than specific allergic sensitivities) to warrant the extremely high costs of most proprietary variations.
†Clinicians should monitor the literature closely for availability and cost-risk-benefit analyses of the cyclo-oxygenase-2-inhibitor class of NSAIDs, which should be commercially available soon.
‡Available in liquid form.
§Available in suppository form.
ˡMinimum platelet dysfunction.

TABLE 6.3   Opioid Analgesic Drugs

Drug	Oral equivalent	Starting dosage	Aging effects	Precautions and recommendations
Short-acting drugs				
Morphine sulfate (Roxanol, MSIR)	30 mg	15–30 mg q 4 h	Intermediate half-life; older people are more sensitive than younger people to side effects	Start low and titrate to comfort; continuous use for continuous pain; intermittent use for episodic pain; anticipate and prevent side effects
Codeine (plain codeine, Tylenol with codeine, other combinations)	120 mg	30–60 mg q 4–6 h	Acetaminophen-NSAID* combinations limit dose; constipation is a major issue	Begin bowel program early; do not exceed recommended maximum dose
Hydrocodone (Vicoden, Lortab, others)	30 mg	5–10 mg q 3–4 h	Acetaminophen-NSAID* combinations limit dose; toxicity similar to morphine	Anticipate and prevent side effects; begin bowel program early; do not exceed recommended maximum dose
Oxycodone (Roxicodone, Oxy IR, Percodan, Tylox, Percocet)	20–30 mg	5–10 mg q 3–4 h	Acetaminophen-NSAID* combinations limit dose; toxicity similar to morphine; oxycodone is available as a single agent	Anticipate and prevent side effects; begin bowel program early; do not exceed recommended maximum dose
Hydromorphone (Dilaudid)	7.5 mg	1.5 mg q 3–4 h	Half-life may be shorter than morphine (3 h); toxicity similar	Similar to morphine; start low and titrate to comfort; give continuously

(continued)

TABLE 6.3   *(continued)*

Drug	Oral equivalent	Starting dosage	Aging effects	Precautions and recommendations
				9q 3–4 h) for continuous chronic pain disorders
Long-acting drugs				
Sustained-release* morphine (MS Contin,† Kadian,‡§ Oramorph SR†)	30 mg	15–30 mg q 12 h or 24 h equivalent of total prior analgesics in divided doses q 12 h	Rarely requires more frequent dosing than recommended on package insert	Escalate dose slowly because of possible drug accumulation; immediate-release opioid analgesic often necessary for breakthrough pain
Sustained-release* oxycodone (Oxycontin)	20–30 mg	10–20 mg q 12 h or 24 h equivalent of total prior analgesics in divided doses q 12 h	Similar to sustained-release morphine	Immediate-release opioid often necessary for breakthrough pain
Transdermal fentanyl (Duragesic)	NA (see package insert)	25 µg/h not recommended in opioid-naive patients	Effective activity may exceed 72 h in older patient (transdermal patches designed for 3-day duration of action)	Titrate slowly using immediate-release analgesics for breakthrough pain; peak effects of first dose may take 18–24 h

*These preparations are not to be broken, crushed, or dissolved. They must be used as formulated to provide continuous-release activity.
†Every 24 hours dosing.
‡Every 8–12 hour dosing.
§Capsules can be opened and contents sprinkled on applesauce for easier ingestion without altering activity of the drug.

or a short-acting analgesic. Data were collected using five instruments to measure demographics, pain intensity and experience, function, and quality of life. The researchers concluded that through appropriate pain management with pain therapies such as controlled-release analgesics, nurses can greatly enhance quality of life (QOL) for cancer patients. In addition, nurses should work with patients to control medication side effects so that the maximum benefit is obtained from the narcotics.

It is important to note that in a double-blind, cross-over study designed to test the response to graded doses of 8 mg and 16 mg of morphine and morphine plasma levels of 715 postoperative patients, older patients responded to morphine as if they were given a larger dose. In addition, an experimental study comparing 13 subjects age 24–28 with 7 subjects age 60–69 after a single IV dose of 10 mg/70 kg morphine showed that plasma clearance was reduced in older subjects, resulting in an increase in drug concentration. This suggests the need to decrease morphine dosages in older subjects. Therefore, it is recommended that older patients be managed on an individual basis, titrating dose and frequency according to requirements of patient. Age should be used as a factor in choosing initial dosing frequency (Kaiko, Wallenstein, Rogers, Grabinski, & Houde, 1982).

In an ex post facto study of 1010 subjects under the age of 70, charts were reviewed to determine which factors contribute to the determination of morphine dosage. The conclusions of this investigation suggest that initial morphine dose should be guided by patient age and not weight. However, subsequent doses must still be titrated according to effect on pain control (Macintyre & Jarvis, 1996).

Despite the effectiveness of morphine in managing pain among older adults, the medication has frequent side effects in this population. In a descriptive study of 4500 older adult residents of Saskatchewen, Canada, who had sustained a hip fracture between 1977 and 1985, the findings suggest that the subjects' use of medication during the time of hip fracture indicated the need for further study on the psychomotor effects of opoid analgesics in older adults (Shorr, Griffin, Daughterty, & Ray, 1992).

Nonpharmacological Pain Management

Nonpharmacological pain management has received much interest among nurses. Nonpharmacological pain management includes relaxation, biofeedback-assisted relaxation, exercise, education, transcutaneous electrical nerve stimulation (TENS), cognitive-behavioral group therapy, and other creative techniques. In a quasi-experimental study of 20 subjects age 56–89, subjects were randomly assigned to experimental and control groups. The experimental group was taught the Jacobson relaxation technique. The effectiveness of the relaxation technique was evaluated through a pain sensation tool and intake of analgesics. The researchers concluded that relaxation is an effective means of increasing postoperative comfort level in this age group.

Middaugh, Woods, Kee, Harden, and Peters (1991) tested biofeedback-assisted relaxation in a quasi-experimental study of 37 subjects divided into an older age group (55–78 years) and a younger age group (29–48 years). Both groups were treated in a multidisciplinary chronic pain program including biofeedback and relaxation training for a period of 3 to 8 weeks. Subjects were evaluated by skin temperature response and respiratory response. Conclusions show that older patients responded well to the biofeedback and relaxation training component of a multimodal pain program, indicating effectiveness in decreasing pain.

Guided imagery was tested in a quasi-experimental study of 52 adults who had chronic pain of 6 months or more. At baseline, subjects were assessed as to the nature of their pain and pleasant images. Subjects were then taught the Jacobsen relaxation technique and reassessed after each relaxation session using the VAS. Acute pain patients responded better to imagery than did chronic pain patients. Pain relief is enhanced when subjects select a focus of imagery (Raft, Smith, & Warren, 1986).

Exercise has been noted as an effective nonpharmacological pain management strategy used by older adults. In a quasi-experimental study of four subjects age 56–89, subjects were exercised to a quota predetermined by a baseline study. Exercise was increased by one repetition every other session for 4 weeks. Pain was evaluated using the MPQ and analgesic intake at baseline and at the end of the study period. The authors concluded that behavioral strategies with exercise and praise may be effective in decreasing pain in older adults (Miller & LeLieuvre, 1982).

In a descriptive study of one group of older adults with osteoporosis, subjects participated in a preventive program including educational, social, and exercise components. Eighty percent of older adults complied with the program, resulting in improved general well-being, stamina, mobility, and pain tolerance. The type of program is valuable in increasing function and decreasing pain in older adults with osteoporosis (Chow, Harrison, & Dornan, 1989).

Dexter (1992) conducted a descriptive study of 110 community-dwelling older adults with chronic hip or knee pain, or both, that met the criteria for osteoarthritis. Subjects were interviewed to obtain information about their performance of therapeutic joint exercises and exercise-related medical care. The researcher concluded that exercise is an effective method for reducing pain and increasing mobility. However, less than 10% of older adults who were advised to exercise were doing so in a manner that might be expected to achieve maximum therapeutic benefit. Older adults need to be encouraged to participate in a therapeutic exercise program that they enjoy to obtain the best compliance.

In a quasi-experimental study of two groups of older adults with chronic pain conditions, subjects underwent treatment in either an active or a passive physical exercise program. The active approach included physical therapy, occupational therapy, behavior modification, and counseling. The passive approach included functional electric stimulation (FES). Ergonomic assessment of the subject's functional abilities, including static strength and range of motion, was performed. Both methods were effective in physical restoration of the elderly, which may be useful in decreasing painful conditions (Khalil, Abdel, Diaz, Stelle-Rosomoff, & Rosomoff, 1994).

TENS has been studied as a method to control pain in the elderly (Mostowy, 1996). In a case study analysis of one 80-year-old frail elderly woman with pain in right iliac spine, a TENS unit was applied and medication usage was evaluated. The TENS unit was an effective means of pain control in this patient and should be considered for older adults with chronic pain. Thorsteinsson (1987) conducted a double-blind study with 93 subjects age 22–88 with chronic pain. Each subject was given three sessions with a TENS and three sessions with a placebo, and device preference was recorded. The results again showed that TENS is an effective method of pain relief in elderly patients, and it should be integrated into an overall pain management plan.

Puder (1988) conducted a descriptive study of 69 outpatients age 27 to 80. Subjects underwent a 10-week cognitive-behavioral group therapy training program for chronic pain. Pain, activity, coping, the use of medications, and other physical pain control techniques were self-reported at baseline, during therapy, and at 1- and 6-month follow-up periods. Stress inoculation training appears to be an effective method of ameliorating the interference of pain with ADLs and is recommended for adults of all ages.

Ferrell, Ferrel, Ahn, and Tran (1994) conducted a quasi-experimental study testing the effect of a pain education intervention on 66 elderly patients with cancer during three home visits. Response to the intervention was assessed using four instruments to measure demographic variables, QOL, drug and nondrug interventions, and pain. The researchers recommended that structured pain education should become a part of the standard health care plan for pain management of older adults with chronic illness.

SUMMARY, CONCLUSIONS, AND IMPLICATIONS FOR FUTURE RESEARCH

Moving beyond descriptive studies is necessary for further research on pain. Patient involvement is essential. Investigators need to address issues such as patients' perceptions of their pain management, how pain affects their function, mood, general state of well-being, and QOL. Enabling older adults to participate in and provide data regarding their perceptions of the barriers to pain management will provide practitioners with much-needed data.

A major obstacle to improving patient care in this area is the lack of emphasis placed on the education of pain management in nursing and medical schools. (Davis, 1998; Ferrell, 1995). The study conducted by Closs (1996) addressed the problem of nurses' perception of pain and their knowledge of assessment and treatment, but further study in this area is necessary.

A great deal of effort has been placed on the need to be a cautious prescriber of drugs when caring for the elderly because overmedication may lead to side effects such as increased confusion and frequent falls. This has led to a pendulum swing, causing fear and anxiety about prescribing and administering drugs in the elderly. Although careful prescribing is an important part of patient care, neglecting pain management can be equally harmful to the elderly patient.

Evidence exists that demonstrates the importance of nonpharmacological interventions to manage pain in the elderly. Studies are needed to investigate alternative measures of pain management, such as distraction, humor, massage therapy, therapeutic touch, acupuncture, and imagery. Creative solutions, including the use of computers to create artwork and be connected to the outside world through the Internet, need to be explored.

In conclusion, the problem of pain in older adults must be investigated through further nursing research. Maintaining comfort and promoting independent function are the cornerstones of gerontological nursing. Additional research focusing on the refinement and development of reliable and valid assessment tools, pharmacological studies to determine the safe use of analgesic drugs, and nonpharmacological interventions need to be explored.

Although experts on pain in the elderly recognize the need for a multidisciplinary approach to this complex problem, nursing must take the lead to coordinate a systematic approach to study pain in older adults. Providing a framework that involves all the dimensions of pain, including the physiological aspects of this pervasive health problem, will strengthen research and help to improve patient outcomes.

REFERENCES

American Geriatric Society Panel on Chronic Pain in Older Persons. (1998). The management of chronic pain in older persons. *Journal of the American Geriatrics Society, 46,* 635–651.

Bombardier, C., Melfi, C. A., Paul, J., Green, R., Hawker, G., Wright, J., & Coyte, P. (1995). Comparison of a generic and a disease-specific measure of pain and physical function after knee replacement surgery. *Medical Care, 33* (4 suppl), AS131–AS144.

Casten, R. J., Parmelee, P. A., Kleban, J. H., Powell Lawton, M., & Katz, I. R. (1995). The relationships among anxiety, depression, and pain in a geriatric institutionalized sample. *Pain, 61,* 271–276.

Chakour, M. C., Gibson, S. J., Bradbeer, M., & Helme, R. D. (1996). The effect of age on A delta and C-fibre thermal pain perception. *Pain, 64,* 143–152.

Chang, B. L. (1995). Nursing diagnoses and construct validity of pain, self-care deficit and impaired mobility. *International Journal of Nursing Studies, 36,* 556–567.

Chow, R., Harrison, J., & Dornan, J. (1989). Prevention and rehabilitation of osteoporosis program: Exercise and osteoporosis. *International Journal of Rehabilitation Research, 12,* 49–56.

Chrischilles, E. A., Lemke, J. H., Wallace, R. B., & Drube, G. A. (1990). Prevalence and characteristics of multiple analgesic drug use in an elderly study group. *Journal of the American Geriatrics Society, 38,* 979–984.

Closs, J. (1996). Pain and elderly patients: A survey of nurses' knowledge and experiences. *Journal of Advanced Nursing, 23,* 237–242.

Collins, G., & Stone, L. A. (1965). Pain sensitivity, age and activity level in chronic schizophrenics and in normals. *British Journal of Psychiatry, 112,* 33.

Dalton, J. A. (1989). Nurses' perceptions of their pain assessment skills, pain management practices, and attitudes toward pain. *Oncology Nursing Forum, 16,* 225–231.

Davis, G. C. (1998). Nursing's role in pain management across the health care continuum. *Nursing Outlook, 46,* 19–23.

Dexter, P. A. (1992). Joint exercises in elderly persons with symptomatic osteoarthritis of the hip or knee. Performance patterns, medical support patterns, and the relationship between exercising and medical care. *Arthritis Care Research, 5,* 36–41.

Escalante, A., Lichtenstein, M. J., White, K., Rios, N., & Hazuda, H. P. (1995). A method for scoring the pain map of the McGill pain questionnaire for use in epidemiologic studies. *Aging (Milano), 7,* 358–366.

Farrell, M. J., Gibson, S. J., & Helme, R. J. (1996). Chronic nonmalignant pain in older people. In B. R. Ferrell & B. A. Ferrell (Eds.), *Pain in the elderly: A report of the task force on pain in the elderly.* Seattle, WA: International Association for the Study of Pain.

Ferrell, B. A. (1995). Pain evaluation and management in the nursing home. *Annals of Internal Medicine, 123,* 681–687.

Ferrell. B. A., Ferrel, B. R., Ahn, C., & Tran, K. (1994). Pain management for elderly patients with cancer at home. *Cancer, 74,* 2139–2146.

Ferrell, B. A., Ferrell, B. R., & Osterweil, D. (1990). Pain in the nursing home. *Journal of the American Geriatric Society, 38,* 409–414.

Ferrell, B., Wisdom, C., & Wenzl, C. (1989). Quality of life as an outcome variable in management of cancer pain. *Cancer, 63,* 2321–2329.

Ferrell, B. A., Ferrell, B. R., & Rivera, L. (1995). Pain in cognitively impaired nursing home patients. *Journal of Pain and Symptom Management, 10,* 591–598.

Greipp, M. E. (1992). Undermedication for pain: An ethical model. *Advances in Nursing Science, 15* (1), 44–53.

Haley, W. E., Turner, J. A., & Romano, J. M. (1985). Depression in chronic pain patients: Relation to pain, activity, and sex differences. *Pain, 23,* 337–343.

Harkins, S. N., & Chapman, C. R. (1977). The perception of induced dental pain in young and elderly women. *Journal of Gerontology, 32,* 428–435.

Herr, K. A., & Mobily, P. R. (1992). Geriatric mental health: Chronic pain and depression. *Journal of Psychosocial Nursing, 30* (9), 7–11.

Herr, K. A., & Mobily, P. R. (1993). Comparison of selected pain assessment tools for use with the elderly. *Applied Nursing Research, 6,* 39–46.

Hurley, A. C., Volicer, B. J., Hanrahan, P. A., Houde, S., & Volicer, L. (1992). Assessment of discomfort in advanced alzheimer patients. *Research in Nursing and Health, 15,* 369–377.

Kaiko, R. F., Wallenstein, S. L., Rogers, A. G., Grabinski, P. Y., & Houde, K. W. (1982). Narcotics in the elderly. *Medical Clinics of North America, 66,* 1079–1089.

Khalil, T. M., Abdel, M. E., Diaz, E. L., Stelle-Rosomoff, R., & Rosomoff, H. L. (1994). Efficacy of physical restoration in the elderly. *Experimental Aging Research, 20,* 189–199.

Levasseur, S. A., Gibson, S. J., & Helme, R. D. (1990). The measurement of capsaicin-sensitive sensory nerve fiber function in elderly patients with pain. *Pain, 41,* 19–25.

Lewis, B., Lewis, D., & Cumming, G. (1995). Frequent measurement of chronic pain: An electronic diary and empirical findings. *Pain, 60,* 341–347.

Macintyre, P. E., & Jarvis, D. A. (1996). Age is the best predictor of postoperative morphine requirements. *Pain, 64,* 357–364.

Magni, G., Schifano, F., & DeLeo, D. (1985). Pain as a symptom in elderly depressed patients. Relationship to diagnostic subgroups. *European Archives of Psychiatry and Neuroscience, 235,* 143–145.

Melzack, R. (1975). The McGill pain questionnaire: Major properties and scoring methods. *Pain, 1,* 277–299.

Melzack, R., & Wall, P. D. (1982). *The challenge of pain.* New York: Basic Books.

Middaugh, S. J., Woods, S. E., Kee, Hardin, R. N., & Petors, J. R. (1991). Biofeedback assisted relaxation training for the aging chronic pain patient. *Biofeedback Self Regulation, 16,* 361–377.

Miller, J., Neelon, V., Dalton, J., Ng'andu, N., Bailey, D. Jr., Layman, E., & Hosfeld, A. (1996). The assessment of discomfort in elderly confused patients: A preliminary study. *Journal of Neuroscience Nursing, 28,* 175–182.

Miller, M., & LeLieuvre, B. (1982). A method to reduce chronic pain in elderly nursing home residents. *The Gerontologist, 22,* 314–317.

Mobily, P. R., Herr, K. A., Clark, K., & Wallace, R. B. (1994). An epidemiologic analysis of pain in the elderly. *Journal of Aging and Health, 6,* 139–155.

Mosier, R., Nusser-Gurlach, B., Manz, B., & Bergstrom, N. (1998). Pain assessment in cognitively impaired and non-impaired elderly. Presented at the 22nd Annual Midwest Nursing Research Society, Columbus, Ohio.

Mostowy, D. E. (1996). An application of transcutaneous electrical nerve stimulation to control pain in the elderly. *Journal of Gerontological Nursing, 22* (2), 36–38.

Nesher, G., Sonnenblick, M., & Dwolatzky, T. (1995). Protective effect of misoprostol on indomethacin induced renal dysfunction in elderly patients. *Journal of Rheumatology, 22,* 713–716.

Parmalee, P. A., Smith, B., & Katz, I. R. (1993). Pain complaints and cognitive status among elderly institution residents. *Journal of the American Geriatrics Society, 41,* 517–522.

Popp, B., & Portenoy, R. K. (1996). Management of chronic pain in the elderly: Pharmacology of opoids and other analgesic drugs. In B. R. Ferrell & B. A. Ferrell (Eds.), *Pain in the elderly: A report of the task force on pain in the elderly* (pp. 21–34). Seattle, WA: International Association for the Study of Pain Press.

Porter, F. L., Malhotra, K. M., Wolf, C. M., Morris, J. C., Miller, J. P., & Smith, M. A. (1996). Dementia and response to pain in the elderly. *Pain, 68,* 413–421.

Puder, R. S. (1988). Age analysis of cognitive-behavioral group therapy for chronic pain outpatients. *Psychology of Aging, 3,* 204–207.

Raft, D., Smith, R., & Warren, N. (1986). Selection of imagery in the relief of chronic and acute pain. *Journal of Psychosomatic Research, 30,* 481–488.

Raway, B. (1994). Pain behaviors and confusion in elderly patients with hip fracture (Doctoral dissertation, Catholic University of America, 1994). *Dissertation Abstracts International, 55,* 02B. (University Microfilms No. AAI94-18593).

Schludermann, E., & Zubeck, J. P. (1962). Effect of age on pain sensitivity. *Perceptual Motor Skills, 14,* 295–301.

Shorr, R. I., Griffin, M. R., Daughterty, J. R., & Ray, W. A. (1992). Opioid analgesics and the risk of hip fracture in the elderly: Codeine and propoxyphene. *Journal of Gerontology, 47,* M111–M115.

Skander, M. P., & Ryan, F. P. (1988). Non-steroidal anti-inflammatory drugs and pain free peptic ulceration in the elderly. *British Medical Journal, 297,* 833–834.

Thorsteinsson, G. (1987). Chronic pain: Use of TENS in the elderly. *Geriatrics, 42* (12), 75–82.

Turk, D. C., & Melzack, R. (1992). *Handbook of pain assessment.* New York: Guilford Press.

Turk, D. C., Okifuji, A., & Scharff, L. (1995). Chronic pain and depression: Role of perceived impact and perceived control in different age cohorts. *Pain, 61,* 93–101.

U.S. Department of Health and Human Services, Public Health Service, Agency for Health Care Policy and Research. (1992). *Acute pain management: Operative of medical procedures and trauma* (Publication No. 92-0032) Washington, DC: U.S. Government Printing Office.

Weiner, D., Pieper, C., McConnell, E., Martinez, S., & Keefe, F. (1996). Pain measurement in elders with chronic low back pain: Traditional and alternative approaches. *Pain, 67,* 461–467.

Weiner, D. K., Ladd, K. E., Pieper, C. F., & Keefe, F. J. (1995). Pain in the nursing home: Resident versus staff perceptions. *Journal of the American Geriatrics Society, 43,* SA2.

7

Nutrition

Donna Fick and Lori B. Schumacher

> Every careful observer of the sick will agree in this that thousands of patients are annually starved in the midst of plenty, from the want of attention to the ways which alone make it possible for them to take food. . . . How often have we known a patient eat nothing at all in the day, because one meal was left untasted. . . . A patient who cannot touch his dinner at two, will often accept it gladly if brought to him at seven . . . remember how much he has had, and how much he ought to have today.—Florence Nightingale

As Florence Nightingale pointed out more than 100 years ago, nowhere is individualized care more essential than in assessing and caring for the nutritional status and feeding of the hospitalized and critically ill older adult. However, little attention is given in research, education, and clinical practice to individualizing nursing care to maintain and improve nutrition and hydration in the acute and critical care setting.

The majority of medical intensive care unit (ICU) patients are more than 65 years of age. Problems with eating, feeding, and undernutrition are of great significance for the critically ill older adult. Patients 65 and over receive half of the enteral nutrition feedings in the hospital (Fedullo & Swinburne, 1983; United States Congress, 1987). Elders who present with critical illness and are malnourished or unable to eat are at significantly increased risk for poor outcomes, including increased morbidity, mortality, functional and mental decline, falls, pressure ulcer development, and nursing home placement (Elic, Cole, Primeau, & Bellavance, 1998; Herrmann, Safran, Levkoff, & Minaker, 1992; McMurtry & Rosenthal, 1995; Mentes, Culp,

Maas, & Rantz, 1999; Sullivan & Walls, 1994; Sullivan, Walls, & Bopp, 1995). A study of intensive care found that as albumin levels decrease, mortality increases. The researchers found a 12-fold increase in mortality with albumin levels of less than 2 g/dL (Boosalis et al., 1989). A recent study of 214 older adults living in the community found low body mass index (BMI) was associated with dependency in activities of daily living (ADLs) and 1-year survival (Landi et al., 1999).

The epidemiology of malnutrition in elders in the hospital and community setting has been investigated in several studies. The prevalence of malnutrition ranges from 21–60% in hospitalized elders, 5–40% in community-living elders, and up to 85% of nursing home patients (Constans et al., 1992; Covinsky et al., 1999; Incalzi et al., 1996; Mion, McDowell, & Heaney, 1994). This variability in the prevalence of malnutrition is due in part to differences in measurement as well as in definition of malnutrition.

The Nutrition Screening Initiative (NSI) is one of the most recent and largest studies, jointly conducted by the American Academy of Family Physicians, American Dietetic Association, and National Council on Aging (1991). The main goal of this initiative is to promote nutrition screening and improve nutritional care of older adults. This initiative has three steps to nutrition screening. Step one is a "determine your nutritional health checklist" that is designed to be self-administered and easy to complete. The checklist includes statements such as "I eat fewer than two meals a day, and I eat alone most of the time." It provides a score and three levels of nutritional risk: good, moderate, and high. Step one emphasizes nine warning signs using the acronym DETERMINE (Disease, Eating poorly, Tooth loss/mouth pain, Economic hardship, Reduced social contact, Multiple medicines, Involuntary weight loss/gain, Needs assistance in self-care, and Elder years above 80). Step two is designed for use by health professionals and is the basic Level 1 nutrition screen that includes sections on weight, eating habits, living environment, and nutritional status. The screen refers a patient to the physician if he or she has gained or lost 10 pounds unexpectedly in the past 6 months or if BMI is above 27 or below 24. Step three is a Level 2 screen that is for persons identified as having potentially serious nutritional or medical problems and includes anthropometric measurements (Nutrition Screening Initiative [NSI], 1991; Morrisson, 1997).

Few studies have examined successful nursing interventions for eating and feeding problems in the acute and critical care setting. Nurses play an integral role in the identification, management, and prevention of nutritional problems in older adults in all settings and must be involved.

The focus of this chapter is the assessment of eating, feeding, and hydration in the hospitalized older adult and the effects of common aging changes and disease processes on eating, feeding, and hydration. Last, the challenges and interventions to optimize nutrition and hydration in the critically ill patient are described.

AGING CHANGES AND COMMON GERIATRIC
PROBLEMS: IMPLICATIONS FOR MAINTAINING
NUTRITION AND FEEDING OLDER ADULTS
IN THE ICU SETTING

Several factors place older adults at increased risk for malnutrition and complicate the process of feeding and hydrating critically ill older adults. These include normal changes associated with aging, common geriatric problems, the presence of multiple chronic diseases and their treatment, and psychosocial and ethical issues. These factors are detailed in Table 7.1. Additionally, when making decisions about feeding critically ill older adults, several issues are critical. These include the patients' mental state, the presence and quality of a surrogate decision maker, ageism and ethical issues, end-of-life care, the use of physical restraints, and the prognosis of the patient.

Simply consuming enough food becomes a major challenge for older adults. Chronological age alone is not a precise indicator of the rate or degree of age-related changes that may be influenced by the presence of chronic diseases and other personal and environmental factors. However, aging is associated with changes in several physiological systems and an increased incidence of disease processes that often negatively influence the utility of nutrients, profoundly affecting nutritional health in the critically ill patient. Even though our knowledge about "normal" age-related changes is constantly in flux, several common aging changes are important when assessing and treating nutritional problems in critically ill older adults.

Body Composition

As one ages, there are several changes in body hydration, including a decrease in total body water and lean body mass with a subsequent increase in total body fat and its distribution. Because of a decrease in body mass, basal metabolic rate also declines with age. Because of these changes, malnutrition is often not suspected in an older person because they may appear "well nourished," altering the assessment of anthropometrics (both height and skinfold measures) (Kerstetter, Hothausen, & Fitz, 1992).

Loss of lean body mass also results in decreased serum creatinine levels so that a low normal value may not reflect impaired renal function (Lerstetter et al., 1992). In addition, blood urea nitrogen levels also increase because of age-related decreases in the glomerular filtration rate and decreased cardiac output. Therefore, when concerned about hydration and before prescribing medications excreted by the kidneys, a creatinine clearance should be calculated for all critically ill older adults (Lamberta & Wyman, 1999).

There may be a slight decrease seen in albumin levels with age, but total serum protein should remain unchanged. Both albumin and total protein are important indicators of nutritional status.

TABLE 7.1 Factors Related to Nutritional Status in the Critically Ill Older Adult

Age-related changes	Chronic disease	Common geriatric problems	Psychosocial	Environmental	Ethical issues
Body composition ($\downarrow$ lean body mass, $\uparrow$ in SQ fat and changes in distribution of fat, $\downarrow$ total body water)	Cancer	Polypharmacy	Fixed income	Being NPO for tests or surgery	Use of surrogate decision makers
Gastrointestinal ($\downarrow$ colonic motility and absorption of nutrients)	COPD	Poor dentition and oral health	Inability to shop	Dietary restrictions	End-of-life care
Renal, endocrine, and hepatic ($\downarrow$ in GFR, renal and hepatic blood flow, $\downarrow$ serum albumin)	Dementia and depression	Swallowing problems	Isolation	Lack of personnel	Use of restraints
Loss of total body water	Arthritis	Alcoholism	Cultural food preferences	Unappetizing food	

(continued)

TABLE 7.1 *(continued)*

Age-related changes	Chronic disease	Common geriatric problems	Psychosocial	Environmental	Ethical issues
Sensory/neuro (↓ in number of taste buds, ↑ in presbyosis and presbycusis, ↓ in number of neurons and delayed reaction time)	CAD, diabetes	Decreased appetite and alterations in taste		Staff knowledge of aging issues	
Multiple disease processes (Increased incidence of delirium, dementia, depression, and stroke with age)	Osteoporosis	Complications of enteral feedings and parenteral nutrition ↓ Dexterity/mobility			

CAD, coronary artery disease; COPD, chronic obstructive pulmonary disease; GFR, glomerular filtration rate

Loss of total body water is an important consideration when assessing and treating nutritional alteration in the critically ill older adult. Total body water declines to less than 60% and may lead to dry mouth, constipation, poor appetite, and difficulties with swallowing. In addition, dehydration and hypovolemia occur frequently in older adults.

Alterations in the gastrointestinal system and oral and dental health may have a significant effect on nutritional status. Dental health is a concern for both those who are dentate and those wearing dentures. Dentate older persons are at risk for gum disease and dental caries; denture-wearing persons often have ill-fitting or broken dentures that interfere with the ability to eat. The assessment of oral and dental health is an important but frequently overlooked part of a nutritional assessment (Dolan, Monopoli, Kaurich, & Rubenstein, 1990; Kayser-Jones & Schell, 1997).

A decrease in the number of taste buds along with the use of multiple medications may lead to a decreased taste sensation. Aging changes in the salivary glands result in atrophy and decreased saliva, making it difficult to break down protein and starches, leading to dry oral membranes. The incidence of extremely dry oral membranes or dry mouth (xerostomia) increases with age and may be related to medications, radiation therapy, or disease (Dolan et al., 1990). Because many older adults take multiple medications, xerostomia becomes an important nutrition issue.

Gastrointestinal changes such as gastric motility, reflux, stasis, and hyperchlorhydria also may alter the absorption of some drugs and nutrients. These changes may lead to prolonged gastric emptying, decreased blood supply, and decrease in the absorption of micronutrients. In addition, gastric acid production decreases, resulting in decreased absorption of vitamin B_{12}, iron, calcium, and zinc (Morrisson, 1997). There is also an increased incidence of swallowing and constipation problems, both of which may lead to a decreased appetite or desire to eat.

Other factors that affect nutrient intake include the presence of multiple chronic diseases, especially cancer, diabetes, cardiac and pulmonary disorders, dementia, depression, delirium, alcoholism, polypharmacy, dietary restrictions, and refusal to eat (Morrisson, 1997). Each of these factors should be assessed routinely in all hospitalized older adults.

Chronic Illness and Nutrition in the Geriatric Patient

Primary medical conditions may also have ramifications for the nutritional status of the geriatric patient. Dementia and altered neurological status have many nutrition implications. Delirium, dementia, and depression have been found to be associated with decreased oral intake and weight loss. Patients with dementia are often malnourished. Weight loss is common at all stages of dementia and may be related to the decreased ability to shop for, prepare, recognize, and respond to food. More than half of all nursing home patients have impaired cognition. Inadequate staffing and the lack of individualized care have been shown to influence the nutritional state of nursing home residents, in whom the incidence of malnutrition is also highest (Kayser-Jones & Schell, 1997). Assessment and differentiation of these conditions requires a careful assessment of mental status with standardized measures and a history of functioning and living arrangements before the hospitalization.

A geriatric patient with an altered mental status may not have the full ability to chew and swallow, may not cooperate, may forget to eat, or may not be able to cognitively rationalize why they need to eat. This all makes it difficult for the health care provider to get the patient to eat (Johnson & Chernoff, 1998; Lamberta & Wyman, 1999; Marcus & Berry, 1998).

Depression is another reason why the geriatric patient may not want to eat. Depression may be a part of the elder's underlying illness or a result of his or her loss of independence or self-destructive behavior reflecting a desire to die (Johnson & Chernoff, 1998; Marcus & Berry, 1998). Therefore, it is critical to screen for depression and other psychosocial issues that may be the reason for the patient not eating.

Patients with altered mental status or confusion may be placed in physical restraints, which may further complicate their ability to take in nutrients because of a decreased mobility and the need to be fed or supervised by the health care provider. It is important to discuss restraint use with patients and families because restraints are a frequent complication associated with the use of enteral feedings (Kayser-Jones & Schell, 1997).

Chronic diseases such as cancer, diabetes, cardiac and pulmonary disorders, alcoholism, delirium, dementia, and depression all present challenges for maintaining nutritional health and place patients at greater risk of malnutrition. Many chronic diseases and their treatments cause patients to have increased energy expenditures and catabolic rates coupled with decreased nutrient intakes. These chronic energy imbalances lead to patient fatigue, muscle wasting, weight loss, and decreased immune function.

Long-term alcohol use may replace necessary nutrients and lead to suppressed appetite and vitamin and mineral deficiencies. For an older adult, alcohol use may be hidden and has been found to be less likely to be assessed.

Polypharmacy

Persons more than 65 years of age represent 12% of the population, yet they receive 30% of all prescription medications and purchase 40% of over-the-counter (OTC) drugs. The elderly take an average of 5 medications at any one time, and 13–15 different prescriptions over the course of a year. Thirty percent of hospital admissions in the elderly are related to adverse drug reaction (ADR) or drug toxicity (Schwartz, 1997; Health Care Financing Administration, 1990). Medication side effects and adverse reactions may be related to preventable problems in the elderly such as weight loss, depression, constipation, falls, immobility, confusion, and hip fractures (Lindley, Tully, Paramosothy, & Tallis, 1992; Montamat, Cusak, & Vestal, 1989; Schneider, Mion, & Frengley, 1992).

Polypharmacy contributes to malnutrition and poor appetite through several pathways, including the interaction of drugs and common foods, the side effects of drugs (decreased taste, xerostomia, nausea, vomiting, drowsiness, confusion), and a diminished appetite. Many common medications contribute to both poor appetite and altered nutrient absorption. The most common medications that have significant nutritional side effects are digoxin, anticholinergics, laxatives, corticosteroids, antipsychotics, sedative-hypnotics, and cancer chemotherapy medications. Parkinson's disease drugs (L-dopa) and digoxin commonly lead to decreased appetite in an older person. Parkinsonian drugs and other anticholinergic drugs (diphenhydramine [Benadryl], antihistamines) may suppress appetite directly or lead to poor conditions for eating, such as xerostomia, nausea, vomiting, or loss of taste (Kerstetter et al., 1992). Digoxin has a very narrow margin of safety, and typically toxicity results in profound loss of appetite and in weight loss. Other drugs, such as laxatives, antacids, corticosteroids, and H_2 blockers, affect the absorption of nutrients.

The use of antipsychotics in the elderly may lead to excess sedation and loss of contact with the environment, resulting in decreased ability to prepare and eat food independently. These drugs should not be used in older adults unless the individual presents a safety threat to himself or herself or to other persons (Rader, 1995).

Dietary Restrictions and Environmental Factors

Many of the reasons for poor dietary intake and altered nutritional health in the hospitalized older adult are preventable or iatrogenic, such as ordering a patient to take nothing by mouth (NPO) while waiting for surgery, putting a patient who is already malnourished on inappropriate dietary restrictions, and a lack of staffing and individualized care in feeding (Kayser-Jones & Schell, 1997). If possible, nutrition should be maintained in a manner that protects the dignity and independence of the patient and involves them in the decision-making process about the type of nutritional intervention used. Factors to consider include psychosocial, financial, and ethical issues. The presence and quality of a surrogate decision maker, ageism, end-of-life care, the use of physical restraints, and the patient prognosis are common ethical issues that arise when caring for the needs of the critically ill older adult.

Frequently, the patient's prognosis is an element in the decision-making process on the overall care that the patient receives. If the prognosis is poor, the patient may express his or her desires through a living will or designate a Durable Power of Attorney who knows and respects the individual's wishes and requests. Nutrition support is included in a living will, and one may decide to receive artificial nutrition or terminate all nutritional substance.

TABLE 7.2   Complications of Malnutrition in the Critically Ill Older Adult

Delayed wound healing
Infection/sepsis
Pneumonia
Failure to wean from ventilator
Altered skin integrity/decubitus ulcers
Impairment of vital organ function
Multisystem organ failure
Bleeding disorders
Difficulties reestablishing normal feeding

BEDSIDE ISSUES IN MAINTAINING NUTRITION IN THE CRITICALLY ILL OLDER ADULT

The admission of a patient into the critical care setting involves priority setting, with immediate life-threatening issues receiving the highest priority. Nutritional intervention tends to be a low priority and usually is considered after the patient has been in the critical care setting more than 24 hours (Schoemaker, Ayres, Grenvik, & Holbrook, 2000). Usually, nutritional assessments and nutrient delivery are not started within the first 24 hours of ICU admission. It is during this time frame that the body undergoes several physiological metabolic alterations occurring regardless of nutrition delivery as a result of the critical illness and stress. During periods of critical illness lean body tissue is systematically catabolized in order for the organism as a whole to survive. Severe catabolic stress utilizes skeletal muscle breakdown preferentially as metabolic fuel. The serum albumin level rapidly falls in critical illness and injury, regardless of the level before injury. Severe catabolic stress can lead to the loss of 20 to 30 g of urinary nitrogen (UN) per day (Sternberg, Rohovsky, Blackburn, & Babineau, 2000).

An individual can initially adapt to being without nutritional intake during the first 24 to 48 hours of critical illness. The body initially uses its glycogen stores as a source of energy. If the patient is malnourished at admission, he or she may not have sufficient glycogen stores to meet the body's basic energy needs. During metabolic stress, multiple alterations lead to use of alternate fuels for energy. Lean body mass is mobilized and converted to glucose via the gluconeogenic pathway. Adipose tissue is catabolized; however, because of hormonal alterations it is not used efficiently for energy (Anding, 1996a; Barton, 1994).

The hypercatabolism that occurs leads to an overloss of lean body mass (Barton, 1994). If patients are nutritionally compromised, then their recovery may be hindered, predisposing them to a number of complications (Table 7.2).

These complications are associated with an increasing morbidity and mortality as well as costs to the individual (Anding, 1996a; Barton, 1994;

Pinchcofsky-Devin & Kaminski, 1996; Preiser et al., 1999; Viall, 1998). There-fore, it is vital that nutritional status is assessed, and patients at nutritional risk are identified in a timely manner.

NUTRITIONAL ASSESSMENT AND TREATMENT OPTIONS IN CRITICAL CARE

The nutritional assessment process for hospitalized patients should begin during admission of the patient. A comprehensive nutritional assessment includes patient diagnosis and patient history (medical, surgical, drug, di-etary, social), anthropometric measurements, physical assessment, and labo-ratory studies. A comprehensive nutritional assessment will not only identify a patient who is already undernourished but can also be useful in determin-ing those at risk for developing nutritional problems. A nutritional assess-ment is multidisciplinary and encompasses the disciplines of medicine, nursing, dietary, pharmacy, and speech therapy. All of these disciplines work together to ensure that a patient's full nutritional needs are met through appropriate interventions.

A dietary history is an integral component in the assessment of a patient's nutritional status. However, in the critical care setting, it may be difficult to obtain this information from patients because of their illness, and the information may be gathered from family members, significant others, or friends. One difficulty in collecting a dietary history is that the information may not be accurate because it typically consists of subjectively recalled information. A dietary history can provide a general outlook of the nutri-tional status of the patient and whether there is a possibility of preexisting malnutrition (Anding, 1996b).

Because a patient's body composition and weight depend on nutrition, anthropometric measurements provide this information for the nutritional assessment of the patient. The most commonly used measurements are patient height, weight, BMI, and skinfold thickness. These are usually exam-ined over a period of time to monitor any changes (Anding, 1996a, 1996b). Because of age-related changes in body composition, malnutrition may not be suspected in an older person who "looks" well-nourished. This is further complicated by the assessment of anthropometric measures (both height and skinfold measures) that are often affected by the hydration status of the older adult. A patient's height is usually a measurement that is obtained at time of admission. Generally, weight is measured on admission and daily in the critical care setting. A patient's weight is monitored and compared for changes, especially to assess fluid balance (Anding, 1996b; Schoemaker et al., 2000). It is important to have a patient's actual body weight along with an estimate of his or her ideal body weight to determine caloric and protein requirements (Anding, 1996b). Also, other variables of the patient's illness affect the accuracy of these measurements, such as fluid shifts. Therefore, weight is usually an important measure for the critically ill patient (Anding, 1996b).

The physical examination of a patient provides essential information for the assessment of nutritional status. Muscle strength and tone can be assessed; if suboptimal, this could suggest possible depletion of a body's protein stores. Also, preexisting deficiencies of essential nutrients, vitamins, and minerals can manifest in numerous physical signs, such as proximal muscle weakness, bleeding, anorexia, fatigue, headache, bruising, skin changes, hair, nails, and so on (Anding, 1996b). Changes in body composition that affect the physical assessment include an increase in subcutaneous fat, a decrease in lean body mass, a decrease in total body water, and changes in the distribution of fat.

Laboratory studies are the final component of a nutritional assessment. Blood work that is most commonly performed to determine a patient's nutritional status is the measurement of serum albumin, serum transferrin, and prealbumin and retinol binding proteins (Anding, 1996b). One major problem with these laboratory studies is their half-life. Albumin has a long half-life of 20 days, and transferrin has a half-life of 8–10 days, which makes it difficult to determine early protein malnutrition (Anding, 1996b). In addition, many factors, such as hydration status, infection, liver conditions, and sepsis can decrease albumin levels (Anding, 1996b). On the other hand, prealbumin has a half-life of 1–2 days, and retinol binding proteins have a half-life of 10–12 hours and are considered an excellent means of monitoring a recent onset of malnutrition and the effectiveness of nutritional support (Anding, 1996b).

Urine laboratory studies also may be performed to assist in determining a patient's nutritional status. A 24-hour urine collection may be obtained to measure a patient's nitrogen balance. A negative nitrogen balance correlates with a catabolic state and warrants further nutrition assessment or readjustment, or both (Anding, 1996b).

SWALLOWING ABILITY AND RISK OF ASPIRATION

A patient's ability to swallow may be impaired because of age-related physiological changes or their underlying disease process. Dysphagia, or the impaired ability to swallow, may cause malnutrition because the patient is not able to consume the required nutrients. Dysphagia places the patient at an increased risk for aspiration. Aspiration may predispose a patient to acquiring pneumonia; it is therefore essential that a patient at risk for aspiration be identified and appropriate precautions to prevent aspiration initiated. Patients at risk for aspiration include individuals with cognitive impairment (delirium, dementia, or depression) and those who have had a stroke, are sedated or on narcotics, have no mobility, are on bedrest, or are otherwise restricted in their ability to chew and swallow (Burrell, Gerlach, & Pless, 1997). Examples of interventions used to prevent aspiration include:

- feeding the patient in an upright sitting position
- maintaining a semiupright position between 30 and 45 degrees for 30 minutes after feeding
- allowing sufficient time for eating so the patient does not feel rushed
- removing distractions during feeding so the patient concentrates on chewing and swallowing
- providing small and frequent feedings to prevent fatigue
- thickening thin liquids to assist in the initiation of swallowing
- avoiding foods that fall apart easily because these can be aspirated (i.e., rice, corn, peas)
- making certain the patient does not take too much food in the mouth (one half of a heaping teaspoon is adequate)
- performing neck flexion during swallowing to enhance swallowing and facilitate glottis closure
- rotating the head toward a weak or paralyzed side to improve swallowing
- checking the patient's mouth and removing any pockets of retained food.

PARENTERAL NUTRITION

Total parenteral nutrition (TPN) is one method of providing nutrient and fluid requirements. There are advantages and disadvantages in using TPN. TPN may be indicated in certain clinical conditions when the gastrointestinal (GI) tract should not be used, for example, in cases of intractable diarrhea and vomiting, bowel obstruction, ileus, and malabsorption (Anding, 1996a, 1996b; Schneider et al., 1992; Viall, 1998). TPN also may be indicated when enteral access cannot be obtained. A disadvantage of TPN is gut atrophy. When nutrients are not provided enterally, the GI mucosa can slough, leading to bacterial translocation and potential systemic infection. TPN also can increase the risk of infection via the central line (Anding, 1996a, 1996b; Sternberg et al., 2000; Viall, 1998). TPN is also more costly than enteral nutrition is (Anding, 1996a).

ENTERAL NUTRITION

When feasible, enteral nutrition is the preferred route of nutrient delivery (Barton, 1994; McQuiggan, Marvin, McKinley, & Moore, 1999; Preiser et al., 1999). Enteral nutrition allows the GI tract to maintain its normal physiological process and is available at a lower cost than is parenteral nutrition. Using enteral nutrition prevents atrophy of the GI mucosa, maintaining a protective immunological barrier against bacterial and endotoxin migration from the mucosa to the mesenteric lymph nodes and into the systemic circulation, which could potentially lead to infections, sepsis, and multisystem organ failure (Anding, 1996b; Keithley & Eisenberg, 1993; Viall, 1998). Also, the use of enteral nutrition promotes the use of the GI tract by maintaining the normal function of the gut and stimulating mucosal growth through the nutrients absorbed (Barton, 1994; Keithley & Eisenberg, 1993; Viall, 1998).

Prior to initiating enteral nutrition, caloric and nutrient requirements must be calculated to ensure that the best formula is selected to support the patient's needs. The adequacy of nutrition by a feeding tube is volume dependent. The calorie content in tube feeding formulas varies but most provide 1 kcal/mL and the recommended daily allowance of vitamins and trace elements once a determined volume is delivered (Anding, 1996b; Viall, 1998). As a general rule, calorie requirements for the critically ill are estimated to be 20–30 kcal/kg. Critically ill patients have elevated protein requirements in the range of 1.5–2 g/kg. Adjustments are made for renal or hepatic dysfunction, or both (Anding, 1996b; Roberts & Zaloga, 2000).

Although enteral nutrition is the preferred method of providing nutrition to the critically ill, there are various complications that may be encountered with its use. The most common complications with the causes and interventions are outlined in Table 7.3 (Anding, 1996a, 1996b; Edes, Walk, & Austin, 1990; Guenter et al., 1991; Roberts & Zaloga, 2000; Viall, 1998). Of the complications listed, diarrhea is the most common and bothersome. The causes of diarrhea are numerous, so, when assessing a patient with diarrhea, it is necessary to consider the entire spectrum of appropriate causes to effectively treat the diarrhea. Frequently, diarrhea is managed by using diapers, fecal incontinence bags, or rectal tubes. Other interventions that are sometimes used are the administration of antidiarrhea medications or opiates (if noninfectious), evaluation of the osmolality of enteral medications, and changing of formula type (Preiser et al., 1999; Roberts & Zaloga, 2000). Usually, the diarrhea will subside and resolve as the patient's condition improves.

SUMMARY

Several factors place older adults at increased risk for altered nutrition, complicating the process of feeding and hydrating them. These include normal changes associated with aging, common geriatric problems, the presence of multiple chronic diseases, and personal and environmental issues. Nutrition assessment of the elderly should include dietary history, physical examination, assessment of height and weight, mental state, concurrent disease processes, the presence and quality of a surrogate decision maker, complications from the use of restraints, patient prognosis, and ethical issues.

TABLE 7.3   Complications of Enteral Nutrition

Complication	Cause	Intervention
Malpositioned feeding tube	Misplaced in the endobronchial tree or pleural space	Confirm feeding tube placement by radiographic study prior to initiation of feedings Check feeding tube placement by auscultation
Aspiration of gastric contents	Improper placement of feeding tube NG tube feeding Gastric reflux Head of bed not elevated	Check feeding tube placement by auscultation Elevate head of bed 30–45 degrees during feeding and for at least 30 minutes after feeding
Clogged feeding tube	Inadequate flushing of tube Medications Congealed formula	Flush tube before and after administration of medications Finely crush medications Unclog tube by using carbonated beverages, meat tenderizer, grape juice, or an enzyme preparation specific for unclogging feeding tubes
Intolerance of feeding as evidenced by distention, cramps, nausea, and high gastric residual	Rapid infusion of feedings Decreased gastric emptying Obstruction	Check residuals every 4 hours. Hold feedings if high for 1 hour and recheck residual Check feeding tube placement by auscultation Decrease rate of infusion Decrease concentration of formula Flush feeding tube Metoclopramide (Reglan) may be ordered
Metabolic dehydration	Insufficient fluid administration Use of formulas that are hyperosmolar and high protein Inability of patient to communicate thirst	Provide adequate fluid intake; usually 25–35 mL/kg/d Monitor intake and output, electrolytes May need to place patient on fluid restrictions

(continued)

TABLE 7.3   *(continued)*

Complication	Cause	Intervention
Overhydration	Excessive infusion of formula and fluids Underlying disease process (i.e., cardiac or renal failure)	Monitor intake and output, electrolytes Weigh patient daily Diuretics may be ordered Formula may be changed to be more calorically dense
Nasal necrosis, rhinitis, sinusitis	Use of stiff tubes Prolonged use of feeding tube Excessive pressure of tube on nares	Use small-bore silicone or polyurethane feeding tube Secure feeding tube without pressure to the nares Change position of the tube, daily Consider alternative measure for feeding tube (i.e., gastrostomy, PEG, etc.)

Diarrhea	Gut atrophy from prolonged bowel rest causes increased intestinal permeability
	Hyperosmolar formula (osmolarity > 500 mOsm/kg and predigested elemental products)
	Medications
	  Antibiotics sterilize the gut and contribute to pseudomembranous colitis and the overgrowth of *Clostridium difficile*
	  Drugs that have a sorbitol base (many elixirs) can cause osmotic diarrhea (i.e., acetaminophen, aminophylline, vitamins, codeine, cimetidine, lithium, theophylline)
		Initiation of early enteral feedings
		Use an isotonic formula
		Administration of *Lactobacillus acidophilus* cultures to assist in restoring normal gut flora
		Substitution of pills for elixirs containing sorbitol when possible
		Use a continuous feeding pump
		Stool cultures
		Addition of fiber
		Digitally check for impaction and manually remove stool if necessary

TABLE 7.3   *(continued)*

Complication	Cause	Intervention
	H₂ antagonists and antacids (containing magnesium) may indirectly cause diarrhea by buffering the stomach and hindering its bacteriostatic properties Impaired digestion and absorption caused by the rapid dumping of formula from the stomach into the small intestine Gut failure manifests as diarrhea in the patient with multisystem organ failure Gut infection (*Clostridium difficile, Vibrio cholerae, Salmonella*) Hypoalbuminemia (albumin levels <2.5 g/dL) causes diarrhea by decreasing colloid osmotic pressure Lack of fiber Fecal impaction	

NG, nasogastric; PEG, percutaneous endoscopic gastrostomy.

Adapted from *Maintaining Nutrition*, p. 49, by C. D. Viall, 1998, St. Louis, MO: Mosby.

ACKNOWLEDGMENTS

The authors would like to thank Gail Cresci, Registered Dietician, Department of Surgery, Medical College of Georgia, Augusta, Georgia, for her review of this chapter.

REFERENCES

Anding, R. (1996a). Nutrition support for the critically ill older patient. *Critical Care Nursing Quarterly, 19* (2), 13–22.

Anding, R. H. (1996b). *Nutritional support of the critically ill patient* (2nd ed.). Philadelphia: F. A. Davis Company.

Barton, R. G. (1994). Nutrition support in critical illness. *Nutrition in Clinical Practice, 9,* 127–139.

Boosalis, M. G., Ott, L., Levine, A. S., Slag, M. F., Morley, J. E., Young, B., & McClain, C. J. (1989). Relationship of visceral proteins to nutritional status in chronic and acute stress. *Critical Care Medicine, 17,* 741–747.

Burrell, L. O., & Pless, B. (1996). *Adult nursing acute and community care* (2nd ed.). Stamford: Appleton & Lange.

Constans, T., Bacq, Y., Brechot, F., Guilmot, L., Choutet, P., & Lamisse, F. (1992). Protein-energy malnutrition in elderly medical patients. *Journal of the American Geriatrics Society, 40* (3), 263–268.

Covinsky, K. E., Martin, G. E., Beyth, R. J., Justice, A. C., Sehgal, A. R., & Landefeld, C. S. (1999). The relationship between clinical assessments of nutritional status and adverse outcomes in older hospitalized medical patients. *Journal of the American Geriatrics Society, 45* (5), 532–538.

Dolan, T., Monopoli, M., Kaurich, M., & Rubenstein, L. S. (1990). Geriatric grand rounds: Oral diseases in older adults. *Journal of the American Geriatrics Society, 38* (11), 1239–1250.

Edes, T. E., Walk, B. E., & Austin, J. L. (1990). Diarrhea in tube-fed patients: Feeding formula not necessarily the cause. *The American Journal of Medicine, 88,* 91–93.

Elic, M., Cole, M. G., Primeau, F. J., & Bellavance, F. (1998). Delirium risk factors in elderly hospitalized patients. *Journal of General Internal Medicine, 13,* 204–212.

Fedullo, A. J., & Swinburne, A. J. (1983). Relationship of patient age to cost and survival in a medical ICU. *Critical Care Medicine, 11* (3), 155–159.

Guenter, P. A., Settle, R. G., Perlmutter, S., Marino, P. L., DeSimone, G. A., & Rolandelli, R. H. (1991). Tube feeding-related diarrhea in acutely ill patients. *Journal of Parenteral and Enteral Nutrition, 15* (3), 277–280.

Health Care Financing Administration, Office of National Cost Estimates. (1990). National expenditures 1988. *Health Care Financial Review, 11,* 1–41.

Herrmann, F. R., Safran, C., Levkoff, S. E., & Minaker, K. L. (1992). Serum albumin level on admission as a predictor of death, length of stay, and readmission. *Archives of Internal Medicine, 152,* 125–130.

Incalzi, R. A., Gemma, A., Capparella, O., Cipriani, L., Landi, F., & Carbonin, P. (1996). Energy intake and in-hospital starvation: A clinically relevant relationship. *Archives of Internal Medicine, 156,* 425–429.

Johnson, R. E., & Chernoff, R. (1998). *Geriatric nutrition support.* Philadelphia: W. B. Saunders Company.

Kayser-Jones, J., & Schell, E. (1997). The mealtime experience of a cognitively impaired elder: Ineffective and effective strategies. *Journal of Gerontological Nursing, 23* (7), 33–39.

Keithley, J. K., & Eisenberg, P. (1993). The significance of enteral nutrition in the intensive care unit patient. *Critical Care Nursing Clinics of North America, 5* (1), 23–29.

Kerstetter, J. E., Hothausen, B. A., & Fitz, P. A. (1992). Malnutrition in the institutionalized older adult. *Journal of the American Dietetic Association, 92* (9), 1109–1116.

Lamberta, H., & Wyman, J. F. (1999). Failure to thrive. In J. Stone, J. Wyman, & S. Salisbury (Eds.), *Clinical gerontological nursing: A guide to advanced practice* (pp. 313–319). Philadelphia: W. B. Saunders.

Landi, F., Zuccala, G., Gambassi, G., Incalzi, R. A., Manigrasso, L., Pagano, F., Carbonin, P., & Bernabei, R. (1999). Body mass index and mortality among older people living in the community. *Journal of the American Geriatrics Society, 47*, 1072–1076.

Lindley, C. M., Tully, M. P., Paramosothy, V., & Tallis, R. C. (1992). Inappropriate medication is a major cause of adverse drug reactions in elderly patients. *Age & Ageing, 21* (4), 294–300.

Marcus, E., & Berry, E. M. (1998). Refusal to eat in the elderly. *Nutrition Reviews, 56* (6), 163–171.

McMurtry, C. T., & Rosenthal, A. (1995). Predictors of 2-year mortality among older male veterans on a geriatric rehabilitation unit. *Journal of the American Geriatric Society, 43* (10), 1123–1126.

McQuiggan, M. M., Marvin, R. G., McKinley, B. A., & Moore, F. A. (1999). Enteral feeding following major torso trauma: From theory to practice. *New Horizons, 7* (1), 131–146.

Mentes, J., Culp, K., Maas, M., & Rantz, M. (1999). Acute confusion indicators: Risk factors and prevalence using MDS data. *Research in Nursing & Health, 22*, 95–105.

Mion, L. C., McDowell, J. A., & Heaney, L. K. (1994). Nutritional assessment of the elderly in the ambulatory care setting. *Nurse Practitioner Forum, 5*, 46–51.

Montamat, S. C., Cusak, B. J., & Vestal, R. E. (1989). Management of drug therapy in the elderly. *New England Journal of Medicine, 321*, 303–309.

Morrisson, S. G. (1997). Feeding the elderly population. *Nursing Clinic of North America, 32* (4), 791–812.

Nightingale, F. (1992). *Notes of nursing*. Philadelphia: J. B. Lippincott Company.

Nutrition Screening Initiative: Nutrition screening manual for professionals caring for older Americans. (1991). Washington, DC.

Pinchcofsky-Devin, G. D., & Kaminski, M. V. (1996). Correlation of pressure sores and nutritional status. *Journal of the American Geriatrics Society, 34*, 435–440.

Preiser, J. C., Berré, J., Carpentier, Y., Jolliet, P., Pichard, C., Van Gossum, A., & Vincent, J. L. (1999). Management of nutrition in European intensive care units: Results of a questionnaire. *Intensive Care Medicine, 25*, 95–101.

Rader, J. (1995). *Individualized dementia care: Creative, compassionate approaches*. New York: Springer Publishing Company.

Roberts, P. R., & Zaloga, G. P. (2000). Enteral nutrition. In A. Grenvik, S. M. Ayres, P. R. Holbrook, & W. C. Shoemaker (Eds.), *Textbook of critical care* (4th ed., pp. 875–897). Philadelphia: W. B. Saunders Company.

Schneider, J. K., Mion, L. C., & Frengley, J. D. (1992). Adverse drug reactions in an elderly outpatient population. *American Journal of Hospital Pharmacy, 49* (1), 90–96.

Schoemaker, W., Ayres, S., Grenvik, A., & Holbrook, P. (2000). Nutrition for the critically ill geriatric patient. In A. Grenvik, S. M. Ayres, P. R. Holbrook, & W. C. Shoemaker (Eds.), *Textbook of critical care* (4th ed., pp. 898–901). Philadelphia: W. B. Saunders Company.

Schwartz, J. B. (1997). Geriatric clinical pharmacology. In W. Kelly (Ed.), *Textbook of internal medicine* (3rd ed.) (pp. 2547–2554). New York: Lippincott-Raven.

Sternberg, J. A., Rohovsky, S. A., Blackburn, G. L., & Babineau, T. J. (2000). Total parenteral nutrition for the critically ill patient. In A. Grenvik, S. M. Ayres, P. R. Holbrook, & W. C. Shoemaker (Eds.), *Textbook of critical care* (4th ed.) (pp. 989–908). Philadelphia: W. B. Saunders Company.

Sullivan, D. H., & Walls, R. C. (1994). Impact of nutritional status of morbidity in a population of geriatric rehabilitation patients. *Journal of the American Geriatric Society, 42* (5), 471–477.

Sullivan, D. H., Walls, R. C., & Bopp, M. M. (1995). Protein-energy undernutrition and the risk of mortality within one year of hospital discharge: A follow-up study. *Journal of the American Geriatric Society, 43* (5), 507–512.

United States Congress, Office of Technology Assessment. (1987). *Life sustaining technologies and the elderly.* Washington, DC: U.S. Government Printing Office.

Viall, C. D. (1998). *Maintaining nutrition* (4th ed.) (pp. 39–60). St. Louis, MO: Mosby.

8

Injury Prevention in the Elderly

Pamela Stinson Kidd

INCIDENCE AND PREVALENCE

For each decade of life after age 65, the incidence of injury-related death increases. Falls, motor vehicle crashes (MVCs), fires, choking, and poisoning are the major causes of injury death in the elderly (Vernon, 1995). Falls present a serious health risk. One of every three people over the age of 65 fall each year. The cost of fall-related injuries for age 65 and older in 1994 was $20.2 billion (the latest year for which these figures were available) (Centers for Disease Control [CDC], 1999).

THE STUDY OF INJURIES

Injuries are difficult to study for several reasons. Unlike diseases, injuries are not caused by a single organism. Many activities associated with injury are considered a right rather than a privilege (for example gun ownership, driving an automobile). Risk taking is a valued American trait. Some activities associated with injury are considered a cultural rite of passage (such as operating a tractor in a rural community). Injuries are frequently viewed as "accidents," implying that they are out of one's control. This view is perpetuated by the media and insurance companies and can discourage scientific study. Injured patients are referred to by health-care providers as "victims," again implying the person was at the wrong place at the wrong time. Although in some situations the injured person may truly be a victim, often the injury is a result of decisions, such as choosing not to change locks and add deadbolts.

Injury may be viewed as a disease (Houck, 1986). As such, there are increased risks for this disease. Injuries can be predicted based on epidemiological study of patterns of events. The nurse's role is to assess for these patterns in at-risk clients, intervene in a manner that has shown to be effective for the target person or group, and evaluate the outcomes associated with the intervention.

It is difficult to predict or explain safety. Even in cases in which a person engages in good health practices (e.g., not smoking, avoiding fried foods, regular exercising), there is no evidence to support the idea that the person will practice injury avoidance behaviors (e.g., wearing a seat belt, observing the speed limit) (Shinar, Schechtman, & Compton, 1999).

INJURY FROM AN EPIDEMIOLOGIC PERSPECTIVE

Injuries can be viewed from an epidemiological perspective. Haddon (1980) developed and expanded a matrix for classifying factors associated with injuries. In the matrix, three factors—host (the elderly person), agent (the mechanism of injury), and environment (physical as well as sociocultural)—interact simultaneously to cause injury. There are three phases to assess when exploring injury risk. The first phase, pre-event, focuses on variables that interact to increase susceptibility to injury. The second phase, event, addresses variables that help determine whether an injury will result from the dissipation of energy as well as the severity of the injury. The third phase, post-event, focuses on variables that determine what sequelae may result from the injury and the impact on lifestyle. Table 8.1 illustrates application of Haddon's matrix to the elderly person. In addition to creating the matrix, Haddon also developed a series of 10 countermeasures that provides a foundation for injury prevention and control strategies. These countermeasures are customized to the elderly population in Table 8.2.

Nursing interventions may focus on one or all of these phases as well as one or more of the factors. For a comprehensive injury prevention program, the cooperation and collaboration of professionals from multiple disciplines are needed to provide the expertise in designing engineering controls, enforcing public policy, and educating the host.

BEHAVIORAL FACTORS

The prevalence of drinking alcohol and driving declines as one ages. However, drivers age 65 or older have a three times as likely involvement in a MVC after drinking and driving as compared with younger drivers (Kamimoto, Easton, Maurice, Husten, & Macera, 1999). It is not clear how alcohol mediates its effects in older persons. Routes of potential mediation include cognition, motor function, and memory. Prescription drugs may interact with alcohol, and the effects of this interaction in the elderly is not well-studied. In a study of severe injuries in the elderly, failure to use seat belts

TABLE 8.1 Haddon's Matrix Applied to Elderly Injury

Phase	Host	Agent	Environment
Preevent	Slower reflexes Decreased ability to judge distances Decreased visual acuity	Condition of motor vehicle Firearm in the home	Visibility of traffic signals Visibility of hazards Divided highways Voluntary surrender of license encouraged by community Screening by health-care providers for at-risk driving expected
Event	Seat belt use Osteoporosis	Presence of airbag in vehicle Size and type of bullet Number of pills in bottle	Presence of guard rails Median barriers Laws about seat belt use
Postevent	Use of beta blocker drugs Coexisting medical conditions	Fuel system integrity Half-life of drugs taken	Availability of rehabilitation services in rural areas Insurance coverage for follow-up services

(83% of the sample) and alcohol intoxication (1% of the sample) were precipitating factors for greater injury (Schiller, Knox, & Chleborad, 1995).

ANATOMIC AND PHYSIOLOGIC FACTORS

Arthritis is the most prevalent chronic condition among adults age 65 or older (Desai, Zhang, & Hennessy, 1999). Adults aged 65 years and older account for approximately 88% of all health-care expenditures for fractures resulting from bone loss density (Ray, 1997). Hip fractures account for most of the hospitalizations for fractures and are the second major cause of hospitalization for women age 85 and older.

Sensory impairments are more common in the elderly. In adults age 70 years and older, 18% report vision impairments, 33% report hearing

TABLE 8.2   Countermeasures Relevant for Elderly

1. Prevent the creation of the hazard
   Avoid cars without side airbags because elderly are frequently involved in side crashes in intersections
2. Reduce the amount of the hazard
   Voluntary reduction of driving during heavy traffic flow
3. Prevent the release of the hazard
   Make bathtubs less slippery
4. Modify the rate or spatial distribution of the hazard
   Elderly at risk of falls should wear hip pads
5. Separate in time or space the hazard from the person who is to be protected
   Create crosswalks with medians to allow elderly a place to stop safely if crossing signal changes while they are crossing the street
6. Separate the hazard from the person who is to be protected by a material barrier
   Fireproof clothing
7. Modify relevant basic qualities of the hazard
   Construct homes with smoke alarms built into the electrical system
8. Make sure that the person to be protected is more resistant to damage from the hazard
   Nutrition and exercise to prevent osteoporosis
9. Begin to counter the damage already done by the hazard
   Provide emergency care
10. Stabilize, repair, and rehabilitate the object of the damage
    Rehabilitation programs designed for elderly and frail elderly

impairments, and 9% report both vision and hearing impairments (Campbell, Crews, Moriarty, Zack, & Blackman, 1999). Vision loss may be secondary to cataracts, glaucoma, and visual field disturbances. Elderly with vision impairments report difficulty walking, changing positions, preparing meals, and managing medications, all factors that increase risk of injury. Older adults with vision impairments have a higher incidence of falls (Campbell et al., 1999). Falls may result in costly injuries such as hip fractures and spinal cord injuries (Apple, Anson, Hunter, & Bell, 1995). These injuries also affect quality of life. Half of older adults who experience a hip fracture never regain their former level of functioning (Tinetti et al., 1994).

The changing physiology of aging includes systolic hypertension; susceptibility to hypothermia and hyperthermia; decreases in maximal ventilatory capacity, kidney function, and cardiac reserve; and osteoporosis (Baraff, Della Penna, Williams, & Sanders, 1997). These factors increase injury risk through increasing serum concentration and half-life for some drugs, the incidence of syncope, sequelae postinjury (referred to as secondary injury), return to preinjury lifestyle, and the severity of injury with less energy.

Polypharmacy is also a risk factor for injury, particularly when the person visits several health-care providers, none of whom may have the patient's total medication history across providers. Table three lists drugs that are relatively contraindicated (and have a higher injury risk associated with their use) in older persons and possible alternative drugs that may be helpful for the advanced practice nurse. Overall, psychotropic agents are associated with falls in the older population. Cardiovascular agents producing peripheral vasodilation are also implicated. However, there is less proof that analgesics and hypoglycemic agents increase the elderly injury risk (Hanlon, Cutson, & Ruby, 1996).

Fall-related deaths are highest for men in all age categories; this may be because men have a greater number of comorbid conditions. It is important to explore whether a fall is in itself the primary event or the result of an undetected decline in health due to another health condition.

RISK PERCEPTIONS

Although elderly may perceive a general increased risk of injury, particularly falls, as they age and also perceive that injuries are preventable, they still may not consider themselves susceptible for a specific injury event (Braun, 1998).

There is some evidence that once a person has fallen, there is increased anxiety and fear of falling that may lead to increased health care contacts and an overall decreased sense of well-being (Baldwin, Craven, & Dimond, 1996; Luukinen, Koski, Kivela, & Laippala, 1996). Falling is both a consequence of a fall and a risk factor for future falls because it may limit mobility and decrease functional impairment. About one third of elderly persons who fall develop a fear of falling (Vellas, Wayne, Romero, Baumgartner, & Garry, 1997). Fear of falling is also associated with depression (Chandler, Duncan, Sanders, & Studenski, 1996).

It may be that a switch in the living environment of an elderly person (such as moving from a rural to an urban community, or one house to another) requires a reorientation of risk perceptions. Rural elderly may be accustomed to walking in underbrush, around fallen trees, and among animals and may have adapted their movement to accommodate these hazards. However, the same person may not be comfortable crossing a busy street or may underestimate the risk of walking against a crossing light or miscalculate the speed of an oncoming vehicle.

Older people may resist changing habitual behavior or fail to recognize that old habits can pose an injury risk now versus when they were younger. Poor judgment and inappropriate environmental use (e.g., washing your foot in a sink) may result in injury even when the hazards in the environment are minimized (Connell & Wolf, 1997). Personal experience affects perception of risk (Tversky & Kahneman, 1974). History of a previous injury event is associated with greater perceived risks of other activities, such as crossing the street or climbing stairs.

Although the elderly tend to be greater risk aversive, physical decline may counterbalance this attribute with the net effect of greater injury risk (McGwin & Brown, 1999).

ENVIRONMENT

Sociocultural Environment

The growth of a community can influence health status and health stress in the elderly. When community education levels are high, community growth does not negatively affect the health of the elderly (Preston & Bucher, 1996). Therefore, growing communities with higher educational levels tend to have more health resources, such as injury prevention programs.

In rural communities elders are less likely to seek or get formal services to assist them in activities of daily living (ADLs) and household chores (Mainros & Kohrs, 1995). The decision to not use services or the inability to receive these services may be associated with a greater injury rate. Elderly living in rural communities have poorer health, but they do not use more services or report more unmet needs than their urban counterparts do (Clark & Dellasega, 1998; Mainous & Kohrs, 1995). Poorer health is associated with greater injuries.

Family solidarity is an important cause of nonreporting of elder abuse among ethnic groups (Wolf & Li, 1999).

Physical Environment

The physical environment can be made safer for elderly persons. Environmental improvements can be made within the home and the community. Specific improvements are addressed within each injury problem discussed in this chapter.

SAFE AT HOME

Fall-Related Injuries

To adequately prevent hip fractures, interventions need to begin during adolescence and early adulthood. Regular weight-bearing exercise and adequate dietary consumption of calcium are the best preventive factors. However, risks can be reduced in the elderly by modifying behavior (smoking and alcohol consumption) as well as modifying the physical environment. Tai chi has been effective in improving strength, balance, and coordination (Kessenich, 1998; Ross & Presswalla, 1998; Wolson et al., 1996). The performance of regular weight-bearing exercise helps maintain joint mobility.

Persons who fall most frequently attribute being in a hurry as the reason for the fall (Berg, Alessio, Mills, & Tong, 1997). Most older adults believe their falls result from internal factors such as dizziness and poor balance as opposed to external factors such as floor rugs and poor lighting. They also perceive the benefits of therapeutic exercise to be greater than home modifications in preventing falls (Hinman, 1998).

Falls by men often result from slips, whereas women tend to trip and then fall. More research is needed to delineate how risk factors differ by gender, but the implication is that interventions need to be customized to the target group. About 10% of all falls in the elderly occur during an acute illness (Mahoney, 1999).

Falls associated with the greatest injury risk occur in persons with cognitive and neuromuscular deficits while climbing stairs, turning around, or reaching for objects. Heavier individuals tend to have less severe injuries. Falls on hard, nonabsorptive ground surfaces, such as tile, wood, and concrete, are more likely to result in injury. Falls are not only associated with hip fractures. Cervical spine injury occurs with minor energy releases in the elderly. C_2 injuries may occur after minor injury and particularly after falls (Spivak, Weiss, Cotler, & Call, 1994).

Nursing personnel should conduct medication reviews, home safety modifications, and risk factor reduction with elderly clients. A practice guideline has been developed to use in assessment of patients age 65 and older who present to the Emergency Department (ED) for treatment (Baraff et al., 1997). Although designed for use in patients who have fallen, this guideline could be used in primary care or at any point along the hospitalization of a patient with fall-related injury. The purpose of the guideline is to ensure that these patients are treated in a uniform manner reflecting the best standard of care possible based on research findings. The guideline delineates actions appropriate for the caregiver in the ED. However, these responsibilities could be reallocated depending on the assessment practice setting. A helpful section of the guideline addresses referral options for assessed risk factors and areas for further diagnostic work-up. The acronym SPLATT can help health care providers remember key items to assess: Symptoms, Previous falls, Location of fall, Activity at the time of the fall, Time of fall, and Trauma (both psychological and physical).

There are several published assessment tools for screening susceptibility for falls. The discussion of these tools is beyond the scope of this chapter. Balance limitations can be assessed easily by asking the elderly person to get up from a chair without using his or her arms (get up and go test). If the person needs to use his or her arms, it indicates a significant weakness in the hip extensors and quadriceps and an increased chance of falling

(Mahoney, 1999). Asking the patient to walk and talk at the same time can help assess ease of gait and balance. The inability to walk while talking indicates a higher risk of falling and the need to concentrate on motor activities.

The United States Preventative Services Task Force (1990) recommendations advise the elderly or those responsible for older persons to inspect their homes for environmental hazards and to install handrails and traction strips. Clinicians are encouraged to perform visual acuity checks and provide mobility counseling and to monitor the use of drugs associated with falls. Older persons are encouraged to engage in a regular exercise program (United States Preventative Services Task Force, 1990).

A geriatric assessment performed by a geriatric specialist is recommended for an elderly person who has sustained at least one other fall within a 3-month period of the current fall for which the elderly person is seeking care ("ED Management of Falls in the Elderly," 1998). Other referrals to consider are social services, home health, physical therapy (especially if there is a gait or balance problem assessed), optometry or ophthalmology, and a podiatrist (for appropriate footwear).

Treatment of osteoporosis decreases the risk of fall-related fractures. Bone density scans are the best method of assessing bone mineral density. For best effects, antiresorptive therapy using biphosphonates should begin soon after menopause and be continued indefinitely (Beier, Maricic, & Staats, 1998). Yet all women benefit to some degree regardless of their age. All postmenopausal women should take in between 1000 and 1500 mg calcium and 400 to 800 IU of vitamin D every day regardless of any prescriptive therapy for osteoporosis (Meiner, 1999).

Intervention strategies should also address mitigating the effects of a fall by using protective hip pads or impact-absorbing floor materials. Physical exercise is associated with decreased falls and fracture risk for healthy elderly; however, the dosing of exercise needs more study in relation to elderly persons with some limitations in ADLs (Stevens, Powell, Smith, Wingo, & Sattin, 1997). Weight-bearing exercise in the amount of 20 to 30 minutes every day or for 60 minutes three times a week is recommended in postmenopausal women. Elderly with a history of falling appear to have co-contraction of muscle groups, perhaps resulting from altered motor control. Thus, muscle strength is not decreased but stability is an issue. It may be that the elderly increase the overall stiffness of their musculoskeletal system to promote stability. Thus interventions that focus on dynamic balance rather than static balance (e.g., tai chi) may enhance motor and balance control and decrease falls (Lee & Kerrigan, 1999).

Benzodiazepines and tricyclic antidepressants (TCAs) have been positively related to falls (Cumming, 1998; Leipzig, Cumming, & Tinetti, 1999). The newer selective serotonin reuptake inhibitor (SSRI) agents are also correlated with falls. There are no significant differences between the risk of falls associated with TCAs or SSRIs (Thapa et al., 1995).

Because of the impact of falls on the quality of life in the elderly and the costs associated with these falls, the Centers for Disease Control (CDC) has developed a Tool Kit to Prevent Senior Falls (CDC, 1999). This tool kit addresses falls in nursing homes as well as in community-dwelling elderly. There is a checklist to use to alleviate fall hazards in the home.

Intervention programs are most effective when targeting persons with the greatest chance of falling (Table 8.3). Risk factors differ among disabled elderly versus independent elderly (Koski, Luukinen, Laippala, & Kivela, 1998). The high-risk group includes those with physiological impairments and transfer limitations (McLean & Lord, 1996). Even low levels of environmental risk can pose a significant threat to frail elderly. They are more likely to lose their balance with a minor hazard, and they spend more time at home than do their healthy counterparts, thus increasing their exposure risk. It is also useful to teach the elderly methods of getting up safely once they have fallen (Reece & Simpson, 1996).

Several factors in the external environment predispose the elderly to falls. These are listed in Table 8.4. The home environment can be modified to include better lighting, use of banisters, removal of carpets and rugs that alter the height surface of the walking area.

In skilled nursing facilities, the use of mechanical restraints increases fall risk (Tinetti et al., 1994). Several fall-prevention strategies have been suggested for this setting, including having personal belongings used frequently within adequate reach, keeping furniture in a consistent place, and responding to call lights quickly.

TABLE 8.3   Fall Risk Factors

Gait disturbance

Previous fall

Physically inactive

Balance difficulty

Fear of falling

Urinary incontinence

Change in housing conditions

Poor pulse rate after standing

Parkinsonism

Arthritis

Divorced, widowed, or unmarried

Low body mass index

Incomplete step continuity

Poor distant visual acuity

Long-acting benzodiazepines

Peripheral neuropathy

TABLE 8.4   Fall-Prevention Strategies

Encourage use of assistive devices through proper fitting and effective teaching

Eliminate household obstacles (floor rugs, books and objects on the floor, furniture that requires walking around)

Have handrails and lights on all staircases (light switch should be at top and bottom of stairs)

No loose tread on stairs

Install bathroom grab bars for toilet and tub

Use no-slip mats in bathtub and on shower floors

Get up slowly from a sitting or lying position

Wear shoes with good support and thin nonslip soles

Wear hip pads if at high risk for fall

Improve the lighting in the home (use 60-watt bulbs or higher and frosted bulbs to reduce glare)

Have vision checked regularly

Ask for a medication review

Begin a regular exercise program, engage in balance training (tai chi), and strengthen muscles around hip, ankle, and knee, increase flexibility of the trunk and lower limbs (yoga)

Keep items used in kitchen on lower shelves

Get a steady step stool with a bar to hold onto

Light pathway between bed and bathroom

Paint doorsills a different color to prevent tripping

Place a phone near the floor in case you fall and cannot get up

Homicides

The rate of homicides among adults age 65 and older decreased 36% from 1987 to 1996 (Stevens et al., 1999). The most frequently used agent was firearms. Perceived risk of being a "victim" of violence might be greater than actual risk. This fear can diminish a person's quality of life. Teaching conflict resolution can be a protective factor against homicide at all ages.

Suicide

Although, overall, the suicide rate for individuals age 65 and older has decreased, it is still the greatest rate of all age groups (Stevens et al., 1999). The highest increase in suicide occurred among persons age 80–84 years. The rate for men increased 35% in this age group (CDC, 1996). Rates are higher for divorced and widowed men. One reason for these higher rates may be that older women are twice as likely as men to be treated with antidepressants (Brown et al., 1995). Older persons make fewer attempts per completed suicide. Thus, calls for help must be quickly noticed and acted upon. The use of a firearm is the most frequently used method of completing suicide in both elderly men and elderly women (Stevens et al., 1999). Because suicide attempt rates are higher among younger adults today than when their grandparents were young adults and because a previous attempt is positively correlated with future completed suicide, it may be that suicide will increase as a public health problem among the elderly in the future (Blazer, Bachar, & Manton, 1986). Other risk factors for suicide are listed in Table 8.5.

There may be a neurobiological tendency for suicide. For example, a vulnerability to suicide may be genetic and brought in time to expression through the aging process. Expression of suicide behavior at an earlier age may be an indicator of premature aging related to neurotransmitter changes in reuptake sites (Conwell, Raby, & Caine, 1995).

The elderly may also engage in homicide-suicide behavior, usually targeted toward a spouse or consort. In these cases, most couples are over age 55, Caucasian, both in poor health with indicators of depression or alcohol abuse in 50% of cases (Cohen, Llorente, & Eisdorfer, 1998). The role of culture in this phenomenon is yet to be explored.

Passive suicide may also manifest itself in the elderly. The elderly lose the will to live and stop caring for themselves. They may stop taking medications and eating and drinking (Devons, 1996). Some elderly suicides may be regarded as a rationale, particularly if the person was suffering from a chronic or terminal illness. The history of cancer is a risk factor for suicide in the elderly (Grabbe, Demi, Camann, & Potter, 1997). Alcoholism is also a risk factor for suicide in the elderly (Arbore, 1998). Most elderly suicides are not related to chronic illness but are the result of depression (Pearson,

TABLE 8.5   Risk Factors for Suicide in the Elderly

Social isolation
Male
Caucasian
Restricted interests
Tendency to hypochondriasis
Irritability, hostility in face of physical illness
Past history of suicide attempt
Lives alone
Significant change in one's life (such as death of spouse, move to a nursing home)
New onset of physical illness of a chronic nature
History of depression
History of alcoholism
Unemployed
Institutionalization of a spouse

Conwell, & Lyness, 1997). Because of social isolation, older adults are less likely to be discovered in time to receive needed health services after the attempt, increasing their mortality rates (Conwell, 1997). Participation in religious services is a protective factor against suicidal behavior. Participation in peer-counseling programs may be a protective factor.

The best way to assess suicide potential is to ask the patient directly about suicidal thoughts (Callhan, Hendrie, Nienaber, & Tierney, 1997). Most elderly people who commit suicide have seen a primary care provider within 30 days of death (Conwell, 1997). Screening for depression by using a standardized form, such as the Geriatric Depression Scale, can help identify elderly persons at high risk for suicide. Asking if the person believes he or she is a burden to the family and the family might be better off without him or her is a good way of leading into asking about suicidal ideations. Ask if the person has access to the means of killing himself or herself (such as a firearm). Ask what he or she might have done to prepare for death. Eighty percent of persons who threaten to commit suicide eventually do it (Osgood, 1985). However, the elderly give fewer warnings of their plans to others (Conwell, 1997). Assessment forms can be used, such as the Modified Scale for Suicidal Ideation or Hopelessness Scale, and can help quantify the risk present (Osgood, 1985).

Once suicide risk is deemed to be present, the health care provider should negotiate removal of firearms from the home, assess the person's medication profile for quantities of medications and their potential toxicities, treat underlying depression carefully, and provide counseling resources. An elderly person is more at risk of committing suicide if there is a firearm in the house.

Community interventions have included training service personnel such as meter readers, postal service workers, and police, personnel from banks, and pharmacies to recognize elderly persons who may be at high risk of suicide. Multidisciplinary in-home services are then initiated.

Elder Abuse

The most common form of elder mistreatment is neglect. Neglect can be an active process (deciding not to get a parent's medication refilled) or passive (not recognizing the need for the elder to take the medication). Older persons tend to not report mistreatment because of denial, embarrassment, fear of retaliation, fear of nursing home placement, or desire to protect the abuser, who may be a close relative (Rosenblatt, 1997). An estimated 4% of the elder population is thought to be mistreated. However, the true incidence and prevalence is not known because of underreporting. Several reasons are given for elder mistreatment, including caregiver stress, isolation, and dependency of the elderly person, transgenerational violence, and psychopathology of the caregiver. In some cases the caregiver may think the elderly person is ignoring the caregiver deliberately, heightening the frustration of the caregiver. In actuality, the elderly may have vision and hearing impairments and not be able to participate in the communication.

Abuse tends to be recurrent. Physical abuse usually results in fractures, burns, abrasions, and wounds. Psychological abuse may accompany physical abuse. It involves threats, humiliations, and treating the elderly person like a child. Financial abuse involves stealing the resources of the elderly person or persuading the elderly person to change his or her will. Sexual abuse also occurs. The perpetrator tends to be the grown-up son of the abused (Hindmarch, 1999). Institutional abuse also occurs in skilled nursing facilities. Signs of this form of abuse are regimented daily routine, denying access to personal belongings, not dressing residents in their own clothes, insufficient toileting or bathing of residents, and theft of property and prescribed drugs from the resident.

Health care providers need to screen for elder mistreatment. Table 8.6 includes screening questions approved by the American Medical Association. History of missed appointments, physician hopping, repeated hospital admissions, and failure to get prescriptions filled are signs that greater care should be taken in the screening process. The following health problems are most frequently associated with abuse: dementia, depression, stroke, and arthritis (Cupitt, 1997). The provider should interview the patient away from family members. The diagnosis of abuse should always be considered when the patient presents with multiple injuries in various stages of healing or when injuries are unexplained or the explanations given are not realistic (Lachs & Pillemer, 1995). Adult Protective Services should be notified. The caregiver may benefit from participating in disease-specific support groups.

Prevention strategies include rapid reporting of suspected cases to proper authorities, encouraging elderly persons to use direct deposit banking services, and providing adequate home care support. Agencies that provide chore social services (meals, housecleaning) can decrease the stress and resentment of the caregiver. Communities can develop respite programs

TABLE 8.6 AMA's Screening Questions

Has anyone at home ever hurt you?
Has anyone ever touched you without your consent?
Has anyone ever made you do things you didn't want to do?
Has anyone taken anything that was yours without asking?
Has anyone ever scolded or threatened you?
Have you ever signed any documents you didn't understand?
Are you afraid of anyone at home?
Are you alone a lot?
Has anyone ever failed to help you take care of yourself when you needed help?

From Aravanis R: *Diagnostic and Treatment Guidelines on Elder Abuse and Neglect*. Chicago. American Medical Association, 1992: Reprinted with permission.

to provide caregivers with personal time. Several national resources are available (Table 8.7).

Fire-Related Injuries

The elderly represent a disproportionate percentage of fire-related deaths (Barillio & Goode, 1996). About 90% of all fire-related deaths in the elderly occur in the home. Scalds represent 20% of burn injuries (Vernon, 1995). Clothing is a risk factor because elderly persons are frequently burned when their clothing catches fire during cooking. Statistics from burn centers indicate that 80% of the elderly survive their injuries, but 50% of those discharged require home assistance postburn. Preexisting pulmonary disease can increase the likelihood of complications from smoke inhalation.

Older persons who die from house fires tend to be nonsmokers and do not have alcohol involvement as compared with persons younger than age 75 (Elder, Squires, & Busuttil, 1996). They also tend to live alone. Frequently, electrical items start the fire. Social isolation, cognitive or physical impairment, and poverty may contribute to the use of faulty appliances, heaters, and equipment. Risk factors for fire-related injuries include problems with vision, hearing, smell, cognition, and mobility. Few elderly persons understand or believe that a scald burn can occur in 30 seconds from hot tap water.

Preventive strategies include developing fire-resistant clothing for the elderly. The use of fire-resistant bed linens and upholstery may decrease incidence of injury. Smoke detectors are an essential home furnishing. Households without smoke detectors have a 50% greater risk of fire-related fatalities than do households with smoke detectors. Homes should also be equipped with fire extinguishers. The hot water heater temperature should be decreased to 110° F. The elderly should be encouraged to use microwave ovens rather than stoves. Elderly persons should have an escape route planned and practice fire drills and use the route frequently.

Poisonings

Most poisoning deaths in the elderly are related to unintentional misuse of prescribed medications. Changes in cognition, failure to use the con-

---

TABLE 8.7   Resources for Elder Mistreatment

National Center on Elder Abuse 202-682-2470 (interinc.com/NCEA)
National Committee for the Prevention of Elder Abuse (Institute of Aging)
Administration on Aging (www.aoa.dhhs.gov)
Commission on Legal Problems of the Elderly 202-662-8690
National Resource Center on Aging and Injury 619-594-0986 (Note: This center
   has information about all injuries in the elderly not just elder mistreatment)

tainer in which the drug was dispensed, and vision problems all contribute to these deaths. The elderly are more vulnerable to toxicity when an overdose is taken. Cardiovascular drugs account for 40% of poisoning deaths in the elderly.

Prevention strategies include limiting the amount of prescribed medication, using clearly marked pill dispensers, and having proper lighting where medication is kept and used.

SAFE ON THE ROAD

Motor Vehicle–Related Injuries: Motor Vehicle Crashes

Drivers over the age of 65 years, have the highest rate of MVC-related deaths except for the youngest drivers (National Highway Traffic Safety Administration [NHTSA], 1999). They are disproportionately involved in MVCs, with older adults representing 13% of the U.S. population but accounting for 17% of all MVC-related deaths. When the fatality rate is adjusted for miles driven, 70-year-old drivers have three times the rate of fatal crashes than 20-year-old drivers have (Vernon, 1995). The rates of MVC-related injuries vary drastically across states. Physical frailty increases susceptibility to injury during a MVC. The number of older adults who drive is expected to increase as the U.S. population ages (Stevens et al., 1999). Yet, maintaining independence is one marker of successful aging (O'Neill, 1996). Continued driving is a sign of independence. Higher levels of life satisfaction, less loneliness, and better perceived control are associated with driving one's own vehicle (NHTSA, 1999).

There is some evidence to suggest that older drivers will be safer in the future because they will have acquired their basic driving experience in a more motor vehicle–dominated time (Stamatiadis & Deacon, 1997). As a group, elderly drivers tend to drive slower, leave greater space between their car and the vehicle in front of their car, and drive in the outer lane (Mori & Mizohata, 1995). Older drivers, even though they acknowledge functional limitations during driving, do not want to quit driving. Nearly half of all Alzheimer's disease patients have been in a crash after the onset of severe cognitive symptoms (Murray, 1997). There is some evidence that suggests older drivers may experience increased age discrimination and tend to be cited more frequently as a consequence of a crash, even when crash severity and other contributing factors have been considered (Dulisse, 1997).

Older adults have difficulty estimating gaps in traffic when crossing or entering traffic, sharing attention between driving and looking at street signs, remembering a series of directions, and maintaining spatial orientation when driving around a block (McKnight & McKnight, 1999). It is difficult for older drivers to assess vehicle velocity and react to unexpected vehicles, probably because of decreased visual processing speed; light sensitivity; and declines in near vision, dynamic vision, and visual search. Arthritic changes in cervical vertebrae, changes in muscle tone, and neurological conditions contribute to difficulty in turning one's head as one ages. This failure to turn the head may account for the higher incidence of intersection crashes in the elderly (Isler, Parsonson, & Hansson, 1997).

Older drivers tend to wear their seat belts more often and drive after drinking alcohol less often than do younger drivers (Nelson, Bolen, & Kresnow, 1998; Lui et al., 1997). Elderly drivers are more likely to get traffic citations for failure to yield, turning improperly, and running stop signs and red lights (Insurance Institute for Highway Safety [IIHS], 1999).

Prevention strategies can address helping the older driver to drive safely. It is possible that unnecessarily stopping older people from driving increases their risk of pedestrian injuries. Helping the older driver may include discussing routes used to necessary destinations, the time of day when driving occurs, vehicles used and their options (such as mounting of mirrors, adjustment of seats). Community interventions can include safe driving sessions in public places, voluntary driving check point where one's driving abilities can be evaluated by an outsider, better street lighting and signage, and mandatory vision testing for license renewal. The physical environment for driving can be made safer for older drivers by installing traffic signals with protected left turns, four-way stop signs, and one-way streets (Preusser, Williams, Ferguson, Ulmer, & Weinstein, 1998).

Health care providers should assess driving risk by administering a screening test, such as the Driving Practices Questionnaire (Kidd & Huddleston, 1994) or the Driving Habits Questionnaire (Owsley, Stalvey, Wells, & Sloane, 1999). Simple tests that examine visuospatial ability, such as the copy design task of the Mini-Mental State Exam, can provide valuable information about driving risk (Gallo, Rebok, & Lesikar, 1999). The amount of driving completed by the patient should be assessed prior to prescribing medication. Benzodiazepines, TCAs, and antihistamines have the potential to impair driving ability. Hip disease may also affect driving ability. The provider should review the patient's driving history, including crashes and citations, episodes of getting lost, and the observations of family members. Primary-care providers can screen elder drivers for visual, auditory, and cognitive impairments. Drivers can be assisted in assessing their own driving abilities; most older drivers self-regulate by altering the situations in which they will drive. Stroke patients and others with disabilities should be referred to rehabilitation specialists for techniques that can be used for driving safely. The 55 Alive Mature Driver course developed by the American Association of Retired Persons offers a positive atmosphere for learning new coping skills for driving.

The design of motor vehicles can be changed to improve the visual field of the older driver and to make it easier to steer and control acceleration and braking. Instrumentation panels can be better illuminated to increase visibility. Traffic intersections can be modified to enhance visibility, and traffic density can be controlled better through use of signals. An area of active research is the use of in-vehicle human support systems that involves technology to facilitate driving.

Motor Vehicle–Related Injuries: Pedestrian Injuries

The number of older adults dying from a pedestrian-related MVC decreased 23% from 1990 to 1997 (Stevens et al., 1999). Most vehicular pedestrian deaths in the elderly occur at intersections. Decreased vision and hearing along with an increased reaction time probably contribute to these injuries. Visual correction, walking aids, and changing crossing styles and walking routes may decrease the incidence of pedestrian-related injuries. Communities can install median strips to allow a person to rest in the center while crossing the road (Oxley, Fildes, Ishen, Charlton, & Day, 1997).

SAFE AT WORK

Occupational injury rates in the elderly are high. Workers age 65 and older have a fatality rate of 14 per 100,000 employed, higher than for any other age group of workers (United States Department of Labor, 1997). As the age of retirement increases, it is anticipated that the number of occupational injuries in the elderly will increase. Older workers tend to be self-employed or employed by small companies. Frequently, these work situations are not under federal safety regulations. There is less likelihood that formal safety training is available in these work situations. Injuries to older workers are most frequently in the form of fractures and dislocations resulting from falls (Layne & Landen, 1997). Service industries have the highest number of injuries for older workers; agriculture and fishing has the highest injury rate.

In some occupations, such as farming, one seldom retires. Older farmers may help their children or friends during peak seasons of planting and harvest even after stopping full-time farming. Injuries sustained by older farmers tend to be more severe and result in a greater number of fatalities and hospitalizations than they do in younger farmers. Older farmers' injuries are usually caused by machines, especially tractors, and overexertion (Gelberg, Struttmann, & London, 1999). Older farmers who sustain injuries tend to be in debt, and they tend to be using prescription medications (Xiang, Stallones, & Chiu, 1999). These injuries may occur because of decreased vision, hearing, and reaction times and because of joint stiffness. Unsafe habits learned in youth may still be performed, but because of physical changes, they may not be performed without injury as one ages.

Injured older farmers are more likely to sustain another injury in the near future. Thus, there may be a "teachable moment" when health care services are obtained for the original injury (Browning, Truszczynska, Reed, & McKnight, 1998). General safety programs targeting proper footwear, clothing, tractor rollover protection structures, maintenance of power take-off shields, and use of personal protection equipment (ear plugs, goggles, etc.) may prevent future injury.

Poor vision and hearing as well as self-reported disability are associated with occupational injury in the elderly (Zwerling, Whitten, Davis, & Sprince, 1998). Injury prevention efforts should encourage workers to have regular physical examinations with vision and hearing screening. Workplace safety training should include identification of knowledge and skills required for particular tasks (Castillo & Rodriquez, 1997).

SAFE AT PLAY

Many of the physical changes of aging predispose the elderly to recreational injury. Decreased bone density; decreased connective tissue elasticity; and decreased muscle mass, volume, and strength all contribute to injury. Older athletes more commonly suffer from chronic overuse injuries of the knee and shoulder (Cummings, Overend, & Vandervoort, 1996). The majority of these injuries are inflammatory in nature. Injuries are more frequently associated with running, racquet sports, walking, and golf in the older person. However, the older person may also experience the same acute sport-related injuries seen in a younger person.

Prevention strategies should focus on reducing the stress on the person and increasing the person's capacity. The older person should engage in warm-up activities to promote stretching. Mild aerobic activity can be used for the warm-up period. This increases the muscle temperature and contributes to more effective muscular contractions. It also decreases the stiffness of connective tissue. The elderly should be encouraged to use protective gear appropriate for the activity. Proper footwear and equipment are also important. The surface used for the activity (such as clay instead of asphalt surface in tennis) should be as shock absorbing as possible. Regular activity is very important. There should be no abrupt increases in intensity. Older persons may have been using improper form and poor technique for years. They can always benefit from sport instruction.

SUMMARY

The elderly are at increased risk of injury from multiple sources and behaviors. Yet, once risk factors are recognized and acted upon, an elder person's susceptibility for injury decreases as for any another disease when risk reduction is attempted. Often the elderly person is a grandparent. More than 5 million grandparents in the United States serve as primary child-care providers, usually for their working children. In this role, they frequently transport children in their motor vehicles. However, 21% of those polled said they never use a child safety seat or seat belt for their grandchildren (AAA Foundation for Traffic Safety, 1999). Safe behaviors benefit the elderly person directly and those around the person indirectly. There is much left to be done in decreasing injuries across the life span, and particularly in the elderly.

REFERENCES

AAA Foundation for Traffic Safety. (1999). Grandparents! Buckle those kids! *Progress Report, 6* (5), 1.

Anonymous. (1998). ED management of falls in the elderly: Avoiding a downward spiral. Clinical update. *Journal of Critical Illness, 13* (2), 105–107.

Apple, D. F., Anson, C. A., Hunter, J. D., & Bell, R. B. (1995). Factors associated with spinal cord injury in the elderly. *Gerontology and Geriatrics Education, 16,* 15–27.

Arbore, P. (1998). Assessing the risk for suicide in the elderly. *Home Healthcare Consultant, 5* (5), 23–27.

Baldwin, R. L., Craven, R. F., & Dimond, M. (1996). Falls: Are rural elders at greater risk? *Journal of Gerontological Nursing, August, 22* (8), 14–21.

Baraff, L. J., Della Penna, R., Williams, N., & Sanders, A. (1997). Practice guidelines for the ED management of falls in community dwelling elderly persons. *Annals of Emergency Medicine, 30,* 480–492.

Barillio, D. J., & Goode, R. (1996). Fire fatality study: Demographics of fire victims. *Burns, 22* (2), 85–88.

Beier, M., Maricic, M., & Staats, D. (1998). Management of osteoporosis and risk assessment for falls in long term care. *Annals of Long Term Care, 6* (suppl. D), 1–16.

Berg, W. P., Alessio, H. M., Mills, E. M., & Tong, C. (1997). Circumstances and consequences of falls in independent community dwelling older adults. *Age and Ageing, 26,* 261–268.

Blazer, D. G., Bachar, J. R., & Manton, K. G. (1986). Suicide in later life: Review and commentary. *Journal of the American Geriatrics Society, 34,* 519–525.

Braun, B. L. (1998). Knowledge and perception of fall related risk factors and fall reduction techniques among community dwelling elderly individuals. *Physical Therapy, 78,* 1262–1276.

Brown, S., Salive, M. E., Guralnik, J. M., Pahor, M., Chapman, D. P., & Blazer, D. (1995). Antidepressant use in the elderly: Association with demographic characteristics, health-related factors, and health care utilization. *Epidemiology, 48,* 445–453.

Browning, S. R., Truszczynska, H., Reed, D., & McKnight, R. (1998). Agricultural injuries among older Kentucky farmers: The farm family health and hazard surveillance study. *American Journal of Industrial Medicine, 33,* 341–353.

Callhan, C., Hendrie, H., Nienaber, N., & Tierney, W. (1996). Suicidal ideation among older primary care patients. *Journal of the American Geriatrics Society, 44,* 1205–1209.

Campbell, V. A., Crews, J. E., Moriarty, D. G., Zack, M. M., & Blackman, D. K. (1999). Surveillance for sensory impairment, activity limitation, and health-related quality of life among older adults, U.S. 1993–1997. *MMWR. Morbidity and Mortality Weekly Report, 48* (SS08), 131–156.

Castillo, D., & Rodriquez, R. (1997). Follow back study of oldest workers with emergency department treated injuries. *American Journal of Industrial Medicine, 31,* 609–618.

Centers for Disease Control. (1996). Suicide Among Older Persons—United States, 1980–1992. *MMWR. Morbidity and Mortality Weekly Report, 45,* 3–6.

Centers for Disease Control. (1999). A tool kit to prevent senior falls. NCIPC, Division of Unintentional Injury Prevention. Atlanta, GA: U.S. Department of Health and Human Services.

Chandler, J. M., Duncan, P., Sanders, L., & Studenski, S. (1996). The fear of falling syndrome: Relationship to falls, physical performance, and activities of daily living in frail older persons. *Topics in Geriatric Rehabilitation, 11* (3), 55–63.

Clark, D., & Dellasega, C. (1998). Unmet health care needs. *Journal of Gerontological Nursing, 24*(12), 24–33.

Cohen, D., Llorente, M., & Eisdorfer, C. (1998). Homicide-suicide in older persons. *American Journal of Psychiatry, 155* (3), 390–396.

Connell, B. R., & Wolf, S. (1997). Environmental and behavioral circumstances associated with falls at home among healthy elderly individuals. *Archives of Physical Medicine and Rehabilitation, 78,* 179–186.

Conwell, Y. (1997). Management of suicidal behavior in the elderly. *The Psychiatric Clinics of North America, 20* (3), 667–683.

Conwell, Y., Raby, W., & Caine, E. (1995). Suicide and aging. II: The psychobiological interface. *International Psychogeriatrics, 7* (2), 165–181.

Cumming, R. (1998). Epidemiology of medication-related falls and fractures in the elderly. *Drugs & Aging, 12* (1), 43–53.

Cummings, I. P., Overend, T. J., & Vandervoort, A. A. (1996). Musculoskeletal injury in the older athlete. *Physical Therapy Review, 1,* 59–69.

Cupitt, M. (1997). Identifying and addressing the issues of elder abuse: A rural perspective. *Journal of Elder Abuse and Neglect, 8* (4), 21–30.

Desai, M. M., Zhang, P., & Hennessy, C. H. (1999). Surveillance for morbidity and mortality among older adults, U.S., 1995–1996. *MMWR. Morbidity and Mortality Weekly Report, 48* (SS08), 7–25.

Devons, C. (1996). Suicide in the elderly: How to identify and treat patients at risk. *Geriatrics, 51* (3), 67–72.

Dulisse, B. (1997). Driver age and traffic citations resulting from motor vehicle collisions. *Accident Analysis and Prevention, 29* (6), 779–783.

Elder, A., Squires, T., & Busuttil, A. (1996). Fire fatalities in elderly people. *Age and Ageing, 25,* 214–216.

Gallo, J. J., Rebok, G. W., & Lesikar, S. E. (1999). The driving habits of adults aged 60 years and older. *Journal of the American Geriatrics Society, 47,* 335–341.

Gelberg, K., Struttmann, T., & London, M. (1999). A comparison of agricultural injuries between the young and the elderly: New York and Kentucky. *Journal of Agricultural Safety & Health, 5* (1), 73–81.

Grabbe, L., Demi, A., Camann, M., & Potter, L. (1997). The health status of elderly persons in the last year of life: A comparison of deaths by suicide, injury, and natural causes. *American Journal of Public Health, 87* (3), 434–437.

Haddon, W. (1980). Advances in epidemiology of injuries as a basis for public policy. *Public Health Report, 95*, 411–421.

Hanlon, J. T., Cutson, T., & Ruby, C. M. (1996). Drug related falls in the older adult. *Topics in Geriatric Rehabilitation, 11* (3), 38–54.

Hindmarch, V. (1999). Elder abuse. *Professional Nurse, 14*, 249–252.

Hinman, M. R. (1998). Causal attributions of falls in older adults. *Physical & Occupational Therapy in Geriatrics, 15* (3), 71–84.

Houck, T. (1986). Injuries are not accidents. *Public Health Reports, 124.*

Insurance Institute for Highway Safety. (1999). *Fatality facts.* Alexandria, VA: IIHS.

Isler, R., Parsonson, B., & Hansson, G. (1997). Age related effects of restricted head movements on the useful field of view of drivers. *Accident Analysis and Prevention, 29* (6), 793–801.

Kamimoto, L. A., Easton, A. N., Maurice, E., Husten, C. G., & Macera, C. A. (1999). Surveillance for five health risks among older adults: U.S. 1993–1997. *MMWR. Morbidity and Mortality Weekly Report, 48* (SS08), 89–130.

Kessenich, C. (1998). Tai chi as a method of fall prevention in the elderly. *Orthopaedic Nursing* (July/August), 27–29.

Kidd, P., & Huddleston, S. (1994). Psychometric properties of the driving practices questionnaire: Assessment of risky driving. *Research in Nursing and Health, 17*, 51–58.

Koski, K., Luukinen, H., Laippala, P., & Kivela, S. L. (1998). Risk factors for major injurious falls among the home dwelling elderly by functional abilities. *Gerontology, 44*, 232–238.

Lachs, M. S., & Pillemer, K. (1995). Abuse and neglect of elderly persons. *New England Journal of Medicine, 332* (7), 437–443.

Layne, L. A., & Landen, D. D. (1997). A descriptive analysis of nonfatal occupational injuries to older workers using a national probability sample of hospital emergency departments. *Journal of Occupational and Environmental Medicine, 39* (9), 855–865.

Lee, L., & Kerrigan, C. (1999). Identification of kinetic differences between fallers and nonfallers in the elderly. *American Journal of Physical Medicine and Rehabilitation, 78*, 242–246.

Leipzig, R., Cumming, R., & Tinetti, M. (1999). Drugs and falls in older people: A systematic review and meta analysis: I. Psychotropic drugs. *Journal of the American Geriatrics Society, 47*, 30–39.

Lui, S., Siegal, P. Z., Brewer, R. D., Mokdad, A. H., Sleet, D. A., & Serdula, M. (1997). Prevalence of alcohol impaired driving: results from a national self reported survey of health behaviors. *Journal of the American Medical Association, 277*, 122–125.

Luukinen, H., Koski, K., Kivela, S. L., & Laippala, P. (1996). Social status, life changes, housing conditions, health, functional abilities and life style as risk factors for recurrent falls among the home dwelling elderly. *Public Health, 110*, 115–118.

Mahoney, J. (1999). Falls in the elderly: Office based evaluation, prevention, and treatment. *Cleveland Clinic Journal of Medicine, 66* (3), 181–189.

Mainous, A., & Kohrs, F. (1995). A comparison of health status between rural and urban adults. *Journal of Community Health, 20* (5), 423–431.

McGwin, G., & Brown, D. B. (1999). Characteristics of traffic crashes among young, middle-aged, and older drivers. *Accident Analysis and Prevention, 31*, 181–198.

McKnight, A. J., & McKnight, A. S. (1999). Multivariate analysis of age-related driver ability and performance deficits. *Accident Analysis and Prevention, 31,* 445–454.

McLean, D., & Lord, S. (1996). Falling in older people at home: Transfer limitations and environmental risk factors. *Australian Occupational Therapy Journal, 43,* 13–18.

Meiner, S. (1999). An expanding landscape: Osteoporosis treatment options today. *Advances for Nurse Practitioners, 7* (7), 27–31, 80.

Mori, Y., & Mizohata, M. (1995). Characteristics of older road users and their effect on road safety. *Accident Analysis and Prevention, 27,* 391–404.

Murray, S. L. (1997). Driving and the elderly. *Journal of the American Academy of Nurse Practitioners, 9,* 133–136.

National Highway Traffic Safety Administration. (1999). *Literature review examines research on older women's transportation needs* (p. 208). Washington, DC: National Highway Traffic Safety Administration.

Nelson, D. E., Bolen, J., & Kresnow, M. J. (1998). Trends in safety belt use by demographics and by type of state safety belt law, 1987–1993. *American Journal of Public Health, 88,* 245–249.

O'Neill, D. (1996). The older driver. *Reviews in Clinical Gerontology, 6,* 295–302.

Osgood, N. (1985). *Suicide in the elderly.* Rockville, MD: Aspen.

Owsley, C., Stalvey, B., Wells, J., & Sloane, M. (1999). Older drivers and cataract: Driving habits and crash risk. *Journal of Gerontology, 54A* (4), M203–M211.

Oxley, J., Fildes, B., Ishen, E., Charlton, J., & Day, R. (1997). Differences in traffic judgements between young and old adult pedestrians. *Accident Analysis and Prevention, 29* (6), 839–847.

Pearson, J., Conwell, Y., & Lyness, J. (1997). Late life suicide and depression in the primary care setting. *New Directions for Mental Health Services, 76* (Winter), 13–38.

Preston, D., & Bucher, J. (1996). The effects of community differences on health status, health stress, and helping networks in a sample of 900 elderly. *Public Health Nursing, 13* (1), 72–79.

Preusser, D., Williams, A., Ferguson, S., Ulmer, R., & Weinstein, H. (1998). Fatal crash risk for older drivers at intersections. *Accident Analysis and Prevention, 30* (2), 151–159.

Ray, W. A., Taylor, J. A., Medor, K. G., Thapa, P. B., Brown, A. K., Kajihara, H. K., Davis, C., Gideon, P., & Griffin, M. R. (1997). A randomized trial of a consultation service to reduce falls in nursing homes. *Journal of the American Medical Association, 278,* 557–562.

Reece, A., & Simpson, J. (1996). Preparing older people to cope after a fall. *Physiotherapy, 82,* 227–235.

Rosenblatt, D. E. (1997). Elder mistreatment. *Critical Care Nursing Clinics of North America, 9,* 183–192.

Ross, M. C., & Presswalla, J. L. (1998). The therapeutic effects of tai chi for the elderly. *Journal of Gerontological Nursing, 24* (2), 45–47.

Schiller, W., Knox, R., & Chleborad, W. (1995). A five year experience with severe injuries in elderly patients. *Accident Analysis and Prevention, 27,* 167–174.

Shinar, D., Schechtman, E., & Compton, R. (1999). Trends in safe driving behaviors and in relation to trends in health maintenance behaviors in the U.S.A.: 1985–1995. *Accident Analysis and Prevention, 31,* 497–503.

Spivak, J., Weiss, M., Cotler, J., & Call, M. (1994). Cervical spine injuries in patients 65 and older. *Spine, 19,* 2302–2306.

Stamatiadis, N., & Deacon, J. (1997). Trends in highway safety: Effects of an aging population on accident propensity. *Accident Analysis and Prevention, 27,* 443–459.

Stevens, J., Powell, K., Smith, S., Wingo, P., & Sattin, R. (1997). Physical activity, functional limitations, and the risk of fall related fractures in community dwelling elderly. *Annals of Epidermiology, 7,* 54–61.

Stevens, J. A., Hasbrouck, L. M., Durant, T. M., Dellinger, A. M., Batabyal, P. K., Coosby, A. E., Valluru, B. R., Kresnow, M., & Guerrero, J. L. (1999). Surveillance for injuries and violence among older adults. *Morbidity and Mortality Weekly Reports, 48* (SS-8), 27–50.

Thapa, P. B., Gideon, P., Fought, R. L., & Ray, W. A. (1995). Psychotropic drugs and risk of recurrent falls in ambulatory nursing home residents. *American Journal of Epidemiology, 142,* 202–211.

Tinetti, M. E., Baker, D. I., McAvay, G., Claos, E. B., Garrett, P., Gottschalk, M., Loch, M. L., Trainor, K., & Horwitz, R. I. (1994). A multifactorial intervention to reduce the risk of falling among elderly people living in the community. *New England Journal of Medicine, 331,* 821–827.

Tversky, A., & Kahneman, D. (1974). Judgement under uncertainty: Heurtistics and biases. *Science, 185,* 1124–1131.

United States Bureau of the Census. (1997). *Statistical abstract of the United States, 1997* (117th ed.). Washington, DC: Department of Commerce, Economics and Statistics Administration.

United States Department of Labor. (1996). *Employment and earnings* 43(1). Washington, DC: U.S. Department of Labor, Bureau of Labor Statistics.

United States Preventative Services Task Force. (1990). Counseling to prevent household and environmental injuries. *American Family Practice, 42* (1), 135–142.

Vellas, B., Wayne, S., Romero, L., Baumgartner, R., & Garry, P. (1997). Fear of falling and restriction of mobility in elderly fallers. *Age and Ageing, 26,* 189–193.

Vernon, M. (1995). *Accidents in the elderly population* (4th ed.). Baltimore: Williams & Wilkins.

Wolf, R. S., & Li, D. (1999). Factors affecting the rate of elder abuse reporting to a state protective services program. *Gerontologist, 19,* 222–228.

Wolfson, L., Whipple, R., Derby, C., Judge, J., King, M., Amerman, P., Schmidt, J., & Smyers, D. (1996). Balance and strength training in older adults: Intervention gains and tai chi maintenance. *Journal of the American Geriatrics Society, 44,* 498–506.

Xiang, H., Stallones, L., & Chiu, Y. (1999). Nonfatal agricultural injuries among Colorado older male farmers. *Journal of Aging and Health, 11* (1), 65–78.

Zwerling, C., Whitten, P. S., Davis, C. S., & Sprince, N. L. (1998). Occupational Injuries among older workers with visual, auditory, and other impairments. *Journal of Occupational and Environmental Medicine, 40,* 720–723.

PART II

Nursing Assessment and Management

9

The Clinical Approach

Catherine M. Eberle and Richard W. Besdine

The increasing number of people who reach old age challenge many commonly held notions of what aging entails and what expectations concerning the later years of life should be. The elderly are not universally disabled, dependent, sick, or demented but instead are a highly diverse group of individuals whose care requires an appreciation of the important physiological changes of aging as well as an appreciation for a person's continued capabilities. There are important changes that occur in most organ systems because of the aging process. Many changes previously attributed solely to aging are, in fact, due to disease; lifestyle exposures, such as dietary, smoking, and alcohol habits; or environmental and occupational exposures. These "external" phenomena interact with the usual changes of aging and influence the overall health of the individual. Our experience as health care providers frequently results in a skewed view of the elderly. It may be hard to believe that only 5% of those over age 65 reside in nursing homes or that almost 50% of those over 85 years remain independent, with activities of daily living.

This chapter addresses the interaction of disease and aging. We examine the older person's perception of health and how this affects the older person's reporting of symptoms, the presentation of illness in old age (typical and atypical), the effect of comorbidity, and the importance of multidimensional assessment of health and physical function in treatment planning.

PERCEPTION OF HEALTH

People of all ages visit a physician or other health care provider when they think they are ill, and they need a health care provider's intervention.

Accordingly, their perception of illness and their ability to recognize and respond to signs and symptoms become crucial factors in the decision to seek care. Self-perception of health is highly correlated with morbidity and mortality (Connelly et al., 1991; Idler & Angel, 1990; Idler & Benyamini, 1997; Idler & Kasl, 1991; Mossey & Shapiro, 1982; Kaplan, Bavell, & Lusky, 1988).

Most older persons accurately assess their health (Blazer & Houpt, 1979). When asked to rate their general health, approximately 70% of those over 65 rate their health as good to excellent (Figure 9.1). Additionally, although most persons of all ages consider their health to be the same as or better than that of others their age, *fewer* in the 60- to 80-year-old category (compared to those <60) consider themselves to be in "worse health" than others their age (Cockerham, Sharp, & Wilcox, 1983). Yet, disease and health conditions are common in those over age 60 years (Figure 9.2). This optimism in the face of increased disability (numbers and severity) suggests that older persons have lower expectations of their health and increased acceptance of disability as a normal part of aging. For this reason, they may not recognize the significance of signs or symptoms of illness and may fail to report the signs and symptoms. Failure to report symptoms may result in missed opportunities to treat and in disease progression and further disability.

SYMPTOM REPORTING

Multiple studies (Brody & Kleban, 1981; Ford et al., 1988; Musil et al., 1998; Williamson et al., 1964) have shown that a large proportion of the

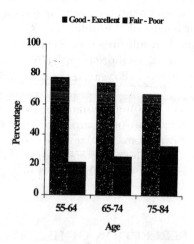

FIGURE 9.1   Self-assessed health. (From Administration on Aging, *Profile of Older Americans, 1999.* Available: www.aoa.dhhs.gov/aoa/stats/agetrend/two1-1.html)

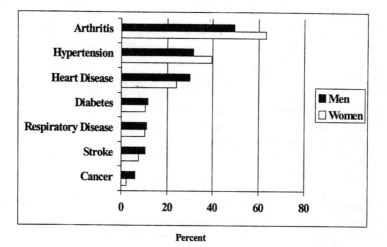

FIGURE 9.2   Percentage of persons 70 years of age and over who reported selected chronic conditions by sex: United States, 1995.

(From the *Health and Aging Chartbook* from *Health, United States, 1999.* From Centers for Disease Control and Prevention, National Center for Health Statistics, 1994 National Health Interview Survey, Second Supplement on Aging. Available: www.cdc.gov/nchswww/products/pubs/pubd/hs/hus.htm)

elderly underreport symptoms and problems. Whereas failure to recognize symptoms is one reason for failure to report symptoms, other reasons include an assumption that symptoms are normal changes of aging, that the complaint was reported previously but ignored, or that "the doctor already knows."

Brody and Kleban (1981) surveyed a group of community-dwelling elderly and found that large numbers of potentially life-threatening symptoms were not reported to health care providers. For example, 31% of those suffering chest pain or discomfort with activity did not tell anyone of their symptoms. Of the reasons given for not reporting symptoms, 17% were attributed to "normal aging" in this group of older individuals. These individuals assumed, possibly incorrectly, that investigation and treatment of the symptom would not be beneficial.

Leventhal and Prohaska (1986) found that older respondents were less likely than were young respondents to use nonspecific symptoms (such as "weakness" or "aches") as signs of illness. This same group of elderly individuals, when given a specific health scenario, were significantly more likely than were the younger individuals in the study to consider the illness as due to aging, even in the case of an acute severely disabling condition.

Twenty percent of the older group stated that even acute and severely disabling symptoms could result from normal aging. It is not surprising, then, that older persons may fail to report such symptoms. (Please note: this also means that 80% of the elderly group did recognize the acute and disabling symptoms as signs of illness.)

When the elderly think symptoms are due to aging, they tend to

1. wait and monitor symptoms
2. accept the symptoms and learn to live with the problem(s) they cause
3. deny or minimize the problem
4. postpone or avoid contacting their physician or family (Leventhal & Prohaska, 1986).

It is important, then, for health-care workers to make specific inquiries regarding the most common and serious signs and symptoms of illness and to educate patients regarding signs and symptoms to be reported.

Most older persons accurately report their health status, but a substantial minority underreport and overreport illness. Either inaccuracy puts them at risk of worsening health from failure to receive timely care or from adverse effects of unnecessary investigations.

ILLNESS IN THE ELDERLY

Because of the decline in normal organ function, older patients may have symptoms earlier in the course of disease than a younger person would have. This presents an opportunity for treatment at an earlier stage of illness. Unfortunately, if signs, symptoms, and disability are accepted as normal aging and go unreported, this opportunity is lost. The decreased physiological reserve of older persons also leads to an increased sensitivity to medications and an increased incidence of adverse drug effects.

Dependency and Disability

Illness in the elderly is highly associated with disability. In a study of hospital deaths in patients over the age of 65, Isaacs and colleagues (1971) noted a pattern of decreasing functional ability prior to hospital admission and long stays for those who eventually died. Increasing dependency in mobility, toileting, and cognitive functioning before the hospitalization preceded a high percentage of deaths. Others have found increased disability prior to death (Incalzi et al., 1992; Lentzner et al., 1992). Recognition of this period of premorbid dependency may enable health care providers to intervene early enough to prevent the downward spiral to death.

There is ongoing research of the patterns of disability and dependency of older persons. Is an illness associated with loss of function in a specific domain or in a specific sequence of loss of function unique to that illness? These investigations may guide future treatments of illnesses or add to our current armamentarium in avoiding disability associated with illness (Ettinger et al., 1994; Guralnik, 1994).

Comorbidity

Multiple conditions, or comorbidity, are common in the elderly (see Figure 9.2). In any individual who does not appear to be ill, the presence of an underlying disease may be unappreciated, whether the person is young or old. Older individuals are more likely (1) to have an unrecognized condition or (2) to already be receiving treatment for another condition. Health care providers must be able to distinguish between a new condition and a progression, or complication, of a known condition. Symptoms may have more than one cause. Failure to recognize or treat associated or concurrent conditions may lead to worsening health and further loss of function, resulting in dependence. The presence of multiple disease conditions may lead to an accumulation of disability that may ultimately result in a partial or total loss of independence. This accumulation of disability can occur in at least one of two ways: either disease-disease interactions or treatment-disease interactions (Besdine, 1988). Disease–disease interaction is exemplified by the woman with unrecognized diabetes mellitus, causing urinary frequency, and with moderately severe osteoarthritis, causing slow, painful ambulation. One evening while hurrying to the bathroom, she is incontinent, slips on the wet floor, falls, and fractures a hip. Treatment of the osteoarthritis might have permitted this woman to ambulate pain free and avoid the incontinent episode that led to her fall and fracture. Investigation of her urinary frequency might have uncovered her diabetes mellitus, treatment could have reduced her urinary frequency, and she could have avoided the rush to the bathroom and the resultant fracture. It may be that treatment of either one of these conditions could have avoided the fracture, but it also might have taken treatment of both (osteoarthritis and urinary frequency) to avoid the accident.

In treatment-disease interaction, the treatment of one condition may interact with a second condition, thereby multiplying problems and disabilities. For example, an elderly gentleman develops a cold and takes an over-the-counter cold preparation (antihistamine and codeine) to treat his symptoms. As a consequence of the medication, he develops acute urinary retention. The role of the drug is not recognized, and his urinary retention is attributed to his benign prostatic hypertrophy and is treated by a transurethral resection of his prostate. He has just suffered an unnecessary hospitalization and surgery with the multitude of risks associated with hospitalization and surgery in the elderly (Warshaw et al., 1982).

As can be seen by these two examples, failure to appreciate the presence of multiple disorders and their interactions, both pathological and therapeutic, can lead to disease progression, disability, and even death by either inappropriate intervention or failure to intervene.

Atypical Presentation

It is a basic tenet of geriatric medicine that many diseases present differently in than elderly than they do in the young (Hodkinson, 1973; vanWeel & Michels, 1997). Whereas older persons may present with usual and classic signs and symptoms of an illness (vanWeel & Michels, 1997), it is one of the challenges of geriatric medicine to recognize and diagnose the aged individual who presents in an atypical manner. The signs and symptoms of illness may be atypical or nonspecific for a single illness (such as a urinary tract infection presenting with confusion, falls, or anorexia), or they can be typical and classic (a urinary tract infection presenting with incontinence and dysuria).

Nonspecific manifestations of illness include any problem that is not commonly recognized as a marker of disease and that does not point to a specific etiologic pathology. The new onset of confusion, incontinence, falls, loss of appetite, weight loss, change in behavior or activity level, dizziness, or change in ability to perform usual tasks (especially activities of daily living [ADLs] and instrumental ADLs [IADLs]) are just such signs. (See Table 9.1 for ADLs and IADLs.) These herald an illness without pinpointing the responsible organ system. The health care provider must

TABLE 9.1   Examples of ADLs and IADLs

Activities of daily living
   Feeding oneself
   Maintaining continence
   Transferring oneself
   Toileting oneself
   Dressing oneself
   Bathing oneself

Instrumental Activities of Daily Living
   Using a telephone
   Doing shopping
   Preparing food and meals
   Keeping house
   Doing laundry
   Arranging transportation
   Managing medication(s)
   Managing finances

have a high index of suspicion and be thorough in searching for cause(s) of any of these nonspecific signs or symptoms. Examples of illnesses that commonly present in an atypical fashion in the elderly include pneumonia (without cough, sputum production, or fever, as commonly seen in the young), which may present with anorexia, decreased activity level, or confusion, and myocardial infarction (without chest pain), which may only be evidenced by breathlessness or decreased activity level.

Another mode of atypical presentation is that of a specific symptom complex for a particular disease in the elderly that is different from the typical presentation of a younger person. Diabetes mellitus, thyrotoxicosis, pulmonary tuberculosis, and depression all can show specific atypical presentation. For example, it is not uncommon for an elderly individual with thyrotoxicosis to present with apathetic hyperthyroidism (withdrawn, mildly confused) rather than the nervousness, weight loss, and tachycardia typical of younger individuals.

Chronicity

Although some people acquire chronic conditions prior to the age of 65, many first experience chronic disease later in life. Prior to this, most experiences are with acute illness, in other words, infection or injury. For the first time, one must cope with a chronic rather than an acute disease, and the behaviors that work in an acute illness may be maladaptive in chronic illness. For example, missing some antibiotic doses when being treated for an infection likely will not cause problems. It is not surprising then that some people have learned that there are no adverse consequences to missing medications when symptoms cease. However, this becomes a dangerous behavior with a chronic condition such as hypertension, heart failure, or lung disease.

In an acute illness, an individual can anticipate a limited duration of symptoms and dependence and a return to prior roles and function in society (Kassbaum & Baumann, 1965). The individual expects a cure and a return to home, family, and work. The chronically ill individual may have ongoing symptoms and not be able to return to the prior level of functioning or to home, family, or work. The loss of a sense of control and dependence on a medical regimen (dietary, exercise, or medication) or on another person as caretaker may be life long and may lead to loss of hope and depression.

Four out of five community-dwelling elderly have at least one chronic condition; 50 to 70% have two or more chronic conditions (Guralnick, LaCroix, & Everett, 1989; Musil et al., 1998; vanWeel, 1996). The most common chronic conditions are arthritis, hypertension, heart disease, and hearing impairment. As shown in Figure 9.3, the risk of functional disability from chronic disease increases with an increasing number of chronic conditions as well as with increasing age over 65 (Guralnick et al., 1989; National

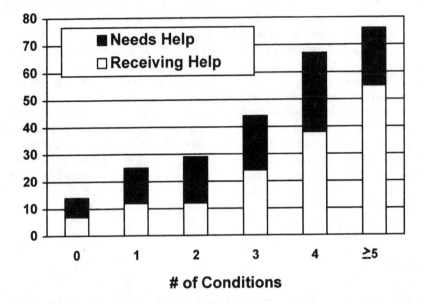

FIGURE 9.3   Prevalence of difficulty and help in ADLs in women ages 60–69 years.

(From *Aging in the eighties: The prevalence of comorbidity and its association with disability*, by J. Guralnick et al., 1989, p. 7, Hyattsville, MD: National Center for Health Statistics.)

Center for Health Statistics, 1999). It is often the accumulation of chronic conditions and their impact on function, rather than one specific diagnosis, that result in disability.

COMPREHENSIVE GERIATRIC ASSESSMENT

When cure is not possible, then stopping or slowing disease progression, relief from functional impairment, and maintenance of independence may become the focus of an older individual's health care. Comprehensive geriatric assessment (CGA) is a means of doing this. CGA has been defined as "a multidisciplinary evaluation in which the multiple problems of older persons are uncovered, described, and explained, if possible, and in which the resources and strengths of the person are catalogued, need for services assessed, and a coordinated care plan developed to focus interventions on the person's problems" (Solomon, 1988, p. 342). Elements of CGA are listed in Table 9.2. To identify impairments objectively, avoiding the biases of both examiner and older person, CGA should use well-defined test items

TABLE 9.2   Elements of Comprehensive Geriatric Assessment

Physical health
  Medical diagnoses and prognosis
  Preventive health care and education
  Patient expectation and goals
  Special issues
    Polypharmacy
    Special senses (vision, hearing)

Psychologic health
  Cognitive function
  Affective health
  Behavioral function

Social health
  Social network
  Economic status (resources and needs)

Functional health
  Activities of daily living (ADL)
  Instrumental activities of daily living (IADL)

Environmental health
  Physical barriers and safety
  Access to, and desire for, social and recreational activities

Modified from "The Clinical Effectiveness of Multidimensional Geriatric Assessment" by L. Z. Rubenstein, 1983, *Journal of the American Geriatrics Society, 31*, p. 760.

or instruments. The choice of instrument or group of instruments is beyond the scope of this chapter. Instruments are selected according to the purpose, the setting, and the person who administers the instrument (Kane & Kane, 1981; Gallo, Fulmer, Paveza, & Reichel, 2000). CGA performed well fosters interaction among disciplines, leads to interdisciplinary solutions, and provides a means to judge the success of any intervention.

When practiced in either a combined geriatric assessment and rehabilitation unit or an inpatient geriatric assessment unit, CGA has been shown to (1) improve diagnostic accuracy (Cheah & Beard, 1980; Rubenstein, Abrass, & Kane, 1981), (2) prolong survival (Rubenstein et al., 1984), (3) reduce medical care costs (Rubenstein et al., 1984), (4) reduce use of acute hospitals (Rubenstein et al., 1984), and (5) reduce nursing home use (Lefton, Bonstelle, & Frengley, 1983; Rubenstein et al., 1984). CGA has also increased health and social services use, decreased medication use, improved placement location, improved affect and cognition, and improved functional status. Which component of CGA results in these improvements remains a focus of research (Reuben, Fishman, McNebney, & Wolde-Tsadik, 1996).

An example is a frail elderly widow who has mobility-limiting arthritis, has had a 5% weight loss, is on a complicated medication regimen for organic heart disease (congestive heart failure and hypertension), and has difficulty taking her medications as instructed. Her comprehensive evaluation reveals the following (by discipline): the physician confirms the need for diuretic and antihypertensive therapy but does not find any reason for her weight loss; the physician also notes some cognitive losses. The nurse finds that the patient has poor understanding of her medications, difficulty with memory, and poor endurance but safe ambulation and good personal hygiene. The social worker finds that the woman has modest financial resources and that she has difficulty with transportation to shopping and appointments. The three team members agree that the patient should be able to manage a medication regimen of once or twice daily medication and that she will benefit from services in her apartment. Initially, services include a home health nurse to monitor medications, blood pressure control, and signs of congestive heart failure and to continue patient education; a housekeeper to do heavy housecleaning; a daily meal prepared and delivered by a community agency; and transportation to shopping and other appointments. Because she can ambulate safely within her home, maintains good personal hygiene, and states she does not want it, she is not referred for physical therapy, and a bath aide is not instituted at the time. Other services, such as senior housing and an adult day program, are discussed with the patient.

Repeated examination of one, some, or all domains of CGA provides objective data on which to judge the success of the team's treatment plan and the need for change in treatment or services. Continuing the previous case as an example, we find that this woman did well for the initial 6 months, but then her physical endurance markedly decreased to the point that she stopped leaving her apartment. Medical evaluation determined that worsening heart failure resulting from the end stages of heart disease was the cause. Medication adjustments were made, and more services were provided in the woman's apartment: a home health aide for personal hygiene because she no longer had adequate endurance for tub or shower bathing, and the housekeeper's responsibilities were increased to include grocery shopping and meal preparation. Her medical diagnostic categories remained unchanged (organic heart disease, hypertension, and osteoarthritis), yet she required changes in service because of changes in her functional abilities.

SUMMARY

Because the changes that occur with aging diminish an individual's physiological reserve, the addition of any disease that further compromises organ system function may result in significant disability and dependence for the older person. Although most older persons assess their health accurately, a large minority are optimistic regarding their health and do not recognize or report signs and symptoms of illness, nor do they report disability. Older individuals are likely to have multiple chronic diseases (conditions) that interact and may present in an atypical manner. Most often, presentation is as an acute loss or decrement in ADL or IADL function, but decline in physical, cognitive, psychological, or social capabilities is also common. Unfortunately, the loss of independence and the disability that results from insidious and chronic disease may often be attributed to aging, rather than recognized as evidence of underlying illness. CGA provides health care workers a means to recognize disease in early stages, make appropriate interventions, and judge the efficacy of treatment.

REFERENCES

Anonymous. (1991). Nutrition screening manual for professionals caring for older Americans: Nutrition screening initiative. Washington, DC: Greer Margolis Mitchell Grunwald & Associates.

Besdine, R. W. (1988). *Functional assessment.* Boston: Little, Brown.

Blazer, D. G., & Houpt, J. L. (1979). Perception of poor health in the healthy older adult. *Journal of the American Geriatrics Society, 27,* 330–334.

Brody, E., & Kleban, M. (1981). Physical and mental health symptoms of older people: Who do they tell? *Journal of the American Geriatrics Society, 29,* 442–449.

Cheah, K., & Beard, O. (1980). Psychiatric findings in the population of a geriatric evaluation unit: Implications. *Journal of the American Geriatrics Society, 28,* 153–158.

Cockerham, W., Sharp, K., et al. (1983). Aging and perceived health status. *Journal of Gerontology 38,* 349–355.

Ettinger, W. H., Fried, L. P., et al. (1994). Self-reported causes of physical disability in older people: The cardiovascular health study. *Journal of the American Geriatrics Society, 42,* 1035–1044.

Ford, A. B., Folmar, S. J., Salmon, R. B., Medalie, J. H., Roy, A. W., & Galazka, S. S. (1988). Health and function in the old and very old. *Journal of the American Geriatrics Society, 36,* 187–197.

Gallo, J. J., Fulmer, T., Paveza, G. J., & Reichel, W. (2000). *Handbook of geriatric assessment.* Gaithersburg, MD: Aspen.

Guralnik, J. M. (1994). Understanding the relationship between disease and disability. *Journal of the American Geriatrics Society, 42,* 1128–1129.

Guralnick, J., LaCroix, A., et al. (1989). *Aging in the eighties: The prevalence of comorbidity and its association with disability* (Advanced data from Vital and Health Statistics, No. 170). Hyattsville, MD: National Center for Health Statistics.

Hodkinson, H. (1973). Non-specific presentation of illness. *British Medical Journal, 4,* 94–96.

Idler, E., & Benyamini, Y. (1997). Self-rated health and mortality: A review of 27 studies. *Journal of Health and Social Behavior, 38,* 21–37.

Idler, E. L., & Angel, R. (1990). Self-rated health and mortality in the NHANES-I epidemiologic follow-up study. *American Journal of Public Health, 80* (4), 446–452.

Idler, E. L., & Kasl, S. (1991). Health perceptions and survival: Do global evaluations of health status really predict mortality? *Journal of Gerontology, 46,* S55–S65.

Incalzi, A. R., Capparella, O., Gemma, A., Porcedda, P., Raccis, G., Sommella, L., & Carbonin, P. O. (1992). A simple method of recognizing geriatric patients at risk for death and disability. *Journal of the American Geriatrics Society, 40* (1), 34–38.

Isaacs, B., Gunn, J., et al. (1971). The concept of pre-death. *Lancet, 1,* 1511–1518.

Kane, R., & Kane, R. (1981). *Assessing the elderly: A practical guide to measurement.* Lexington, MA: Lexington Books.

Kaplan, G., Barell, V., & Lusky, A. (1988). Subjective state of health and survival in elderly adults. *Journal of Gerontology, 43,* S114–S120.

Kassbaum, G., & Baumann, B. (1965). Dimensions of the sick role in chronic illness. *Journal of Health and Human Behavior, 6,* 16–27.

Lefton, E., Bonstelle, S., & Frengley, J. D. (1983). Success with an inpatient geriatric unit: A controlled study of outcome and follow-up. *Journal of the American Geriatrics Society, 31* (3), 149–155.

Lentzner, H., Pamuk, E., Rhodenhiser, E. P., Rothenberg, R., & Powell-Griner, E. (1992). The quality of life in the year before death. *American Journal of Public Health, 82* (8), 1093–1098.

Leventhal, E., & Prohaska, T. (1986). Age, symptom interpretation, and health behavior. *Journal of the American Geriatrics Society, 34,* 185–191.

Mossey, J., & Shapiro, E. (1982). Self-rated health: A predictor of mortality among the elderly. *American Journal of Public Health, 72* (8), 800–808.

Musil, C., Ahn, S., Haug, M., Warner, C., Morris, D., & Duffy, E. (1998). Health problems and health actions among community-dwelling older adults: Results of a health diary study. *Applied Nursing Research, 11* (3), 138–147.

National Center for Health Statistics. (1999). *Health, United States, 1999: Health and aging chartbook.* Washington, DC: U.S. Department of Health and Human Services.

Reuben, D. B., Fishman, L. K., McNabrey, M., & Wolde-Tsadik, G. (1996). Looking inside the black box of comprehensive geriatric assessment: A classification system for problems, recommendations, and implementation strategies. *Journal of the American Geriatrics Society, 44* (7), 835–838.

Rubenstein, L., Abrass, I., & Kane, R. L. (1981). Improved care for patients on a new geriatric evaluation unit. *Journal of the American Geriatrics Society, 29,* 531–536.

Rubenstein, L., Josephson, K., Wieland, G. D., English, P. A., Sayre, J. A., & Kane, R. L. (1984). Effectiveness of a geriatric evaluation unit. *New England Journal of Medicine, 311,* 1664–1670.

Solomon, D. (1988). National Institutes of Health Consensus Development Conference statement: Geriatric assessment methods for clinical decision-making. *Journal of the American Geriatrics, Society, 36,* 342–347.

vanWeel, C. (1996). Chronic disease in general practice: The longitudinal dimension. *European Journal of General Practice, 2,* 17–21.

vanWeel, C., & Michels, J. (1997). Dying, not old age, to blame for costs of health care. *Lancet, 350,* 1159–1160.

Warshaw, G., Moore, J., Friedman, S. W., Currie, C. T., Kennie, D. C., Kane, W. J., & Mears, P. A. (1982). Functional disability in the hospitalized elderly. *Journal of the American Medical Association, 248,* 847–850.

Williamson, J., Stokoe, I., Gray, S., Fisher, M., Smith, A., McGhee, A., & Stephenson, E. (1964). Old people at home: Their unreported needs. *Lancet, 1,* 1117–1120.

10

Pharmacological Therapy

Todd Semla

The elderly are the largest consumers of prescription and nonprescription medications in the United States. Adverse effects and other medication-related problems contribute to or are the cause for a substantial percentage of hospital admissions for the elderly. Medication therapy usually does not become simplified during a hospitalization; rather, it becomes more complex. This complexity often carries over after discharge; in other words, the patient goes home on more medications than prior to admission. Thus, the risk for a new medication-related problem is increased or the patient may cycle back into the cascade, resulting in another admission for a medication-related problem.

Health care providers must understand how the physiological changes that accompany aging and disease states can alter a patient's pharmacokinetic and pharmacodynamic response to medications, whether to adjust a medication's dose or interval for these changes, monitor for the desired effect or adverse events, or screen for drug interactions. It is the intent of this chapter to address these practice adjustments in the context of the elderly patient in the critical care or hospital setting.

PHARMACOKINETIC AND PHARMACODYNAMIC CHANGES ASSOCIATED WITH AGING

Pharmacokinetics is defined as the study of the time course of a drug and its metabolites throughout the body as it relates to absorption, distribution, metabolism, and elimination (DeVane, 1998). *Pharmacodynamics* is the study of the relationship of the time course and intensity of a drug's pharmacological effect (DeVane, 1998). Aging can affect a drug's pharmacokinetics and pharmacodynamics.

Absorption

Absorption refers to the rate and extent that a drug enters the body. Rate of absorption is expressed as k_a^{-hr} and extent of absorption is expressed as the area under the concentration versus time curve for 0 to 24 hours (AUC_{0-24}) or 0 to infinity ($ACU_{0-\infty}$). Drugs can be administered via a variety of routes, including parenteral, oral, transdermal, inhaled, rectal, and other topical routes. Bioavailability, F, refers to the fraction of drug that reaches the circulation. When a drug is given parenterally, its absorption or bioavailability is usually 100% (F = 1). Drugs given by intravenous (IV) infusion or push achieve their peak (highest) blood concentration after the end of the infusion. Exceptions are prodrugs, drugs that require metabolic conversion to their active form, such as fosphenytoin. When a drug administered intramuscularly (IM) will reach its peak concentration depends on the site of injection (muscle size, vascular supply) and the chemical properties of the drug (water or fat solubility, vehicle). When a drug is administered by mouth, its rate and extent of absorption are influenced by many factors, including whether it is taken with other medications, the volume of fluid it is taken with, the pH of the gastrointestinal (GI) tract, the product formulation (enteric coated, sustained release), its solubility, and whether it's metabolized by enzymes in the intestines or subject to first-pass metabolism by the liver (refers to a drug's extraction by the liver during its first pass through the liver via the portal circulation). The influence of these variables explains why the parenteral dose of some drugs is much smaller than when the drug is given orally (e.g., enalapril, verapamil, l-evothyroxine, propranolol, nitroglycerin). However, some drugs' bioavailability is similar when given IV or orally (F = ~1), hence the same dose is given for both routes of administration (e.g., levofloxacin). Drugs such as insulin are not bioavailable orally and must be given by an alternative route. Other drugs, alendronate for example, have such poor oral bioavailability that they must be taken in a specific way to be absorbed at all.

Changes in the GI tract that accompany aging have generally not been found to affect the absorption of drugs. In older patients, the rate of absorption may be slower, with a lower peak concentration, but the total amount (extent) absorbed is the same as for a younger person (DeVane & Pollock, 1999). How the drug is taken and other medications the person is taking are likely to affect bioavailability. Food delays gastric emptying and acts as a buffer (raising the pH). Drugs that are unstable in an acidic environment (e.g., erythromycin) may degrade less when taken with food. Conversely, drugs that require a more acidic environment for dissolution may not be as well absorbed if exposed to a higher pH during dissolution (e.g., penicillin VK). In theory, drugs that stimulate gastric emptying or GI motility may decrease the time of exposure to another drug's site of absorption or decrease its time in an environment necessary for dissolution, resulting in decreased absorption. Examples of such drugs include stimulant laxatives, erythromycin, cisapride, and metoclopramide. Drugs that delay gastric emptying or GI motility (e.g., anticholinergic drugs or opiates) may increase a drug's time in the environment needed for dissolution or time at its site of absorption, thus increasing its absorption. Drugs may also bind to nonabsorbable medications such as psyllium-containing laxatives and cholestyramine, thus reducing their absorption.

In summary, the effects of aging are usually of little consequence on drug absorption. Of greater importance are concurrent medications taken, route of administration, and habits of the elderly person taking the medicine. Insufficient information is available about the effects of aging on other routes of administration (rectal, transdermal, buccal, intranasal) to draw any firm conclusions on how drugs administered by these routes might be absorbed by older patients.

Distribution

The pharmacokinetic parameter of distribution refers to the time course and to where in the body a drug is distributed. Distribution is expressed as the volume of distribution (Vd) with units as volume (e.g., liters) or volume per weight (e.g., liters per kilogram). A drug's real distribution volume is related to body water and cannot exceed this amount. However, the Vd is not an actual volume but rather an apparent volume that relates drug concentration in the blood or plasma to the amount of drug in the body (Gibaldi & Perrier, 1982). A drug's Vd is determined by the extent of its binding to plasma proteins and tissues and its preference for distribution to water (hydrophilic) or fat (lipophilic). Drugs that are hydrophilic (aminoglycosides, lithium) tend to have a smaller volume distribution than drugs that are lipophilic have. The increase in the weight-based percentage of body fat and a decrease in lean body mass and body water that accompanies aging can affect a drug's Vd. An example of this change as it relates to a drug has been shown with ethanol. After a constant weight-based infusion of ethanol, men age 50 years and greater had a significantly greater peak blood-water ethanol concentration than men less 50 years of age had (Vestal et al., 1977). The clinical relevance of this change is that older persons will have higher blood alcohol concentrations after the same number of drinks as when they were younger and may experience greater impairment. Digoxin is an example of a drug with a very large Vd, due to extensive tissue binding, that is reduced in older patients compared with younger patients (Cusack et al., 1979). The opposite is seen with lipophilic drugs: their volume of distribution increases because of the increase in body fat. This, in part, explains why the elimination half-life of lipophilic benzodiazepines (e.g., diazepam, flurazepam) increases with aging. The larger volume of distribution, in part, prolongs the time to steady-state concentrations as well as the time it takes for the drug to be completely eliminated from the body. Similar changes have been seen for other lipophilic drugs such as thiopental, tolbutamide, trazodone, and amitriptylline.

The Vd also reflects the extent of protein binding for a drug. Albumin is the primary plasma protein to which drugs bind. Albumin has been shown to be decreased in older patients, thus a greater fraction of drug will be unbound (free) and pharmacologically active (Greenblatt, 1979). Examples of drugs that bind to albumin and whose unbound fraction has been shown to be increased in the elderly include ceftriaxone, diazepam, lorazepam, phenytoin, valproic acid, and warfarin (Vebeeck, Cardinal, & Wallace, 1984). Normally, the hepatic or renal route clears additional unbound drug; however, age-related decreases in these organ systems may result in increased unbound drug in the body. An example of how an increase in unbound drug can lead to an unnecessary and potentially harmful dosage increase is phenytoin. Table 10.1 contains information for three patients. Patient A is a young and healthy with a normal serum albumin. Patient B is older, and her albumin is also normal. Patient C is older and has a low serum albumin that was most likely due to poor nutrition and chronic disease. All three patients were taking phenytoin in the doses shown, and their seizure disorders were controlled. Based on total (bound + unbound) phenytoin concentrations, Patients A and B are within the therapeutic range (10–20 mg/L), whereas Patient C is subtherapeutic. The initial reaction of some clinicians would be to increase Patient C's dose; however, the patient's free fraction (percent unbound) is increased and her free (unbound) phenytoin concentration is within the acceptable range (1–2 mg/L). An increase in Patients C's dose could result in toxicity.

Another plasma protein that increases with aging is α1-acid glycoprotein, which binds to drugs that are lipophilic and basic (cationic). In addition, α1-acid glycoprotein is an acute phase reactant and will increase with malignancy and inflammatory conditions and after a myocardial infarction. These conditions result in a larger increase in α1-acid glycoprotein than that seen with aging. Drugs that bind to α1-acid glycoprotein include lidocaine, propranolol, salicylic acid, quinidine, erythromycin, amitriptyline, imipra-

TABLE 10.1   Effect of Albumin on Total and Unbound Phenytoin Concentrations

Patient	Daily phenytoin dose (mg/day)	Total phenytoin conc. (mg/L)	Serum albumin (gm/dL)	Unbound phenytoin conc. (mg/L)	Percent unbound
A	300	15	4.2	1.5	10
B	250	12.6	3.3	1.6	12.7
C	200	7.8	2.8	1.0	12.8

mine, and desipramine (Abernethy, Greenblatt, & Shader, 1985; Abernethy & Kerzner, 1984; Nation, Trigg, & Selig, 1977; Vebeeck et al., 1984).

To summarize, drug distribution may be altered as a result of age-related changes in body composition, blood flow, or plasma protein concentrations. Disease, other drugs, and nutrition may augment these changes.

Metabolism

Metabolism is the third pharmacokinetic parameter. In general, the purpose of metabolism is to convert lipophilic drugs into water-soluble compounds that can be eliminated renally. The liver is the most common site of drug metabolism, but metabolic conversion can also take place in the intestinal wall, lungs, skin, and other organ systems. Aging affects the liver by decreasing liver blood flow as well as decreasing liver size and mass (Woodhouse & Wynne, 1988; Wynne et al., 1989). Consequently, the metabolic clearance of drugs by the liver can be reduced. This is the case for drugs that are subject to the Phase I pathways such as hydroxylation, oxidation, dealkylation, and reduction. Most drugs that go through these pathways are converted to active metabolites (of lesser, equal, or greater pharmacological effect than the parent compound). Examples are shown in Table 10.2. Drugs that go through the Phase II pathways are converted to inactive compounds through glucuronidation, conjugation, or acetylation. Medications subject to Phase II metabolism are generally preferred for

TABLE 10.2 Examples of Drugs That Undergo Phase I or Phase II Metabolism

Phase I
Alprazolam, diazepam, chlordiazepoxide, flurazepam, midazolam, clonazepam
Desipramine, nortriptyline, imipramine, amitriptyline, trazodone, nefazodone
Selective serotonin reuptake inhibitors (SSRIs)
Phenytoin, carbamazepine, valproate, phenobarbital
Theophylline
Most nonsteroidal anti-inflammatory drugs (NSAIDs)
Lidocaine, quinidine, metoprolol, propranolol
Verapamil, diltiazem, nifedipine, other calcium channel blockers
Warfarin
Cisapride

Phase II
Lorazepam, oxazepam
Morphine, acetaminophen, aspirin
Valproate, phenobarbital
Labetolol

older patients because their metabolites are not active and will not accumulate (Table 10.2).

The exception to this rule may be the frail elderly. Limited pharmacokinetic investigation has included the frail elderly. Wynne and colleagues (1993) studied metoclopramide's pharmacokinetics in young subjects, fit older subjects, and frail older subjects. Neither liver volume nor bioavailability was different among the three groups. Metoclopramide is metabolized via conjugation pathways (Phase II). Clearance did not differ significantly between the young and the fit elderly but was significantly reduced in the frail elderly compared with the young subjects. These results suggest that in frail elderly patients, drug clearance by conjugation pathways may be reduced (Wynne et al., 1993). Differences have been reported between the genders; for example, elderly men metabolize oxazepam faster than elderly women do.

A drug's metabolism can be altered by other conditions besides age. For example, hepatic congestion due to heart failure will decrease the metabolism of warfarin, resulting in an increased pharmacological response. Smoking stimulates monooxygenase enzymes and increases the clearance of theophylline even in older patients (Cusack, Kelly, Lavan, Noel, & O'Malley, 1980). Hence, nonaging influences can exaggerate or override the effects of aging.

The metabolic clearance of drugs by the elderly is an excellent example of the heterogeneity of the elderly. In general, accounting for smoking status as well as concurrent disease and drug therapy are probably more reliable guides for dosing.

Elimination

Elimination or excretion refers to a drug's final route(s) of exit from the body. For most drugs this involves elimination by the kidney as either the parent compound or a metabolite(s). Terms used to express elimination are half-life and clearance. A drug's half-life is the time it takes for its plasma or serum concentration to decline by 50%, for example, from 20 mg/L to 10 mg/L. Half-life is usually expressed in hours. It takes five half-lives for a drug to reach 95% of steady-state in the body. Steady-state means that the amount of drug entering the system circulation is equal to the amount being eliminated. Clearance is usually expressed as volume per unit of time (e.g., liter per hour or milliliter per minute) and represents the volume of plasma or serum from which the drug is removed (i.e., cleared) per unit of time. Clearance rates may also be expressed as volume per weight per unit of time (liter per kilogram per hour).

The effects of aging on renal function have been studied to a greater extent than they have for hepatic function. Age-related decline in glomerular filtration is attributed to changes in kidney size, renal blood flow, and a decrease in functioning nephrons. In the Baltimore Longitudinal Study on Aging, individuals renal function began to decline when they were in their mid-30s, with an average decline of 6 to 12 mL/min per 1.73 m² per decade (Rowe, Andres, Tobin, Norris, & Shock, 1976). It must be emphasized that this is an average rate of decline. Subsequent follow-up studies in men followed over 10 to 15 years found three normally distributed groups: one whose creatinine clearance declined to the extent that it was clinically significant, a second group whose creatinine clearance declined but was not considered clinically significant; and a third group whose creatinine clearance did not change (Lindeman, Tobin, & Shock, 1985).

An elderly patient's serum creatinine is not an accurate reflection of creatinine clearance. Because of the age-related decline in lean muscle mass, the production of creatinine (by-products of muscle breakdown) is reduced. The decrease in glomerular filtration counterbalances the decreased production of creatinine (less is filtered); thus, serum creatinine stays within the normal range, suggesting no change in creatinine clearance.

When treating an elderly patient, the conservative approach is to dose medications that are renally eliminated as if the patient's renal function had declined with aging. Measuring a patient's 24-hour creatinine clearance would be the most accurate way to determine the dose, but this is time consuming and requires an accurate 24-hour urine collection. An 8-hour collection time has been shown to be accurate but has not been widely accepted to date (O'Connell, Wong, Bannick-Mohrland, & Dwinell, 1993). To estimate a patient's creatinine clearance initially, the clinician can use the equation developed by Cockroft and Gault (1976):[*]

$$\text{Estimated creatinine clearance} =$$

$$\frac{(140 - \text{age}) \times (\text{weight, kg})}{72 \times (\text{serum creatinine, mg/dL})} \times 0.85 \text{ for women}$$

Although the preceding equation is useful and widely applied, there are limitations to consider. First, as mentioned earlier, not all patients experience a significant age-related decline in renal function, and the creatinine clearance estimated by the equation would be an underestimate. Second, the creatinine clearance of patients whose muscle mass is reduced beyond that of normal aging will be overestimated. For example, an 82-year-old nursing home patient who has not been ambulatory for 2 years, weighs 45 kg, and has a serum creatinine of 0.4 mg/dL would be estimated to have a creatinine clearance of 90 mL/min. In these cases it has been advocated that a normal creatinine value, 1 mg/dL, be substituted for the low serum creatinine; thus, the patient's creatinine clearance would be estimated to

---

Note: If the patient's actual body weight is more than 20% of his or her ideal body weight (IBW), then the IBW should be substituted in the equation. $IBW_{(men)} = 50 \text{ kg} + (2.3 \text{ kg})(\text{each inch} > 5 \text{ feet})$, $IBW_{(women)} = 45 \text{ kg} + (2.3 \text{ kg})(\text{each inch} > 5 \text{ feet})$.

be 36 mg/dL. Normalizing the serum creatinine to 1 mg/dL has not been shown to be a very precise estimate because it generally underestimates the actual creatinine clearance (Smythe, Hoffman, Kizy, & Dmuchowski, 1994).

In cases in which estimates of the patient's renal function are in question, consider the following: (1) avoid drugs that are entirely dependent on renal elimination and would accumulate, resulting in toxicity (e.g., imipenem, ceftriaxone); (2) if the use of such an agent cannot be avoided, then an accurate measure of renal function should be obtained (e.g., a 24-hour creatinine clearance); and (3) if available, serum or plasma concentrations of the drug and important metabolites should be monitored (e.g., aminoglycosides).

The tendency is for renal function to decline with age; however, the rate of decline is not uniform. Doses of drugs eliminated by the kidney should be based initially on the patient's estimated creatinine clearance and not solely on the patient's serum creatinine. Medications that are renally eliminated and may require a dose adjustment in the elderly are provided in Table 10.3.

PHARMACODYNAMICS

Pharmacodynamic changes can arise because of or independent of changes in pharmacokinetics. When accompanied by changes in pharmacokinetics,

TABLE 10.3   Renally Eliminated Medications That May Require a Dosage Adjustment in Elderly Patients

Aminoglycosides
Penicillins
Most cephalosporins
Most quinolones
Cotrimoxazole
Imipenim
Vancomycin
Acyclovir, famcyclovir
Amantidine, rimantidine
Fluconazole
Allopurinol
Atenolol, nadolol, soltalol
Codeine, morphine, tramadol, ketorolac
Digoxin
Angiotensin converting enzyme Inhibitors (captopril, lisinopril)
Verapamil
Lithium
Venlafaxine
H_2 antagonists (ranitidine, cimetidine, nizatidine)
Gabapentin

pharmacodynamic changes generally result from increased plasma or blood concentrations. These changes present as an exaggerated response, therapeutic or toxic, to the usual dose of the medication. If a medication is known to have pharmacokinetic changes, then a change in pharmacodynamic response can be anticipated. What cannot always be anticipated are pharmacodynamic changes in the absence of pharmacokinetic changes.

An excellent example of pharmacodynamic changes in older persons has been demonstrated with the benzodiazepines. Greenblatt et al. (1991) found elderly subjects to have a greater degree of sedation and reduced performance on the digit symbol substitution test (a psychomotor test) after a single dose of triazolam compared with younger subjects. These pharmacodynamic changes were attributed to significantly higher plasma triazolam concentrations because of reduced clearance in elderly subjects. Castleden, George, Marcer, and Hallett (1977) found no difference in nitrazepam's (an intermediate-acting benzodiazepine similar to lorazepam) pharmacokinetics between young and older subjects after a single 10-mg dose. Twelve and 36 hours after their dose, elderly subjects made significantly more mistakes on a psychomotor test when compared with their performance after taking placebo. Younger subjects did not demonstrate significant impairment at either time. The authors concluded that the elderly have an increased sensitivity to nitrazepam in the absence of pharmacokinetic changes. These results offer some insight into drug-related problems experienced by older patients taking benzodiazepines. Even with acute use, both young and elderly patients may experience impaired balance and posture following a single dose of a benzodiazepine (Fisch, Baktir, Karlaganis, Minder, & Bircher, 1990; Jansen, Wachowiak-Andersen, Munster-Swendersen, Eng, & Valentin, 1985).

Morphine has been found to cause pharmacokinetic changes associated with aging, but it is uncertain whether these changes account for the increased level and prolonged duration of pain relief seen in elderly patients. In the elderly, morphine has been shown to have smaller Vd, higher plasma morphine concentrations after infusion, and reduced clearance when compared with younger adults (Berkowitz, Ngai, Yang, Hempstead, & Spector, 1975; Kaiko, Wallenstein, Rogers, Grabinski, & Houde, 1982; Owen, Sitar, Berger, Brownell, Duke, & Mitenko, 1983). Pharmacodynamically, the elderly achieve pain relief at least equivalent to that of younger patients with half the IM dose and have an increased duration of pain relief (Kaiko, 1980). Thus, the initial dose or frequency of morphine, or both, given IM or by IV infusion should be less in older patients until their exact response is known.

Pharmacodynamic and pharmacokinetic changes, alone or together, signify an increased sensitivity to medications by the elderly. A reduction in dose, longer intervals between doses, and longer periods between changes in dose are ways to successfully initiate and maintain drug therapy in the elderly and may decrease the chances of medication intolerance or toxicity.

Disease- and drug-specific monitoring are also necessary to ensure a success-ful outcome.

DRUG INTERACTIONS

Drug interactions can result in toxicity to one or more drugs or a negative health outcome because of the one drug inactivating or interfering with the therapeutic actions of another drug. An example of the former is a patient stable on digoxin who develops digoxin toxicity after being started on verapamil. One drug can interfere with the actions of another drug by decreasing its bioavailability with physical binding (adsorption), for example, antacids and ciprofloxacin, or cholestyramine and digoxin. Drug interactions can also cause harm when two drugs have duplicative pharma-cological effects. For example, a patient could develop hyperkalemia when an angiotensin-converting enzyme is added to a regimen that includes a potassium supplement or potassium-sparing diuretic. Clinicians must be familiar with the pharmacological effects, both therapeutic and adverse, of all drugs their patients are taking in order to prevent drug interactions.

The risk for drug-drug interactions increases as the number of medica-tions increase. Cardiovascular and psychotropic drugs are most frequently involved in drug-drug interactions. A positive relationship exists between the number of potential drug-drug interactions and the number of side effects experienced by hospitalized older patients (Doucet et al., 1996). The most common side effects are neuropsychological (primarily confusion) or cognitive impairment, arterial hypotension, and acute renal failure due to hypotension (Doucet et al., 1996). Factors associated with drug-drug interactions include the use of multiple medications, more than one pre-scriber, and more than one pharmacy (Tambylyn, McLeod, Abrahamo-wicz, & Laprise, 1996).

Recently, staying abreast with drug interactions has become more of a challenge because of our increased capability to determine which cyto-chrome P450 isozymes (CYP) are involved in a drug's metabolism. A drug can be a substrate, inhibitor, or inducer of one or more isozymes. Some drugs are a substrate for and an inhibitor or inducer of the same isozyme. Seven different (subfamilies) isozymes are involved in human drug metabo-lism: CYP1A2, 2A6, 2C, 2D6, 2E1, and 3A3/4. Cytochrome 3A3/4 and 2D6 are responsible for the metabolism of more than 50% and 25% of drug in current use, respectively (DeVane & Pollock, 1999). These isozymes are found throughout the body, with the largest concentrations being located in the liver. Cytochrome 3A4, located in cells in the lumen of the GI tract, play an important role in drug bioavailability. Thus drugs that are substrates for CYP3A4 can be metabolized before they have a chance to complete the absorption process, in other words, their bioavailability is reduced. If a patient takes one drug that inhibits the isozyme, then the bioavailability of another drug that is a CYP3A4 substrate may be increased. This has been demonstrated with cyclosporine (substrate) and erythromycin (inhibitor). Conversely, isozyme inducers can decrease the absorption of a substrate by increasing its metabolism. These interactions take place not only in the intestines but also in the liver. Therefore, the substrate's clearance can be either increased or decreased.

The effect of aging on the cytochrome P450 system has not been completely determined. Cross-sectional data have shown that cytochrome 450 content declines incrementally, once in the fourth decade and again after the age of 70 years (Sontaniemi, Arranto, Pelkonen, & Pasanen, 1997). In vitro microsomal activity of cytochrome 3A4 is not altered by aging, but in vivo age- and gender-related reductions in drug clearance have been found for CYP3A4 substrates erythromycin, prednisolone, verapamil, alprazolam, nifedipine, and diazepam (Schmucker et al., 1990; DeVane & Pollock, 1999). CYP3A4 accounts for 30% of the cytochrome P450 content in the liver and is also prominent in the intestinal tract. This isozyme can be induced by drugs, such as rifampin, phenytoin, and carbamazepine, and inhibited by many drugs, including the macrolide antibiotics, nefazodone, itraconazole, and ketoconazole, and by grapefruit juice (Sontaniemi et al., 1997; DeVane & Pollock, 1999).

The isozyme 2D6 has been associated with minimal age-related changes (DeVane & Pollock, 1999). CYP2D6 is involved in the metabolism of many psychotropic drugs and can be inhibited by many agents. At least 7% of Caucasians are deficient in this isozyme and have reduced clearance and increased risk of toxicity to 2D6 substrates (de Leon, Barnhill, Rogers, Boyle, Chou, & Wedlund, 1998). Clinically, these patients and those taking 2D6 inhibitors (e.g., quinidine, paroxetine, fluoxetine) will not be able to convert codeine and tramadol to their active metabolite and have a reduced analgesic response (Tseng, Wang, Lai, Lai, & Huang, 1996; Poulsen, Arendt-Nielsen, Brosen, & Sindrup, 1996).

Drug-Disease Interactions

Drug-disease interactions can also affect drug response. Obesity and ascites will increase the volume of distributions of lipophilic and hydrophilic drugs, respectively. Patients with dementia may have increased sensitivity or paradoxical reactions to drugs with central nervous system (CNS) or anticholinergic activity. Renal insufficiency or impaired hepatic function because of cirrhosis or hepatic congestion can impair the clearance of drugs reliant on one of these pathways.

Adverse Drug Events

An adverse drug event (ADE) is an injury from a medication. Adverse drug reactions (ADRs) are a type of ADE. ADRs are estimated to be involved in

TABLE 10.4   Major Drug Classes and the Effects of Aging on Their Use in Older Patients

Class	Effect
Aminoglycosides	Aminoglycoside (e.g., gentamicin, amikacin, tobramycin) doses and dosing interval must be adjusted for renal function. Serum concentrations and serum creatinine must be monitored to reduce the risk of nephrotoxicity and ototoxicity and to make dose adjustments. Peak serum concentrations should be drawn 30 minutes after the end of a 30-minute infusion. Trough serum concentrations should be drawn 30 minutes before the next dose.
Angiotensin-converting enzyme (ACE) inhibitors	Exaggerated hypotensive response has occurred in older patients who have decreased renal function, are receiving concurrent diuretics, or who are volume depleted. As a class, the ACE inhibitors are well-tolerated with little or no impairment of cognitive function. The dose should be titrated to the highest level tolerated based on the indication.
Antidepressants	Selective serotonin reuptake inhibitors (SSRIs) have become the agents of choice because of a more favorable side-effect profile. Some pharmacokinetic changes have been found in the elderly (e.g., paroxetine), and lower doses and slower titration is recommended. The tricyclic antidepressants (e.g., amitriptyline) are associated with cardiovascular and anticholinergic side effects and sedation. They undergo Phase I metabolism and generally have reduced plasma clearance and prolonged half-lives in the elderly. Nortriptyline and desipramine are the preferred tricyclics for the elderly. Limited pharmacokinetic information is available about the newer antidepressants. Prolonged half-lives have been reported for nefazodone, mirtazepine, and bupropion. Venlafaxine is partially renally eliminated, and its dose should be adjusted based on the patient's creatinine clearance.
Anticonvulsants	Phenytoin, phenobarbital, and carbamazepine undergo Phase I metabolism; therefore, lower doses should be used and adjusted based on serum drug concentration and effect. Valproic acid (valproate) undergoes Phase II conjugation, and one study found decreased plasma clearance in the elderly. Carbamazepine, phenytoin, and valproic acid are highly protein bound, and the elderly may have greater unbound concentrations. Gabapentin and topiramate are renally eliminated, thus dose adjustments based on the patient's creatinine clearance are recommended. The anticonvulsants as a class are prone to drug-drug interactions because of metabolic pathways or protein binding.

TABLE 10.4   *(continued)*

Class	Effect
Antipsychotics	Increased sensitivity to antipsychotics by the elderly is well-documented. The newer "atypical" antipsychotics clozapine, risperidone, olanzapine, and quietiapine undergo extensive hepatic metabolism, and prolonged half-lives have been reported for olanzapine, quietiapine, and risperidone.
Barbiturates (excluding phenobarbital)	It is best to avoid these as hypnotics in older patients. Larger Vd, prolonged half-lives, and duration of action result in daytime sedation. Tolerance to the hypnotic effect of barbiturates develops with daily use; they are highly addictive.
Benzodiazepines	Long-acting (e.g., diazepam) and intermediate-acting (e.g., alprazolam) benzodiazepines undergo Phase I metabolism and have decreased clearance and longer half-lives, with or without changes in Vd. Active metabolites significantly prolong their duration of action and accumulate with frequent dosing. They have been associated with falls, fractures, and impaired driving in the elderly. It is best to use shorter-acting agents (e.g., lorazepam or midazolam), which are less likely to accumulate or have clinically significant pharmacokinetic changes.
Calcium channel blockers	As a class, the calcium channel blockers undergo first pass metabolism after oral administration. First pass metabolism is reduced in the elderly. The atrioventricular conduction delay secondary to diltiazem and verapamil is less in elderly patients than it is in younger patients. The decrease in blood pressure due to peripheral vasodilatation is greater in the elderly because of the absence or reduced reflex increase in heart rate.
Furosemide	Potent loop diuretics (furosemide) can cause severe sodium loss and increased blood urea nitrogen, resulting in mental status changes. Monitor electrolytes carefully. Furosemide's peak effect following infusion can be delayed or reduced in the elderly.
Heparin	Expect a "usual" response to a loading dose and maintenance infusion for the first 24–48 hours, then an exaggerated response may occur in older patients. Older women are more likely to have bleeding complications. Osteoporosis is associated with use of greater than 3 months' duration or a total daily dose greater than 30,000 units.
Insulin	Patients with impaired renal function should initially receive lower doses. Assess each patient's ability to accurately draw up a dose and administer injections. Educate patients on the signs and symptoms of hypoglycemia and hyperglycemia.

(continued)

TABLE 10.4   *(continued)*

Class	Effect
Nonsteroidal anti-inflammatory drugs (NSAIDs)	Older patients taking NSAIDs are at increased risk for GI ulcers or bleeding. The COX-2 (cyclooxygenase-2 enzyme) inhibitors (celecoxib and rofecoxib) are associated with less risk for bleeding and ulcers. Use NSAIDs with caution in patients with impaired renal or liver function, congestive heart failure, or hypertension. Indomethacin is more likely to cause central nervous system side effects such as headache.
Oral hypoglycemic agents	Patients are at risk for hypoglycemia if meals are skipped or reduced or if these agents taken with other agents that reduce blood glucose (insulin, metformin). Doses should be held if the patient is taking nothing by mouth. Chlorpropamide should be avoided in the elderly because it is primarily eliminated by the kidneys. Metformin should not be started in patients 80 years of age or older and is contraindicated in patients with renal disease or renal dysfunction because of the risk of lactic acidosis. Patients should be educated on the signs and symptoms of hypoglycemia and hyperglycemia.
Warfarin	As a rule, older patients require lower doses to achieve therapeutic anticoagulation. The risk of bleeding complications decreases with the duration of therapy. It is preferable to initiate treatment with the expected maintenance dose or 5 mg/d rather than a 10-mg "loading" dose for 2 or 3 days. Many drugs can increase or decrease warfarin's anticoagulant effect. Adjust dose and monitor with the International Normalization Ratio (INR).

up to 17% of hospitalizations of older patients (Beard, 1992). In the nursing home, it is estimated that for every $1.00 spent on medications, $1.33 of health care resources is consumed in the treatment of drug-related morbidity and mortality (Bootman, Harrison, & Cox, 1997).

Medications used with the greatest frequency by older patients (e.g., diuretics, digoxin) or that have a narrow margin of safety (e.g., antiparkinson agents) are most often involved in ADEs. Cardiovascular, CNS, and musculoskeletal medications are most commonly involved in ADEs. The majority of ADEs experienced by older patients are considered predictable.

ADEs in older patients can be prevented by reviewing selected patient characteristics and a systematic review of their medications. Lists of potentially inappropriate medications and medication-disease pairs have been published (Beers, 1997; McLeod, Huang, Tamblyn, & Gayton, 1997).

In addition to medications, patients at risk for ADEs have six or more concurrent chronic diagnoses, 12 or more doses of medications per day, 9 or more medications, a prior ADR, low body weight or body mass index, age greater than 85 years, and an estimated CrCl greater than 50 mL/min (Fouts, Hanlon, Pieper, Perfetto, & Feinberg, 1997).

A common pathway for ADEs and polypharmacy has been described as the "prescribing cascade." A cascade can result when a medication results in an ADE that is mistaken for a separate diagnosis and treated with more medications, increasing the patient's risk for additional ADEs and more medications. Examples that have been studied include metoclopramide-induced parkinsonism and the prescribing of antiparkinson medications and patients treated with anticholinergic agents that result in constipation and the use of laxatives (Rochon & Gurwitz, 1995). Another cascade is the prescribing of a benzodiazepine in a person with other risk factors for falls. The addition of the benzodiazepine may be what tips the scale for a fall and resulting fracture.

SUMMARY

Medications are a reliable and economic way to treat acute and manage chronic conditions in the older adult. Age- and disease-related changes in physiology can affect how medications are absorbed, distributed, and cleared from the body. Disregard for these changes and an increased sensitivity to medications places older patients at risk for adverse drug events. Table 10.4 provides comments and precautions about the use of selected classes of medications not addressed in the text.

REFERENCES

Abernethy, D. R., & Kerzner, L. (1984). Age effects on alpha-1-acid glycoprotein concentration and imipramine plasma protein binding. *Journal of the American Geriatrics Society, 32,* 705–708.

Abernethy, D. R., Greenblatt, D. J., & Shader, R. I. (1985). Imipramine and desipramine disposition in the elderly. *Journal of Pharmacology and Experimental Therapeutics, 232,* 183–188.

Beard, K. (1992). Adverse reactions as a cause of hospital admission in the aged. *Drugs & Aging, 2,* 356–367.

Beers, M. H. (1997). Explicit criteria for determining potentially inappropriate medication use by the elderly: An update. *Archives of Internal Medicine, 157,* 1531–1536.

Berkowitz, B. A., Ngai, S. H., Yang, J. C., Hempstead, B. S., & Spector, S. (1975). The disposition of morphine in surgical patients. *Clinical Pharmacology and Therapeutics, 17,* 629–635.

Bootman, J. L., Harrison, D. L., & Cox, E. (1997). The health care cost of drug-related morbidity and mortality in nursing facilities. *Archives of Internal Medicine, 157,* 2089–2096.

Castleden, C. M., George, C. F., Marcer, D., & Hallett, C. (1977). Increased sensitivity to nitrazepam in old age. *British Medical Journal, 1,* 10–12.

Cockroft, D. W., & Gault, M. H. (1976). Prediction of creatinine clearance from serum creatinine. *Nephron, 16,* 31–41.

Cusak, B., Kelly, J., O'Malley, K., Noel, J., Lavan, J., & Horgan, J. (1979). Digoxin in the elderly: Pharmacokinetic consequences of old age. *Clinical Pharmacology and Therapeutics, 23,* 772–776.

Cusak, B., Kelly, J. G., Lavan, J., Noel, J., & O'Malley, K. (1980). Theophylline kinetics in relation to age: The importance of smoking. *British Journal of Clinical Pharmacology, 10,* 109–114.

de Leon, J., Barnhill, J., Rogers, T., Boyle, J., Chou, W-H., & Wedlund, P. J. (1998). Pilot study of the cytochrome P450-2D6 genotype in a psychiatric state hospital. *American Journal of Psychiatry, 155,* 1278–1280.

DeVane, C. L. (1998). Principles of pharmacokinetics and pharmacodynamics. In A. F. Schatzberg & C. G. Nemeroff (Eds.), *Textbook of psychopharmacology* (2nd ed., pp. 155–169). Washington, DC: American Psychiatric Press.

DeVane, C. L., & Pollock, B. G. (1999). Pharmacokinetic considerations of antidepressant use in the elderly. *Journal of Clinical Psychiatry, 60* (suppl. 20), 38–44.

Doucet, J., Chassagne, P., Trivalle, C., Landrin, I., Pauty, M. D., Kadri, N., Menard, J. F., & Bercoff, E. (1996). Drug-drug interactions related to hospital admissions in older adults: A prospective study of 1000 patients. *Journal of the American Geriatrics Society, 44,* 944–948.

Fisch, H. U., Baktir, G., Karlaganis, G., Minder, C., & Bircher, J. (1990). Excessive motor impairment two hours after triazolam in the elderly. *European Journal of Clinical Pharmacology, 38,* 229–232.

Fouts, M. M., Hanlon, J. T., Pieper, C. F., Perfetto, E. M., & Feinberg, J. L. (1997). Identification of elderly nursing facility residents at high risk for drug-related problems. *Consultant Pharmacist, 12,* 1103–1111.

Gibaldi, M., & Perrier, D. (1982). *Pharmacokinetics* (2nd ed., pp. 199–218). New York: Marcel Dekker, Inc.

Greenblatt, D. J. (1979). Reduced serum albumin concentration in the elderly: A report from the Boston Collaborative Drug Surveillance Program. *Journal of the American Geriatrics Society, 27,* 20–22.

Greenblatt, D. J., Harmatz, J. S., Shapiro, L., Englehardt, N., Gouthro, T. A., & Shader, R. I. (1991). Sensitivity to triazolam in the elderly. *New England Journal of Medicine, 324,* 1691–1698.

Jansen, E. C., Wachowiak-Andersen, G., Munster-Swendersen, J., Eng, M., & Valentin, N. (1985). *Anesthesiology, 63,* 557–559.

Kaiko, R. F. (1980). Age and morphine analgesia in cancer patients with postoperative pain. *Clinical Pharmacology and Therapeutics, 28,* 823–826.

Kaiko, R. F., Wallenstein, S. L., Rogers, A. D., Grabinski, P. Y., & Houde, R. W. (1982). Narcotics in the elderly. *Medical Clinics of North America, 66,* 1079–1089.

Lindeman, R. D., Tobin, J., & Shock, N. W. (1985). Longitudinal studies on the rate of decline in renal function with age. *Journal of the American Geriatrics Society, 33,* 278–285.

McLeod, P. J., Huang, A. R., Tamblyn, R. M., & Gayton D. C. (1997). Defining inappropriate practices in prescribing for elderly people: A national consensus panel. *Canadian Journal of Medicine, 156,* 385–391.

Nation, R. L., Triggs, E. J., & Selig, M. (1977). Lignocaine kinetics in cardiac patients and aged subjects. *British Journal of Clinical Pharmacology, 4,* 439–448.

O'Connell, M. B., Wong, M. O., Bannick-Mohrland, S. D., & Dwinell, A. M. (1993). Accuracy of 2- and 8-hour urine collection for measuring creatinine clearance in the hospitalized elderly. *Pharmacotherapy, 13,* 135–142.

Owen, J. A., Sitar, D. S., Berger, L., Brownell, L., Duke, P. C., & Mitenko, P. A. (1983). Age-related morphine kinetics. *Clinical Pharmacology and Therapeutics, 34,* 364–368.

Poulsen, L., Arendt-Nielsen, L., Brosen, K., & Sindrup, S. H. (1996). The hypoanalgesic effect of tramadol in relation to CYP2D6. *Clinical Pharmacology and Therapeutics, 60,* 636–644.

Rochon, P. A., & Gurwitz, J. H. (1995). Drug therapy. *Lancet, 346,* 32–36.

Rowe, J. W., Andres, R., Tobin, J. D., Norris, A. H., & Shock, N. W. (1976). The effect of age on creatinine clearance in men: A cross-sectional and longitudinal study. *Journal of Gerontology, 31,* 155–163.

Schmucker, D. L., Woodhouse, K. W., Wang, R. K., Wynne, H., James, O. F., McManus, M., & Kremers, P. (1990). Effects of age and gender on in vitro properties of human liver microsomal monooxygenases. *Clinical Pharmacology and Therapeutics, 48,* 365–374.

Smythe, M., Hoffman, J., Kizy, K., & Dmuchowski, C. (1994). Estimating creatinine clearance in elderly patients with low serum creatinine concentrations. *American Journal of Hospital Pharmacists, 51,* 198–204.

Sotaniemi, E. A., Arranto, A. J., Pelkonen, O., & Pasanen, M. (1997). Age and cytochrome 450-linked drug metabolism in humans: An analysis of 226 subjects with equal histopathologic conditions. *Clinical Pharmacology and Therapeutics, 61,* 331–339.

Tamblyn, R. M., McLeod, P. J., Abrahamowicz, M., & Laprise, R. (1996). Do too many cooks spoil the broth? Multiple physician involvement in medical management of elderly patients and potentially inappropriate drug combinations. *Canadian Medical Association Journal, 154,* 1177–1184.

Tseng, C-Y., Wang, S-L., Lai, M-D., Lai, M-L., & Huang, J-D. (1996). Formation of morphine from codeine in Chinese subjects of different CYP2D6 genotypes. *Clinical Pharmacology and Therapeutics, 60,* 177–182.

Vebeeck, R. K., Cardinal, J. A., & Wallace, S. M. (1984). Effect of age and sex on plasma binding of acidic and basic drugs. *European Journal of Clinical Pharmacology, 27,* 91–97.

Vestal, R. E., McGuire, E. A., Tobin J. D., Andres, R., Norris, A. H., & Mezey, E. (1977). Aging and ethanol metabolism. *Clinical Pharmacology & Therapeutics, 21,* 343–354.

Woodhouse, K. W., & Wynne, H. A. (1988). Age-related changes in liver size and hepatic blood flow: The influence on drug metabolism in the elderly. *Clinical Pharmacokinetics, 15,* 287–294.

Wynne, H. A., Cope, L. H., Mutch, E., Rawlins, M. D., Woodhouse, K. W., & James, O. F. (1989). The effect of age upon liver volume and apparent liver blood flow in healthy man. *Hepatology, 9,* 297–301.

Wynne, H. A., Yelland, C., Cope, L. H., Boddy, A., Woodhouse, K. W., & Bateman, D. N. (1993). The association of age and frailty with the pharmacokinetics and pharmacodynamics of metoclopramide. *Age and Aging, 22,* 354–359.

11

Patient Education

Margret S. Wolf

Patient education is an integral part of nursing practice. In 1975, the American Nurses Association (ANA) published the *Professional Nurse and Health Education* outlining nurses' responsibilities in patient education. The document stated that "The responsibility and accountability (of every professional nurse) includes teaching the patient and family relevant facts about specific health care needs and supporting modification of behavior." (American Nurses Association [ANA], 1975, p. 5). The document specifically identified the following responsibility: "Assessing patients' knowledge about his illness, rehabilitation, and health maintenance . . . including diagnostic preparation and procedures, preoperative and postoperative care, treatment and drugs, and discharge planning and follow-up" (ANA, 1975, p. 5).

In its 1981 *Accreditation Manual for Hospitals,* the Joint Commission for the Accreditation of Hospital Organizations (JCAHO) mandated the following accreditation requirements for hospital-based patient education:

> The following information shall be documented in each patient's medical record . . . patient disposition and any pertinent instructions given to the patient and/or family for follow up care. (Joint Commission for the Accreditation of Hospital Organizations [JCAHO], 1981, p. 68)

> Patient education and patient/family knowledge of self-care shall be given special consideration in the nursing plan. The instructions and counseling . . . must be documented and reflect current standards of nursing practice. The plans shall include . . . patient/family education. (JCAHO, pp. 118, 119)

Although nursing as a profession is committed to health teaching in all settings and to all patients across the life span, there are many issues and challenges confronting the implementation of patient education, especially with the older adult. In an atmosphere of cost containment, staff shortages, and increasing numbers of elderly patients in critical care settings, nurses need the knowledge, strategies, organizational support, and commitment for the provision of health education to patients and their families.

ISSUES RELATED TO EDUCATING THE OLDER PATIENT

As identified by the ANA and JCAHO, patient education is directed toward increasing patients' knowledge about their condition, treatment, and prevention. The goal of patient education for older patients is to increase their ability to make decisions about their health and health care, to cope with specific illnesses, and to improve their health-related behaviors (Falvo, 1994).

Many issues influence effective patient education. The health professional who thinks that patient education is just the transmission of factual information will find that the health care outcomes are not as anticipated. The problems all patients, especially the elderly, have with recall and retention of information during times of stress has been well-documented (Grahn & Johnson, 1990; Robinson, 1992). The emotional turmoil elderly patients endure in critical care settings can impair their ability to retain complex treatment-related information. In repeated studies, patients who were presented with information by physicians or nurses were unable to recall the essential points of the health teaching (Hayes, 1999; McDougall, 1999; Ryan, 1999).

In addition to the issue of retention and recall under stress, the learning needs of patients change as their illness progresses (Brandt, 1991; Grahn & Johnson, 1990; Luker et al., 1995). At the same time, shorter hospital stays restrict the time available for patient education. As a result, patients are often discharged with knowledge deficits that become readily apparent as they attempt independence in self-care and try to control their lives (Hughes, Hodgson, Muller, Robinson, & McCorkle, 2000). Many studies found that patients believed they were inadequately prepared during hospitalization for the problems they encountered at home, and they wished they had been told more of the process of recovery (Glavassevich, McKibbon, & Thomas, 1995; Wehby & Brenner, 1999).

Another issue confronting the patient educator is the inability to accomplish desired health goals with patients of all ages and economic and educational backgrounds. A review of patient education literature reveals many variables that influence patients' choices not to follow suggestions of health professionals (Cameron & Gregor, 1987; Marston, 1970). Such variables as religion, ethnicity, family problems, and prior experiences influence the patients' course of action.

Another factor influencing the outcome of patient education is the patient's coping style and locus of control (Lazarus & Folkman, 1984). Lazarus, a cognitive psychologist working in the area of stress and coping, has recognized coping as either primarily *emotion focused* or *problem focused*. His study of coping found patients who use the problem-focused style in reaction to illness are more open to suggestions related to disease management and necessary lifestyle changes than are patients who use emotion focused coping methods.

TEACHING AND LEARNING

In order to promote successful outcomes in patient education, health professionals need to adequately asses the type of patient teaching required and identify which of the categories of human learning are to be included in the teaching plan. The three categories of human learning identified are cognitive, affective, and psychomotor (Bloom, 1956). All three categories, at varying times, are included in patient education.

The *cognitive domain* refers to intellectual activities, such as recognizing, comprehending, analyzing, applying, and evaluating. This category relates to the actual information the patient needs to know. Whereas cognition involves recall and recognition of information presented, it also refers to comprehension of the material taught. Recall and recognition and the patient's willingness to recite the facts are of little benefit, if the patient is unable to understand the meaning of the facts, how they can be put to use, or why they are important (Falvo, 1994).

The *affective domain* refers to the learner's feelings, emotions, and attitudes. Affective behavior reflects values, beliefs, needs, and emotional responses. This domain addresses the patient's beliefs about his or her illness and the validity of the content being taught. The affective domain is critical to the desired goal of patient education. Before the patient can put the information presented to use, he or she must be willing to listen to what is said. Only when the patient is ready to receive the information can the health professional actually teach.

The third category, the *psychomotor domain*, refers to the physical skills needed to implement a specific behavior. These are the skills needed by the patient to return to a higher level of functioning or maintain current health status. For example, assessment of diabetes and insulin injections would be psychomotor skills. Patient teaching in the psychomotor domain involves helping the patient learn an activity or physical skill associated with cognitive information previously received. This type of learning is the most concrete, the easiest to teach and observe, and the easiest to measure.

Building on contextual theories, in a more recent view of learning in the older adult, psychologists differentiate tacit memory from explicit memory (Mezirow, 1991). *Tacit memory* is memory of culturally assimilated habits of expectation that allows the scanning and censoring of one's senses. *Explicit memory* is memory we can produce on command. Tacit memory plays an indispensable role in making an interpretation. Explicit memory, by contrast, is indispensable in perception and plays an essential role in making an explanation and in reflective action. Tacit memory does not appear to decrease as one ages (Mezirow, 1991).

In a critique of mainstream studies and review of an impressive body of supporting research, Labouvie-Vief and Blanchard-Fields (1982) have suggested a model of cognition in aging. Their research suggests that apparent regression and deficits in cognitive abilities reported in the aging may, in fact, be artifacts of youth-centered models. Many research methods fail to recognize that older adults may exhibit a mode of cognitive functioning qualitatively different from that of youth. Additional research suggests that older adults often move to more mature levels of cognitive differentiation that involves greater awareness of context, especially awareness of psychological factors and individual and collective goals, more analysis of premises, and integration of logic and feelings (Mezirow, 1991).

From a physiological perspective, studies of intelligence and aging find cognitive ability changes with age as permanent cellular alterations occur in the brain, resulting in loss of neurons, which have no regenerative powers. Physiological research has demonstrated that people have two kinds of intellectual ability: fluid and crystallized (Bastable, 1997). *Fluid intelligence* is the capacity to perceive relationships, to reason, and to perform abstract thinking. This kind of intelligence declines as degenerative changes occur. *Crystallized intelligence* is the intelligence absorbed over a lifetime, such as vocabulary, general information, understanding social interactions, arithmetic reasoning, and ability to evaluate experiences. This kind of intelligence actually increases as people age (Theis & Merritt, 1994).

The decline in fluid intelligence results in the following changes:

1. *Slower processing time.* Older persons need more time to process and react to information. However, if the factor of speed is removed from IQ tests, older people can perform as well as younger ones do.
2. *Persistence of stimulus (afterimage).* Older people can confuse a previous symbol or word with a new word or symbol just introduced.
3. *Decreased short-term memory.* Older persons experience some decrease in recent memory and have greater recall for events that occurred at earlier times.
4. *Increased test-anxiety.* Older persons are especially anxious about making mistakes when performing, and when they make an error they become easily frustrated. Because of their anxiety, they may take an inordinate amount of time to respond to questions, particularly on tests that are written rather than verbal.
5. *Altered time perception.* For older persons, the concept of the future alters, and "the here and now" philosophy prevails. This approach can be detrimental to health teaching. (Bastable, 1997, pp. 113–114)

Despite the changes in cognition as a result of aging, most research supports the premise that the ability of older adults to learn is virtually as good as ever if special care is taken to slow the pace of the presenting information, to ensure relevance of material, and to give appropriate feedback when teaching. Specifically, it has been pointed out that short-term memory has limited capacity in all age groups, and short-term memory is vulnerable to the aging process, although there is disagreement in the literature about this time-honored belief (Poon, Rubin, & Wilson, 1989; Selkoe, 1992). Although functional changes in the neurological system occur with aging and the older person's ability to react quickly is slowed, studies suggest that the elderly have the capacity to learn, and strategies must be employed that facilitate this learning.

Assessment

The assessment stage of the teaching process is perhaps the most crucial element of patient education. The systematic and thorough collection of data relevant to the teaching process is the basis from which learning needs are identified, objectives are developed, and a teaching plan is formulated (Whitman, Graham, Gleit, & Boyd, 1992). The ways nurses prioritize learning needs, write behavioral objectives, and organize teaching content are all based on learning theories. In the clinical setting, nurses use a variety of approaches depending on their assessment of the learner, the task to be learned, and the learning environment. Prioritizing needs can help the nurse use the time for teaching more effectively. Staffing patterns, work assignments, short hospital stays for patients, or unexpected emergencies can result in less time for teaching. Therefore, the nurse must prioritize the learning needs of the individual to facilitate client learning.

There are several methods that can be used to prioritize learning needs. One method is applying Maslow's Hierarchy of Needs Theory. Maslow (1970) suggests that humans have five broad categories of needs, and before one can satisfactorily meet higher level needs, such as "affection and belongingness" or "self-actualization," lower needs, such as "physiological and survival needs" and "safety and security" must be at least partially met. Therefore, it is essential to prioritize health teaching to address basic physiological and survival needs before addressing higher level needs.

Another method of prioritizing patient education takes into account, on a daily basis, the client's learning needs and the time the nurse has available to teach (George, 1982). The three categories of needs in this method are:

- *Immediate need* (urgent) versus a *long-range need* (can be met at a later time).
- *Specific need* (related specifically to the learner's condition or treatment plan) versus a *general need* (needs for all learners).
- *Survival need* (the learner's life may depend on it) versus a *well-being need* (helpful, but not essential) (Whitman et al., 1992).

Prioritizing allows the nurse to meet immediate and specific needs and to meet more general needs in the future. With proper planning, teaching can be integrated into routine nursing activities such as giving baths and medications. These integrated teaching activities allow the nurse to maximize the time available and help space teaching and learning sessions, giving the patient more time to process the information. Prioritizing learning needs allows for appropriate goals and objectives designed for patient education.

Goals and Objectives

Adult learners are motivated to learn when they recognize a gap between what they know and what they want to know (Knowles, 1980; Merriam & Cunningham, 1989; Reilly & Oberman, 1999). Assessment of the learner's needs provides information about the knowledge, attitudes, and skills important for optimum teaching. The learning experience is directed by goals and objectives. *Goals* are broad, general, end-product statements about what is desired and expected as the outcome of the individual's learning. Goal setting, whenever possible, is a joint venture between the nurse and the patient. The outcomes of goal setting are usually more successful if the goal is the result of a client's expressed need or interest. *Objectives* provide the specific statements related to the goal and describe the behaviors that will be performed to meet the goals. Objectives are "how to" statements that express in specific, measurable terms *who* will do *what*, as *measured by what* and *by when*. Behavioral objectives are designed to deal with one behavior at a time and are yardsticks for measuring an individual's success as a learner. They also help nurses to acknowledge learner readiness, plan of continuity of care, and appropriately sequence teaching and prioritize learning needs (Redman, 1988).

Both goals and objectives must be clearly stated and agreed on by the patient, his or her family, whenever possible, and the educator, if patient education is to have a focus. Setting specific goals for patient education ensures that learning interventions will be tailored to the situation and the client's needs. Goals offer criteria for evaluation of patient education. When goals and objectives are clearly stated, the learner knows what his or her role is and what is expected (Rankin & Stallings, 1990).

SENSORY CHANGES AND OTHER FACTORS AFFECTING OLDER ADULT LEARNING

Sensory Changes: Vision

There are many sensory and other factors that affect the outcome of patient education. A common sensory factor is the change in vision in the older adult. The lens of the eye in the elderly loses its ability to accommodate as it becomes less elastic, larger, and denser. The increased density plus the accumulation of loosened, degenerated cells on the iris, cornea, and lens results in increasing scattering of light and sensitivity to glare (Babcock & Miller, 1994). The lens becomes progressively yellowed and opaque, resulting not only in visual acuity difficulties but also in the inability to discriminate between blue and green. It is much easier for the elderly to distinguish among the warm colors such as yellow, red, and orange. Use of these colors in teaching materials will make it easier for the older learner to distinguish relevant content (Matteson & McConnell, 1988).

Other visual difficulties influencing learning in the elderly are decreased tolerance of glare, decreased ability to adapt to light and dark, and decreased peripheral vision. Smaller images, which project through shorter light waves into the eye, are harder to distinguish, as are crowded or softly colored images. Larger and more intensely colored print is easier to comprehend. In educational printed materials designed for elderly learners, allowing space between each letter facilitates the ability to distinguish the message.

Because it takes longer for the eyes of older clients to adapt to dark and light, it takes more time for their eyes to adjust if a room is darkened to show a video, film, or slide presentation. When the lights are turned on, it takes longer for the elderly to adjust to the light. Ebersole and Hess (1990) note that older clients need three times the amount of light than they did in their second decade. Therefore high-intensity lighting is best placed directly on the teaching object rather than throughout the room. The level of intensity of the light needs to be balanced against the avoidance of glare.

Sensory Changes: Hearing

Another frequent sensory change that influences patient education is the hearing loss that accompanies the aging process. Presbycusis is associated with aging and is the most common hearing loss. As the client ages, the loss involves the sounds in the higher and middle ranges. It becomes problematic for the client when the upper sounds are missed and only lower sounds are heard. Words sound distorted and conversations are difficult to understand, especially with background noise. With high-tone hearing loss, it is more difficult for the client to discriminate among consonants such as *s, t, g, sh, z,* and *th,* which have higher frequencies (Bates, 1991). As hearing loss progresses, consonants such as *b, k,* and *p,* also become distorted (Miller, 1990).

Clients with hearing loss will need more time to process information. Rapid speech will be difficult for older clients to understand. When teaching older clients, nurses need to lower the pitch of their voices and speak more slowly.

Cognitive Change: Memory Loss

As discussed earlier, memory loss as part of the aging process has been the subject of a great deal of study. Some researchers have suggested that perceived memory loss is actually caused by divided attention and naming problems (Carnevali, 1993). Many authors report that short-term memory declines with age, but long-term memory remains intact with normal aging (Carnevali, 1993; Miller, 1995).

Change in Health Status

Another important factor that influences the accomplishment of teaching goals is the patient's acuity. This is clearly a concern for critically ill older adults. Assessment of the learner's health status is important to determine the amount of energy available as well as the present comfort level. Both of these factors have a heavy impact on readiness to learn. Learners who are acutely ill focus their energies on the physiological and psychological demands of their illness. Learning is at a minimum because most of their energy is needed for the demands of their illness and gaining immediate relief. Any learning that may occur is related to treatments, tests, and minimizing pain and other discomfort (Bastable, 1997). As patients improve and the acute stage of the illness diminishes, they can focus on learning follow-up management and avoidance of complications.

Cognitive Changes: Effects of Medication

In the assessment of readiness for learning, it is necessary to take into account direct effects of medication on cognition. For example, minor tranquilizers are frequently prescribed for elderly patients. Many drugs cause cognitive impairment, which is greater in older people, even in those who do not have evidence of an underlying cognitive disorder (Greenblatt, Avorn, Ross-Degnan, Choodnovski, & Ansell, 1991). Furthermore, the pharmacokinetics of drugs may be altered in older people, so they remain effective for longer periods of time. The impact of medication on the patient's ability to understand treatment programs and adhere to them has not been adequately studied (Halter, 1999).

Special Challenges: Patients with Low Literacy Skills

Literacy is another significant factor influencing patient education. In assessing the older adult's ability to learn, it is important to consider that nearly 20% of Americans lack the necessary literacy skills to benefit from even the simplest handout or videotaped program (Rankin & Stallings, 1990). Despite attempts to simplify written materials from the typical ninth-grade reading level to an improved sixth-grade level, the patient with low literacy skills is still lost. In *Teaching Patients with Low Literacy Skills* (Doak, Doak, & Root, 1985), the authors explain how to test patients' comprehension of written materials and how to write educational materials for these patients. Functionally illiterate adults process information differently than do readers. They may have limited vocabulary, may not understand abbreviations, and usually do not ask questions. Yet they may speak articulately and have average IQs. The authors suggest modifying existing materials for these patients and recommend the following teaching tips for these patients, as well as for all elderly clients:

- Focus information on the core of the knowledge and skills patients need to survive and cope with their problems.
- Teach the smallest amount possible.
- Make points vivid.
- Have the patient restate and demonstrate.
- Review. (Rankin & Stallings, 1990)

DEVELOPING A PLAN FOR PATIENT TEACHING

Once data about the patient are assessed and goals and objectives are developed, the next step is the incorporation of the information into a systematic plan. Falvo (1994) identified the following information to be included in the teaching plan:

- what type of information the patient should be given (cognitive, psychomotor, or affective, or a combination of all three)
- when teaching will be done
- where the teaching will be done
- how the teaching will be done (through individual learning sessions, group sessions, supplementary activities such as pamphlets, videos, films)
- who will do the patient teaching (one individual or a variety of health professionals)

Specifically, a complete teaching plan consists of eight basic parts (Ryan & Marielli, 1990):

1. The purpose
2. A statement of the overall goal
3. A list of objectives
4. An outline of the related content

5. The method(s) of presentation
6. The time allotted for the teaching of each objective
7. The instructional resources (materials/tools) needed
8. The method of evaluation of learning

The method of evaluation should match the domain in which learning is to take place. For example, if the behavioral objective for the learner is to identify two side effects of medication (cognitive), then the evaluation method must test that knowledge by asking the learner to state two side effects of a specific medication. Evaluation methods must measure the desired learning outcomes to determine if and to what extent the learner achieved the expectations for learning.

LEARNING CONTRACTS

In a relatively new concept to patient education, the teaching plan can be in the form of a learning contract that formalizes the agreement between the teacher and the learner. The learning contract clearly states learning behaviors, the responsibility of the teacher and the learner, and the methods for follow-up and evaluation. It is a written (formal) or verbal (informal) agreement between the educator and the learner or family, or both, that delineates specific teaching and learning activities that are to occur within a certain time frame. Learning contracts are mutually negotiated agreements that stress shared accountability for learning between the teacher and the learner. The learning contract specifies what the learner will learn, how learning will be achieved, within what time allotment, and the criteria for measuring the success of the learning (Keyzer, 1986). The learning contract provides an explicit mechanism for communication, identifying the responsibilities of the patient, the patient's family, and the members of the health team (Rankin & Stallings, 1990).

STRATEGIES FOR TEACHING THE ELDERLY PATIENT

The object of patient education is not only to help patients comprehend information but also to help put the information to use in their daily lives. This is most readily accomplished in the context of the relationship between the patient and the health professional. The quality of the relationship will have significant impact on the outcome of teaching and the patient's willingness to carry out recommendations. Although evidence suggests that the one important factor in the relationship may be the professionals' ability to communicate information effectively to patients about their condition and treatment, other findings indicate that health professionals' ability to establish rapport may also be a significant factor (DiMatteo, 1982). The basic aspects of a relationship that facilitate open communication and rapport are acceptance, understanding, empathy, and trust. Although these terms have become platitudes when used by some, they are essential in the building of a relationship that can influence the effectiveness of patient education (Falvo, 1994).

It has been recognized that the health professional's attitude as well as the lack of understanding of the older patient may well be the greatest barrier to effective patient education. Patient education may be viewed by some professionals as a futile task. Aspects of teaching the older adult about prevention may be neglected. The health professional may believe the myths about aging and approach older adults with these stereotypes in mind rather than dealing with them as individuals.

Aging, as viewed by health professionals, is a multidimensional process in which the individual's function and health status are related to multiple factors. When conducting patient education, it is essential that the health professional treat the elderly with the same interest and respect as any other patient with whom education is conducted. For example, addressing the older patient by his or her first name is inappropriate unless invited to do so. Patient education with older adults should be conducted with the same convictions with which it would be delivered to patients of any age (Falvo, 1994). In teaching older persons, it is important to capitalize on the patient's strengths, avoid patronizing behaviors, and speak clearly and concisely. Barriers to independence should be assessed to help the patient find ways to maximize strengths and an optimal health status.

PATIENT EDUCATION WITH THE ELDERLY PATIENT AND THE FAMILY

The role of the family in patient education is considered one of the key variables influencing patient care outcomes. The primary motives for involving family members in the care-delivery and decision-making process are to decrease the stress of hospitalization, reduce costs of care, and effectively prepare the client for self-care management after hospitalization. Family members provide critical emotional, physical, and social support to the patient.

However, illness disrupts the family. Each individual within a family—whether parent or child—plays a certain role that the family incorporates within its basic everyday function (Falvo, 1994). Health professionals will be more successful with patient education if they are able to recognize the impact that illness has on the family and include the family in the teaching process. The impact on the family depends, to some extent, on the seriousness of the illness. It also depends on the level of functioning before the illness, as well as on socioeconomic considerations, the emotional dependence of others, and the extent to which other family members can absorb the role of the person who is ill (Falvo, 1994). Phillips (1989) points out that although there is a great deal of attention given to the way young and adolescent families function, there is minimal attention to the dynamics of the complex interactions that characterize the aging family.

In conducting patient education with the family, it is essential to assess the impact of the illness on the family, because the family's reaction may have significant influence on the patient's motivation to recover and cooperate with the treatment recommended. It is also important to identify what the illness means, not only to the individual but also to the family. It is often the family's perception of the illness that is more important than the type of illness (Falvo, 1994). The health professional, in planning patient education, needs to be alert to family reactions to learning about the condition and the treatment. One area for assessment is how responsive family members are to learning skills to be used in caring for the patient after discharge from the hospital.

Other areas for assessment are stressors verbalized by the family and the family's method of coping with stress in the past. Members of the family who are anxious and under stress often misinterpret or misunderstand what they are told. It is not uncommon for family members to distort information, turning it into what they want to hear.

Therefore, assessment of the family member's understanding of what they have been told is essential so that any misinterpretation can be corrected early. Anticipatory teaching with family caregivers can reduce their anxiety, uncertainty, and lack of confidence. Providing the family with written information and having them return to discuss it may be a helpful strategy. The greatest challenge for caregivers is to develop confidence in their ability to do what is right for the patient. Education is the means to confront this challenge.

DISCHARGE PLANNING

Learning needs for elderly patients during the transition from hospital to home are complex and cannot be adequately addressed during the elderly patient's hospitalization or through the distribution of written discharge instructions. Discharge teaching content includes material about diet, activity patterns, medication names, uses, side effects, and community resources available. Patients need ongoing contact with nurses who have the expertise and clinical experience, and with the wide range of learning needs experienced after hospital discharge. Hughes et al. (2000), in a study of 148 elderly postsurgical cancer patients, concluded that patients needed information regarding the application of specialized knowledge so they could independently respond to problems and symptoms.

Specifically, teaching interventions ranged from providing concrete instructions about wound care to explaining complex and sophisticated information about options for cancer treatment and identifying appropriate community resources. Interventions were focused on providing information to alleviate patients' sense of uncertainty about the diagnosis and their ability to safely care for themselves at home. Emphasis on urgent concerns such as pain management and recognition of events that required physician notification were essential elements of the teaching plan. Teaching at the level of application meant that nurses acted as advisors or consultants, coaching patients and families to make sound decisions and use problem-solving skills to gain independence. Hughes et al. (2000) further recommend that a nurse case manager model may be a cost-effective option for providing informational support that patients need. In this study, 40% of teaching was provided during telephone contacts. They point to the need for knowledgeable and experienced practitioners to provide health teaching. In their study, many generalist practitioners who had limited experiences of working with cancer patients lacked experiential knowledge needed to provide this level of teaching.

DOCUMENTATION OF HEALTH TEACHING

Documentation of all health teaching, including discharge planning, is required in every health care setting. To qualify for Medicare and Medicaid reimbursement, "a hospital has to show evidence that patient education has been a part of patient care" (Boyd, 1992, p. 21). For at least 20 years, the JCAHO has reinforced the federal mandate by requiring evidence (documentation) of patient or family education, or both, in the patient record. Haggard points out that of all the omissions in documentation, patient teaching "is probably the most undocumented skilled service because nurses do not recognize the scope of depth of teaching they do" (1989, p. 144). Written documentation of all aspects of patient care, including patient education, is essential. Documentation is important for communication among the health team members to provide a legal record of patient care activities, to support quality assurance efforts, and to promote reimbursement. Communication between members of the health-care team is necessary if there is to be a coordinated, consistent approach to health teaching. This communication, in the form of documentation in patient records, communicates not only that teaching has been done but also what has been taught, the patient's level of understanding, and what further teaching or reinforcement or information needs to be provided. From a legal perspective, it is important for patient educators to keep in mind that *if it is not documented, it did not happen* (Creighton, 1987). Documentation of health teaching is often the exception rather than the rule. Porter (1990) found that nurses only document health teaching 15% of the time. So much of patient teaching is incidental and is given at "teachable moments;" therefore, nurses may not document spontaneous teaching the way they would document teaching that is more formal.

The guidelines for documentation of health teaching identify that charting should be

1. *Accurate and concise.* Detail enough of the teaching content so there is no ambiguity about what is taught.
2. *Objective.* Use descriptive words that present a detailed picture or account of what occurred and the patient's response.
3. *Prompt.* What is taught can affect the patient's response to treatments, procedures, or medications and how other health professionals approach the patient. Therefore, every effort should be made to chart soon after teaching.
4. *Legible and use only standard abbreviations.*
5. *Complete.* Include health-teaching plans, checklists, anecdotal notes, as well as progress notes in the patient's permanent chart. (Whitman et al., 1992, p. 27)

PATIENT EDUCATION STRATEGIES IN THE 21ST CENTURY

The opportunities and possibilities for patient education are changing in the 21st century. The new millennium brings with it the development of information and communications technology, which facilitates all forms of patient education. Round-the-clock online access to patient records and support on best clinical practices for all clinicians will facilitate the transmission of essential knowledge for maximizing patient health. Electronic libraries and databases will provide up-to-date information for research and teaching. More educated consumers of health care and their families will have access to information, advice, and care through online information services and telemedicine, for example, through a video conference for remote diagnosis, consultation between professionals in different locations, and the provision of care (Clark, 2000).

SUMMARY

Nurses are mandated by nurse practice acts and professional organizations to educate clients and their families in health practices. The elderly patient, the health care environment, the current practice of discharging patients "sicker and quicker," and health professionals' attitudes toward the elderly present multiple challenges to the process of patient education. Yet, patient education is the most powerful tool to ensure maximizing the patient's health practices and providing safer discharge from health-care settings. The nurse who understands the theories and principles of teaching and learning is better able to assist the elderly client in achieving desired health behaviors.

As the field of patient education grows and more technologies and methods for delivering effective patient education are developed, it is important for health professionals to continue to search for ways to improve the quality and the accountability of the practices used. In addition, the role patient education has in reducing health care costs as well as human costs related to illness and disability warrants future study. Effective patient education is a complex process. Through this process the health professional acts as a guide and resource, helping patients and their families adjust to necessary changes with the end goal being assisting patients in gaining responsibility for and control over their own health and optimal well-being (Falvo, 1994).

REFERENCES

American Nurses Association. (1975). *The professional nurse and health education.* Kansas City, MO: ANA.

Babcock, D. E., & Miller, M. A. (1994). *Client education: Theory and practice.* St. Louis: Mosby.

Bastable, S. B. (1997). *Nurse as educator: Principles of teaching and learning.* Sudbury, MA: Jones & Bartlett.

Bates, B. (1991). *A guide of physical examination and history taking* (5th ed.). Philadelphia: J. B. Lippincott.

Bloom, B. S. (Ed.). (1956). *Taxonomy of educational objectives: The classification of educational goals. Handbook I: Cognitive domain.* New York: David McKay.

Boyd, M. D. (1992). Policies, guidelines and legal mandates for health teaching. In N. I. Whitman, B. A. Graham, C. J. Gleit, & M. D. Boyd (Eds.), *Teaching in nursing practice: A professional model* (pp. 17–30). Norwalk, CT: Appleton & Lange.

Brandt, B. (1991). Informational needs and selected variables in-patients receiving brachytherapy. *Oncology Nursing Forum, 18,* 1221–1227.

Cameron, K., & Gregor, F. (1987). Chronic illness and compliance. *Advances in Nursing, 12,* 671–676.

Carnevali, D. L. (1993). *Nursing management for the elderly* (3rd ed.). Philadelphia: Lippincott.

Clark, J. (2000). Old wine in new bottles: Delivering nursing in the 21st century. *Journal of Nursing Scholarship, 32,* 7–9.

Creighton, H. (1987). Legal significance of charting—Part 1. *Nursing Management, 18* (9), 17–20.

DiMatteo, M. R. (1982). *Social psychology and medicine.* Cambridge, MA: Oegleschlager, Gunn and Hain Publishers.

Doak, C., Doak, L., & Root, J. (1985). *Teaching patients with low literacy skills.* Philadelphia: Lippincott.

Ebersole, P., & Hess, P. (1990). *Toward healthy aging: Human needs and nursing response* (3rd ed.). St Louis: Mosby.

Falvo, D. R. (1994). *Effective patient education.* Gaithersburg, MD: Aspen.

George, G. (1982). If patient teaching tries your patience, try this plan. *Nursing, 12,* 50–55.

Glavassevich, M., McKibbon, A., & Thomas, S. (1995). Information needs for patients who undergo surgery for head and neck cancer. *Canadian Oncology Nursing Journal, 5* (1), 9–11.

Grahn, G., & Johnson, J. (1990). Learning to cope and living with cancer: Learning needs assessment in cancer patient education. *Scandinavian Journal of Caring Sciences, 4,* 173–181.

Greenblatt, D. J., Avorn, J., Ross-Degnan, D., Choodnovski, I., & Ansell, J. (1992). Sensitivity to triazolam in the elderly. *New England Journal of Medicine, 324,* 1691–1698.

Haggard, A. (1989). *Handbook of patient education.* Rockville, MD: Aspen.

Halter, J. B. (1999). The challenge of communicating health information. In D. C. Park, R. W. Morrell, & K. Shiffren (Eds.), *Processing of medical information in elderly patients: Cognitive and human perspectives.* Mahwah, NJ: Lawrence Erlbaum Associates.

Hayes, K. S. (1999). Adding medications in the emergency department: Effect on knowledge of medications in older adults. *Journal of Emergency Room Nursing, 25,* 178–182.

Hughes, L. C., Hodgson, N. A., Muller, P., Robinson, L. A., & McCorkle, R. (2000). Information needs of elderly postsurgical cancer patients during the transition from hospital to home. *Journal of Nursing Scholarship, 32* (1), 25–30.

Joint Commission on Accreditation of Healthcare Organizations. (1981). *Accreditation manual for hospitals.* Chicago: JCAHO.

Keyzer, D. (1986). Using learning contracts to support change in nursing organizations. *Nurse Educator Today, 6* (80), 103–108.

Knowles, M. S. (1980). *The modern practice of adult education* (2nd ed.). New York: Cambridge Books.

Labouvie-Vief, G., & Blanchard-Fields, F. (1982). Cognitive ageing and psychological growth. *Ageing and Society, 2,* 183–211.

Lazarus, R. S., & Folkman, S. (1984). *Stress, appraisal and coping.* New York: Springer.

Luker, K. A., Beaver, K., Leinster, S. J., Owens, R. G., Degner, L. F., & Sloan, J. A. (1995). The information needs of women newly diagnosed with breast cancer. *Journal of Advanced Nursing, 22,* 134–141.

Marston, M. V. (1970). Compliance with medical regimens: A review of the literature. *Nursing Research, 19,* 312–323.

Maslow, A. (1970). *Motivation and personality.* New York: Harper & Row.

Matteson, M. A., & McConnell, E. S. (1988). *Gerontological nursing: Concepts and practice.* Philadelphia: W. B. Saunders.

Merriam, S. B., & Cunningham, P. M. (Eds.). (1989). *Handbook of adult education and continuing education.* San Francisco: Jossey-Bass.

Mezirow, J. (1991). *Transformative dimensions of adult learning.* San Francisco: Jossey-Bass.

McDougall, G. (1999). Cognitive interventions among older adults. *Annual Review of Nursing Research, 17,* 219–240.

Miller, C. A. (1990). *Nursing care of older adults.* Glenview, IL: Scott, Foressman/Little, Brown Higher Education.

Miller, C. A. (1995). *Nursing care of older adults: Theory and practice* (2nd ed.). Philadelphia: Lippincott.

Poon, L. W., Rubin, D. C., & Wilson, B. A. (Eds.). (1989). *Everyday cognition in adulthood and late life.* Cambridge: Cambridge University Press.

Phillips, L. R. (1989). Elder-family caregiver relationships: Determining appropriate nursing relationships. *Nursing Clinics of North America, 24,* 795–807.

Porter, Y. (1990). Brief: Evaluation of nurses' documentation of patient teaching. *The Journal of Continuing Education in Nursing, 21,* 134–137.

Rankin, S. H., & Stallings, K. D. (1990). *Patient education: Issues, principles, practices* (2nd ed.). Philadelphia: Lippincott.

Redman, B. (1988). *The process of patient teaching.* Chicago: Mosby.

Reilly, E., & Oberman, M. (1999). *Clinical teaching in nursing education* (2nd ed.). Sudbury, MA: Jones and Bartlett.

Robinson, S. (1992). The learning needs of cancer patients. *European Journal of Cancer Care, 1* (3), 18–20.

Rosoff, A. J. (1981). *Informed consent: A guide for the health care provider.* Gaithersburg, MD: Aspen.

Ryan, A. A. (1999). Medication compliance and older people: A review of the literature. *International Journal of Nursing Studies, 36,* 153–162.

Ryan, M., & Marielli, T. (1990). *Developing a teaching plan.* Unpublished Self-Study Module, College of Nursing, State University of New York Health Science at Syracuse.

Selkoe, D. J. (1992). Aging brain, aging mind. *Scientific American, 267,* 135–142.

Slavin, R. E. (1991). *Educational psychology: Theory and practice* (3rd ed.). Boston: Allyn & Bacon.

Wehby, D., & Brenner, P. S. (1999). Perceived needs of patients with heart failure. *Heart and Lung: Journal of Critical Care, 28* (1), 31–40.

Whitman, N. I., Graham, B. A., Gleit, C. J., & Boyd, M. D. (1992). *Teaching in nursing practice.* Norwalk, CT: Appleton & Lange.

12

Evaluating Outcomes

Ruth M. Kleinpell and Diane J. Mick

As projections of the growing numbers of elderly persons have become a reality, evaluating outcomes in the elderly has become a fundamental necessity in planning for adequate health care. A number of factors have increased the demand for data on outcomes for the elderly, including the expanding older population, the changing health care environment, and the emphasis on patient involvement in medical decision making. Because health outcomes become more important as one ages, information is needed on what impact illness has on the elderly, and on the effectiveness of various therapies.

Although termed "the elderly," the older population has an age range spanning more than 30 years and is quite diverse and heterogeneous (Feasley et al., 1996). Information is needed on the outcomes of health care for all groups of the elderly to ensure the health and well-being of all older persons. The focus of this chapter is on evaluating outcomes in the elderly. Issues in measuring outcomes and in instrument selection and use and issues related to conducting intervention outcomes research in the elderly are addressed.

OVERVIEW OF OUTCOMES RESEARCH

The literature on outcomes is expanding rapidly. Outcomes are being used to describe the impact of care on patients' lives, establish a basis for clinical decision making, evaluate the effectiveness of care, and identify areas for improvement in care (Davies et al., 1994). Although is it clear that measuring outcomes is important, choosing which outcomes are to be measured remains unclear. Outcomes can include familiar clinical measures such as signs and symptoms, or they can be expressed as complications, such as infection (Kane, 1997). The selection of an outcome measure should be based on a clear sense of what is to be measured and why (Kane, 1997). The challenge in outcomes research comes in selecting outcomes that are comprehensive, comparable, meaningful, and accurate in their reflection of areas that are important to the elderly (Kleinpell, 1997).

Outcomes research scientifically evaluates a process and quantifies the results. This type of research determines how key outcomes for the elderly can be used as a measure of quality within a health care system. There are two major components to consider when initiating clinical outcomes assessment: domain and when measurement should occur (Titler & Reitler, 1994). Traditional outcome measures (domains) to evaluate the impact of medical care used to include death, disease, disability, discomfort, and dissatisfaction—all negative outcomes (Lohr, 1988). Today, more positive aspects of health such as satisfaction, physical and emotional health, and quality of life are being used as outcome measures. The goals of outcomes research are avoiding adverse effects of care, improving the patient's physiological status, reducing the patient's signs and symptoms, and improving the patient's well-being (Davies et al., 1994).

OUTCOMES RESEARCH IN THE ELDERLY

For the elderly, assessing outcomes of care is especially important because multiple factors can influence their health care outcomes. Comorbidities, frailty, chronic illness, and limitations in activities of daily living (ADLs) can have an impact on health-care outcomes in ways that can complicate identifying the effect of a treatment or health care intervention. A challenge of health outcomes research involving the elderly is in discovering how to draw generalized conclusions about outcomes while recognizing that each person's circumstances are unique and that some variation is to be expected (Feasley et al., 1996). An outcomes approach that considers risk factors (baseline clinical status, demographic or psychosocial characteristics) and treatment characteristics (treatment and setting) has been proposed as a model for analyzing the outcomes of care (Kane, 1997). In this manner, the effects of other factors can be identified. This becomes important in analyzing outcomes in the elderly, because accurate data are essential in guiding care for the elderly.

Although a number of outcome measures have been used in outcomes research in the elderly, several parameters are essential in capturing areas of life that are important to the elderly. These include functional status, health status, and quality of life. These parameters are briefly discussed, and examples of instruments for measuring them appear in Table 12.1.

Functional Status

The measurement of functional status is recognized as an important outcome measure. Functional status refers to an individual's performance of

TABLE 12.1   Selected Instruments for Outcomes Research in the Elderly

Instrument	Outcome Parameters
Instruments for Measuring Functional Status	
Older Americans Resources and Services Multidimensional Functional Assessment Questionnaire (Fillenbaum & Smyer, 1981)	Physical, psychological, social and economic functioning, self-care capacity, and service evaluation
Sickness Impact Profile (Bergner et al., 1981)	Functioning in physical, psychosocial, and overall dimensions and in 12 categories: sleep and rest, eating, work, home management, recreation and pastimes, ambulation, mobility, body care and movement, social interaction, alertness behavior, emotional behavior, communication
Medical Outcomes Study General Health Survey Short Form (SF-36) (Ware & Sherbourne, 1992)	Physical functioning, role limitations, bodily pain, general mental health, vitality, general health perceptions
Nottingham Health Profile (Hunt et al., 1981)	Physical, social, emotional areas within 2 parts: problems and effect on daily life
Duke University Health Profile (Parkerson et al., 1981)	Symptom status, physical function emotional function, social function
Instruments for Measuring Activities of Daily Living	
Karnofsky Index of Performance Status (Schag, Heinrich & Ganz, 1984)	Ability to work and perform normal activity, need for assistance
Index of ADL (Katz et al., 1963)	Bathing, dressing, toileting, transferring, continence, feeding
Barthel Index (Mahoney & Barthel, 1965)	Bathing, dressing, toileting, transferring, feeding, hygiene/grooming, walking, stair-climbing, bladder & bowel control
Philadelphia Geriatric Center Instrumental Activities of Daily Living Scale (Lawton & Brody, 1969)	Using the telephone, shopping, preparing food, housekeeping, doing laundry, using public transportation, taking medications, handling finances
Instruments for Measuring Quality of Life	
Quality of Life Index (Ferrans & Powers, 1985)	Overall quality of life, and four subscales: health and functioning, psychological-spiritual, social-economic, family
Quality of Life Questionnaire (Young & Longman, 1983)	Quality of life and satisfaction with quality of life

(continued)

TABLE 12.1   *(continued)*

Instrument	Outcome Parameters
QL-Index (Spitzer et al., 1981)	Health, family support, activity, daily living, outlook
Quality of Life Index (Padilla et al., 1983)	Psychological well-being, physical well-being, symptom control

From "Neutralizing ageism in critical care via outcomes research," by D. Mick and M. Ackerman, 1997, AACN Clinical Issues, 8 (4). Copyright 1997 by American Association of Critical Care Nurses. Adapted with permission. Also from "Assessing outcomes in advanced practice nursing," by R. Kleinpell and T. Weiner, 1999, AACN Clinical Issues, 10 (3). Copyright 1999 by American Association of Critical Care Nurses. Adapted with permission.

activities and tasks normally expected of an adult (Richmond, McCorkle, Tulman, & Fawcett, 1997). Assessment of functional abilities becomes especially important when illness or aging compromises functioning. Limitations in functional status often occur with aging, and the measurement of functional abilities is an essential component of an outcomes assessment for the elderly. Issues in the measurement of function include the purpose of the measurement, the match between the theoretical dimension of function, the focus of an instrument, the unique requirements of the population of interest, and methodological concerns (Richmond et al., 1997). These issues must be addressed prior to the design and conduct of a study measuring functional status in the elderly in order to ensure accurate assessment of functional status.

Health Status

Health status is traditionally defined as a comprehensive state of physical, mental, and social well-being and not just the absence of disease. Health status is often used interchangeably with functional status as an outcome measure in clinical research (Richmond et al., 1997). However, health status incorporates aspects of well-being in addition to functional abilities. Measurement of health status involves more than assessing general health attitudes or overall ratings such as good, fair, or poor. Classifications of health measurements include functional, descriptive, and methodological (health indices and health profiles including subjective and objective measures) (McDowell & Newell, 1996).

The measurement of health status is an important component of an outcomes assessment for the elderly, because changes in health status naturally occur with aging. Health status incorporates general aspects of health along with physical, social, and mental aspects, all of which need to be considered in comprehensive health status assessments of the elderly. Measures of physical functioning are important in the elderly and have been cited as the most important measure required for research on the elderly (Kane & Kane, 1981). Physical functioning includes the performance of ADLs (such as bathing, feeding) and performance of instrumental tasks (such as shopping and home maintenance). Measures of physical functioning in the elderly should be inclusive of ADLs and instrumental activities of daily living (IADLs) to capture essential components of physical functioning.

The measurement of social functioning includes such parameters as social activities, social support, and life satisfaction. These activities add to an individual's overall health status and become of increasing importance to the elderly who may be socially distanced from family or friends or whose participation in social activities may change with illness. As an additional component of health status, cognition is also a crucial measure to the elderly, because cognitive changes occur with increasing frequency in the elderly.

Quality of Life

Quality of life is being increasingly addressed in health care outcomes research yet rarely is a precise definition of the term described. To be clinically useful, quality of life must be clearly defined (Ferrans, 1990). Quality of life is a multidimensional concept incorporating an individual's perceptions of various aspects of life, including health status, life satisfaction, lifestyle, and well-being (Padilla & Frank-Stromborg, 1997). The importance of health in determining and impacting overall quality of life is clear (Padilla & Frank-Stromborg, 1997). Measuring quality of life as part of an assessment of outcome status for the elderly is important in providing a comprehensive evaluation of the impact of illness, chronic disease, and treatment interventions on aging.

Although physical functioning, health status, and quality of life are important outcome parameters for the elderly, additional domains such as economic resources, formal and informal services received, and family well-being have also been proposed as essential in comprehensive evaluations of the elderly (Kane & Kane, 1981). Satisfaction, comorbidity, severity of illness, frailty, and vitality should also be included in outcome assessments (Kane, 1997; Mick & Ackerman, 1997). The choice of which parameters to include in an outcomes assessment of the elderly will depend on the purposes and goals of the outcome analysis.

MEASURING OUTCOMES IN THE ELDERLY: FACTORS TO CONSIDER

Goals related to outcomes measurement for aging hospitalized patients include an increased understanding of the effectiveness of various health care interventions; eventual use of this information to aid in health care decision making by patients, physicians, and third-party payers; and a potential for the development of standards for guiding health care providers in optimizing the use of available resources. When sociopolitical discussions related to appropriate use of health care resources take place, there often is an underlying thread of ageism directed against provision of highly technological, and presumably costly, health care for older patients. However, without convincing evidence related to postillness outcomes for aging patients, sound health care decisions are difficult to make, and political discussions related to age-based rationing of health care are groundless.

Influence of Ageism

Some practitioners may associate chronological age with negative patient characteristics and conditions, such as poor prognosis, cognitive impairment, decreased quality of life, limited life expectancy, and decreased social worth (Wetle, 1987). Based on these attributed characteristics, decisions may be made to withhold treatment, resulting in unnecessary illness, suffering, and death. Populations of aging patients, on average, may be more likely to suffer from cognitive impairment, chronic health problems, and decreased function than are younger groups of patients, however, the health and social heterogeneity of persons of all ages make generalized assumptions insupportable. As negative health characteristics commonly attributed to aging patients are examined individually, chronological age becomes less important in planning treatments and predicting outcomes, and ageism becomes the plausible explanation for differences in treatment associated with age.

Loewy (1996) noted that the use of age as an independent variable in medical decision making depersonalizes the elderly ill individual and fails to address the person and his or her needs. He further stated that a natural life span for a species is not necessarily a life span for a singular organism within it. From an ethical standpoint, limitation of care for all elderly above an arbitrarily determined age should not be considered until clinical parameters for all those who can no longer benefit from health care are determined (Loewy, 1996).

Results from two studies (Hamel et al., 1996, 1999) of more than 9100 critically ill patients revealed that covert age-based rationing of intensive care is already taking place. Comparisons of seriously ill older patients with younger patients revealed that older patients receive fewer invasive procedures and hospital care that is less costly. This preferential allocation of hospital resources to younger patients was not based on differences in illness severity or general preferences for life-extending care. According to Blanchette (1995), discussion of resource allocation with the potential for rationing should be guided by an examination of the quality of existing data related to health outcomes for all age groups, and care should be therapeutically appropriate. Provoking intergenerational conflict related to allocation of health care resources is socially counterproductive. Objective assessment without financial incentive or motivation of individuals' needs and probable outcomes of care is necessary to prevent allegations of ageism and tendencies toward covert rationing of health care (Blanchette, 1995).

Physiological Changes Associated with Aging

As a person ages, normal biological senescence occurs. The aging patient experiences a decrease in organ system functional reserve and a concomitant diminished ability to withstand the stress of traumatic injury, unexpected critical illness, or acute exacerbations of underlying chronic illnesses. However, because not all age-related changes are progressive or pathological, an elderly person's body systems are regarded as dysregulated rather than dysfunctional (Resnick, 1998). The immune system suffers dysregulation by the time a person reaches age 50 years, when the thymus has lost 95% of its physiological properties. After this time, the previously normal immune inflammatory response may be insufficient in the case of serious insult or injury. As well, the aging body has a decreased ability to combat and compensate during systemic inflammation and sepsis (Mick, in press). However, it is thought that physiological as well as psychological adaptation helps to influence outcomes from illness events in the elderly (Mick, in press).

Impact of Admission Illness Severity

Research has demonstrated that among patients of all age groups, acute and chronic illness and severity of illness and organ system failure are strongly related to intensive care mortality (Brun-Buisson et al., 1995; Chelluri, Pinsky, Donahoe, & Grenvik, 1993; Ludwigs & Hulting, 1995; Mayer-Oakes, Oye, & Leake, 1991; Oye & Bellamy, 1986; Sage, Hurst, Silverman, & Bortz, 1987). However, measures of illness severity that incorporate age as an element of scoring have a potential of limiting treatment on the basis of an unfavorable total score, jeopardizing acceptable treatment and outcomes for the elderly intensive care unit (ICU) patient (Niskanen & Niskanen, 1994). Measures of illness severity are objectively scored scales of physiological variables and, as such, do not incorporate quality of life considerations or functional abilities. When used in isolation, illness severity instruments are inadequate for clinical decision making across all age groups because intangible factors related to life and personhood are not addressed (Mick & Ackerman, 1997).

Activities of Daily Living

ADLs often are described as basic self-care activities such as eating, dressing, grooming, toileting, and mobility (Law & Letts, 1989). ADL instruments may have one of three purposes: description, prediction, or evaluation (Law & Letts, 1989). A descriptive ADL instrument presents a picture of a person's status at one moment in time and permits comparison with other persons. A predictive ADL sets criteria against which a person's status is compared; an evaluative instrument measures a person's status over time in order to detect any changes in ADL ability (Kirsher & Guyatt, 1985). The Index of ADL (Katz & Akpom, 1976), first developed in 1959 and first published in 1963 (Katz, Ford, Moskowitz, Jackson, & Jaffe, 1963), often is regarded as the "gold standard" of ADL scales. This predictive ordinal scale measures self-care categories of bathing, dressing, toilet use, transferring, continence, and feeding. These categories are hierarchical, in that the ability to bathe independently is the first activity to be affected among the physically impaired, whereas feeding oneself is the last to be affected. The Index of ADL can be used to measure a person's baseline independence or dependence and helps to classify a person as "frail elderly" or "well elderly," depending on the degree of dependence demonstrated by responses to this scale. The components of the Katz ADL and several other selected instruments used in outcomes research in the elderly are outlined in Table 12.1.

Comorbidity Indices

Evaluating the number and type of comorbidities possessed by an individual at the time of hospital admission helps to explain the synergistic relationship of chronic illness conditions and functional status (Greenfield, Bianco, Elashoff, & Ganz, 1987; Mick & Ackerman, 1997). Unless an adjustment is made for the presence of comorbidities, any apparent age bias in clinical decision-making is a reflection of an assumption of poorer general health of older versus younger patients (Greenfield et al., 1987; Mick & Ackerman, 1997). Comorbidity scales are thought to contribute significant additional information to that obtained by illness severity measures and, in doing so, enhance the explanatory power of chronic illness conditions on outcomes from critical illness among elderly patients (Mick & Ackerman, 1997).

Functional Status

Measurement of functional status originated in rehabilitation clinical practice and is a key element in geriatric evaluation. Scales for functional assessment were devised as a means to measure performance, for determination of disability, and as an integral part of clinical management (Frey, 1984). In view of decreased physiological reserves, the older patient is at risk for a significant decline in functional status as a result of acute illness (Hirsch, Sommers, Olsen, Mullen, & Winograd, 1990). Diminished functional capacity may go unrecognized in many older patients, resulting in a potential for increased economic as well as psychological costs of hospitalization via increased length of stay or discharge to a dependent level of care (Hirsch et al., 1990).

Preserving Function While Hospitalized

Frail older adults who are "living on the edge" with marginal functional capacity are at risk for falling off that edge into a cascade of functional decline when admitted to the hospital (St. Pierre, 1998). The decrease in physiological reserve associated with normal aging makes older adults vulnerable to rapid decompensation when faced with catastrophic illnesses. Documented risk factors for in-hospital functional decline include preexisting chronic illnesses, immobility, sleep disturbance, uncontrolled pain, and malnutrition (Bossenmaier, 1982; Fretwell, 1993; Murray et al., 1993). Geriatric syndromes such as impaired gait and balance, falls, incontinence, delirium, and polypharmacy can be causes or effects of functional impairment (St. Pierre, 1998; Tinetti, Inouye, Gill, & Doucette, 1995). Any of these conditions may be associated with increased length of stay, increased morbidity, a need for home care services after discharge, or nursing home placement. Nursing's key role in preventing functional impairment in the hospital and improving posthospital functional outcomes lies in measurement and documentation of baseline function and systematic assessment and intervention to identify risk factors and prevent adverse outcomes.

ISSUES RELATED TO OUTCOME ASSESSMENT IN THE ELDERLY

Aside from determining which outcome measures to use, other issues related to conducting outcome assessments in the elderly relate to instrument selection and study methodology. Because these are key factors that will influence the results of an outcomes assessment, careful attention should be paid to both instrument selection and the study design.

Selecting Appropriate Outcome Instruments

There are many sources for identifying outcome measures, including regulatory agencies (National Commission on Quality Assurance, Joint Commission on Accreditation of Hospital Organizations), government sources (Agency for Health Care Policy and Research), specialty outcome groups, outcome measures manuals, and the literature on outcomes and Internet sources (Kleinpell, 1997). Several books exist that focus on outcome measurement and instruments designed for use with elderly populations (Feasley et al., 1996; George & Bearon, 1980; Kane & Kane, 1981). Specialty groups such as Health Outcomes Institute/Stratis Health (http://www.stratishealth.org), the Medical Outcomes Trust (http://www.outcomes-trust.org/instruments), the Picker Institute (http://www.picker.org), and QualityMetrics (http://www.qmetric.com) can serve as sources for instruments that have been used with elderly persons (SF-36 and specialty condition outcome tools). Several Internet compilations of tools exist that can also provide access to a variety of outcome instruments. Examples include MERLIN (http://laurel.lso.missouri.edu/) and ERIC (http://ericae.net/) (Kleinpell & Weiner, 1999).

Issues to consider in instrumentation selection for the elderly include reliability, validity, sources of error, readability, and clarity in wording. Reliability and validity are fundamental properties of an instrument (Rasin, 1997). Reliability, or consistency of measurement, and validity or the degree to which an instrument measures a concept, are essential psychometric properties. Validity testing validates an instrument with a specific group and not the instrument itself (Rasin, 1997). Therefore, any instrument used with the elderly must be validated for use with elderly populations. Reliability testing is also essential, particularly with instruments not specifically developed and used on elderly subjects. As George and Bearon (1980) relate, when unreliable measures are used, a study will lack significance. One reason that some tools may lack reliability and validity for older persons is that standards might have been established on younger persons (Gueldner & Hanner, 1989). A number of tools exist that do have established reliability and validity with use in elderly persons (see Table 12.1). Psychometrically sound instruments are essential for outcomes research in the elderly if the data collected are to be accurate and meaningful (Rasin, 1997).

Measurement Issues

Sources of error can influence both reliability and validity. Random error threatens measurement reliability and systematic error threatens validity (Rasin, 1997). Sources of error that are of particular importance in studies with the elderly include physiological age changes, readability, and clarity in wording. Physiological age changes include primary age changes that result from the aging process and secondary age changes that result from disease processes (Rasin, 1997).

Primary age changes that can influence measurement in the elderly include vision changes and hearing problems (Foreman, 1997). For interview or qualitative studies, questions directed to elderly subjects should be asked slowly and clearly. Verification of question meaning can also be used to ensure understanding. For questionnaire studies, several strategies can be incorporated to facilitate accurate responses from elderly subjects. The use of large print size, black and white type rather than letter coloring, nonglossy paper, printing of text on only one side of the page, use of adequate white space and vertical flow pattern response choices are factors to consider in questionnaire design to help aid instrument administration. If several tools are being used, pilot testing of the questionnaire packet can help to ensure that questions are clearly outlined and that the packet is user friendly (Kleinpell, 2000). Timing how long it takes pilot test subjects to complete a questionnaire packet is also helpful in determining if changes need to be made to decrease response burden.

Fatigue, frailty, and the need for proxy respondents are issues related to secondary age changes that should also be considered when assessing outcomes in the elderly (Bowsher, Bramlett, Burnside, & Gueldner, 1993; Rasin, 1997). Fatigue is an important consideration for outcomes research in the elderly. Because many elderly tire easily, measures to minimize fatigue, such as pacing questionnaire administration, allowing for breaks, and ensuring adequate room temperature and lighting, can help to minimize fatigue. Limited experience with questionnaires can also make it difficult for the elderly to record accurate written responses (Gueldner & Hanner, 1989). Researchers may need to hire assistants to help subjects who require special attention because of problems with hearing, vision, or writing (Burnside, Preski, & Hertz, 1998). The use of proxy respondents such as a spouse or family member may need to be considered as an option for some elderly subjects. However, the issue of tool administration variation as a source of measurement error in these conditions needs to be considered (Burnside et al., 1998). Research with elderly subjects has found that the elderly tend to overestimate functional abilities, whereas relatives tend to underrate their capabilities (Rubenstein, Schairer, Wieland, & Kane, 1984).

Additional Issues

Readability and clarity of wording are crucial elements to consider in the design and administration of research tools for use with the elderly. Demographic data from studies with the elderly indicate a wide spread in educational levels (Burnside et al., 1998). Determining the readability of a questionnaire is essential prior to use and can provide an objective assessment of the level of item difficulty. Because low readability of items will influence validity, the researcher must estimate the mean educational level of the elderly population of interest to ensure that measurement procedures are neither too difficult nor too basic (Rasin, 1997).

Instrument clarity can be compromised if instructions are not clear or if the instrument is not appropriate for an elderly population (Burnside et al., 1998). Concise and clear directions are essential. Other issues include the measurement of recall. Because memory loss is a common problem for the elderly, several methods may need to be used to obtain recall information (Burnside et al., 1998).

Many factors can have an impact on the reliability and validity of studies being conducted with the elderly, and special attention needs to be given to issues pertaining to instrument appearance, length, readability, and clarity.

Study Methodology

No one set of research designs or methods is uniquely suited for outcomes research (Cherkin, 1992). Several methods to study outcomes include randomized clinical trials, cross-sectional and longitudinal research design, continuous quality monitoring, and clinical practice improvement. An integrated approach to outcomes research that includes domain analysis (structure, process, outcome), evaluation analysis (individual, subunit, organizational), and focus evaluation (outcomes, quality, effectiveness) has been proposed as a comprehensive framework for outcomes research (Marks, Salyer, & Geddes, 1997).

Randomized clinical trials are the preferred study method when comparing treatments or intervention effects. However, they may not always be feasible in the clinical setting. Although cross-sectional studies can enable the study of large samples of subjects, they are limited in their generalizability. Longitudinal studies may be preferred to study changes in outcome measures in the elderly, such as functional status or ADLs. Yet factors such as recurrent illness, rehospitalizations, mortality and subject attrition are issues in longitudinal studies (Kleinpell, 2000). The choice of a research design for an outcomes study in the elderly will be determined by the study purpose and goals.

INTERVENTION RESEARCH RELATED TO OUTCOMES IN THE ELDERLY

Outcome studies examining the impact of interventions for the elderly have focused on a variety of interventions, including discharge planning for the elderly (Naylor et al., 1994), health promotion programs (Heidrich, 1998), acute confusion in hospital and acute care settings (Cronin-Stubbs, 1996), home-based mental health care services for the elderly (Horton-Deutsch, Farran, Loukissa, & Fogg, 1997), use of comprehensive geriatric day hospital care (Morishita et al.,1989), long-term care delivery model of care (Eng, Pedulla, Eleazer, McCann, & Fox, 1997), interventions for cognitive impairment in older adults (Cronin-Stubbs, 1997), home follow-up of hospitalized elders with heart failure (Naylor et al., 1999), and psychosocial nursing interventions provided to geriatric inpatients (Farran, Horton-Deutsch, Meyer, & Bourgard, 1998).

Outcome parameters explored in studies of the elderly have included mortality rates, changes in health-service usage, use of institutional care, functional status, health status, quality of life, ADLs, residential status after hospitalization, social function, emotional behavior, home management, self-care, satisfaction with care, appropriate medication use, rehospitalization rates, hospitalization days, and caregiver burden (Campion, Mulley, Goldstein, Barnett, & Thibault, 1981; Chelluri, Pinski, & Grenvik, 1992; Eng et al., 1997; Le Gall et al., 1982; Naylor et al., 1999; Rauckhorst, 1989; Sage et al., 1987).

Several issues that need to be addressed in conducting intervention research in the elderly include recruitment, retention, and ethical concerns. Personal contact, newspaper and radio advertisement, and flyer distribution at senior centers, community centers, and churches have been identified as successful recruitment strategies for elderly subjects (Bowsher et al., 1993; Gueldner & Henner, 1989). Attrition rates for the elderly have been cited to be higher than for younger subjects participating in research (Bowsher et al., 1993). General retention measures such as adequate communication, participant reward, and monetary or gift incentives have been identified as useful for retention of elderly subjects. Unwillingness to sign a consent form and ensuring cognitive understanding of study components are ethical issues that also need to be addressed when planning and conducting intervention research in the elderly.

Although a variety of outcome studies and measures have been used in interventional research related to outcomes in the elderly, insufficient data on the effects of illness, health-care treatment, interventions, and the trajectory of chronic illness and aging exist. Additional research that explores the responses of general and specific groups of elderly, selected comorbid and chronic illness states, specific interventions for the elderly, and concise strategies for enlisting and retaining elderly subjects in outcomes research remains to be done.

THE FUTURE OF OUTCOMES RESEARCH

The challenges of the future for outcomes research on the elderly are already apparent. Although the aging of individuals and the presence of people living into their 80's and 90's may not be new, this circumstance is becoming increasingly common. As the aging population grows, health promotion and disease prevention and treatment will continue to be priorities in health care for the elderly. Research is needed on the outcomes of care for the elderly to provide accurate data on the elderly. In 1994, the Hastings Center released a statement asserting that "the collection and dissemination of data on the elderly and on social and economic trends that affect their well-being is a role that only government can fill" (Joint International Research Group of the Institute for Bioethics, 1994, p. S4). Nurses and other allied health professionals are in a prime position to fulfill this role. Collaboration with economists as well as with social scientists and public policy experts is realistic and necessary to fully operationalize the process of this type of research. Related areas for research include the effect of treatment on survival, examination of outcomes by diagnostic group, and cost-benefit analyses related to inpatient physical rehabilitation prior to discharge, as well as analyses of inhome physical therapy as an alternative to extended inpatient stays. Study findings have demonstrated that optimal mental health and functioning depend on physical health and functioning. Discharge planning, which incorporates continuing social services contact, will help to ensure that opportunities for both social and physical activity via links to senior centers and adult day services are made available.

Additionally, the traditional health care delivery system may not be able to meet the diverse needs of the aging population (Raukhorst, 1989). It has been proposed that the emphasis on health-related outcomes should be patient centered because the patient is the best judge of outcomes (Davies et al., 1994). Thus far, a predominance of objective indicators have been used in outcomes research in the elderly. Additional studies that include subjective evaluations of outcomes in the elderly are also needed.

As the health care system continues to change, and as the elderly population continues to grow, the importance of conducting outcomes research in the elderly will only escalate. Much work is needed before the state of outcomes research in the elderly is adequate enough to enable informed decision making on health-care issues for the elderly.

REFERENCES

American Association of Retired Persons. (2000). A profile of older Americans: 2000 [On-line]. Available: http://www.aoa.dhhs.gov/aoa/stats/profile/default.htm

Blanchette, P. L. (1995). Age-based rationing of health care. *Hawaii Medical Journal, 54,* 507–509.

Bossenmaier, M. (1982). The hospitalized elderly: A first look. *Geriatric Nursing, 3,* 253–256.

Bowsher, J., Bramlett, M., Burnside, I., & Gueldner, S. (1993). Methodological considerations in the study of frail elderly people. *Journal of Advanced Nursing, 18,* 873–879.

Brun-Buisson, C., Doyon, F., Carlet, J., Dellamonica, P., Gouin, F., Lepoutre, A., Mercier, J. C., Offenstadt, G., & Regnier, B. (1995). Incidence, risk factors, and outcome of severe sepsis and septic shock in adults. *Journal of the American Medical Association, 274* (12), 968–974.

Burnside, I., Preski, S., & Hertz, J. (1998). Research instrumentation and elderly subjects. *Image, 30* (2), 185–190.

Campion, E., Mulley, A., Goldstein, R., Barnett, O., & Thibault, G. (1981). Medical intensive care for the elderly. *Journal of the American Medical Association, 246,* 2052–2056.

Chelluri, L., Pinsky, M., & Grenvik, A. (1992). Outcome of intensive care of the "oldest-old" critically ill patients. *Critical Care Medicine, 20,* 757–761.

Chelluri, L., Pinsky, M. R., Donahoe, M. P., & Grenvik, A. (1993). Long-term outcome of critically ill patients requiring intensive care. *Journal of the American Medical Association, 269,* 3119–3123.

Cherkin, D. (1992). Methods and measurement in patient outcomes research: Universal issues. In *Patient outcomes research: Examining the effectiveness of nursing practice.* Proceedings of the State of the Science Conference sponsored by the National Center for Nursing Research. (NIH Publication No. 93-3411, pp. 154–158). Washington, DC: U.S. Department of Health and Human Services, Public Health Service, National Institutes of Health.

Cronin-Stubbs, D. (1996). Delirium intervention research in acute care settings. *Annual Review of Nursing Research, 14,* 57–73.

Cronin-Stubbs, D. (1997). Interventions for cognitive impairment and neurobehavioral disturbances of older adults. *Annual Review of Nursing Research, 15,* 35–56.

Davies, A., Doyle, M., Lansky, D., Rutt, W., Orsolits, S., & Doyle, J. (1994). Outcomes assessment in clinical settings: A consensus statement on principles and best practices in project management *Joint Commission Journal on Quality Improvement, 20* (1), 6–16.

Eng, C., Pedulla, J., Eleazer, G., McCann, R., & Fox, N. (1997). Program of all-inclusive care for the elderly (pace): An innovative model of integrated geriatric care and financing. *Journal of the American Geriatric Society, 45,* 223–232.

ERIC Clearinghouse on Assessment and Evaluation [On-line]. Available: http://ericae.net/

Farran, C., Horton-Deutsch, S., Meyer, P., & Bourgard, L. (1998). Quantifying psychosocial nursing interventions provided to geriatric inpatients. *Outcomes Management for Nursing Practice, 2,* 167–173.

Feasley, J., and the Committee to Develop an Agenda for Health Outcomes Research for Elderly People. (1996). *Health outcomes for older people: Questions for the coming decade.* Institute of Medicine. Washington, DC: National Academy Press.

Ferrans, C., & Powers, M. (1985). Quality of Life Index: Development and psychometric properties. *Advances in Nursing Science, 8* (1), 15–24.

Ferrans, C. E. (1990). Quality of life: Conceptual issues. *Seminars in Oncology Nursing, 6,* 248–254.

Fillenbaum, C., & Smyer, M. (1981). The development, validity, and reliability of the OARS multidimensional functional assessment questionnaire. *Journal of Gerontology, 36,* 428–434.

Foreman, M. D. (1997) Measuring cognitive status. In M. Frank-Stromborg & S. J. Olsen (Eds.), *Instruments for clinical health-care research* (2nd ed., pp. 86–113). Boston: Jones and Bartlett.

Fretwell, M. D. (1993). Prevention of functional decline in older hospitalized patients. *Rhode Island Medicine, 76,* 13–18.

Frey, W. D. (1984). Functional assessment in the '80s. In A. S. Halpern & M. J. Fuhrer (Eds.), *Functional assessment in rehabilitation* (pp. 11–43). Baltimore, MD: Brookes.

George, L., & Bearon, L. (1980). *Quality of life in older persons,* New York: Human Sciences.

Greenfield, S., Bianco, D. M., Elashoff, R. M., & Ganz, P. A. (1987). Patterns of care related to age of breast cancer patients. *Journal of the American Medical Association, 257,* 2766–2770.

Gueldner, S., & Hanner, M. (1989). Methodological issues related to gerontological nursing research. *Nursing Research, 38,* 183–185.

Hamel, M. B., Phillips, R. S., Teno, J. M., Lynn, J., Galanos, A. N., Davis, R. B., Connors, A. F., Oye, R. K., Desbiens, N., Reding, D. J., & Goldman, L. (1996). Seriously ill hospitalized adults: Do we spend less on older patients? *Journal of the American Geriatrics Society, 44,* 1043–1048.

Hamel, M. B., Teno, J. M., Goldman, L., Lynn, J., Davis, R. B., Galanos, A. N., Desbiens, N., Connors, A. F., Wenger, N., & Phillips, R. S. (1999). Patient age and decisions to withhold life-sustaining treatments from seriously ill, hospitalized adults. *Annals of Internal Medicine, 130,* 116–125.

Heidrich, S. (1998). Health promotion in old age. *Annual Review of Nursing Research, 16,* 173–195.

Hirsch, C. H., Sommers, L., Olsen, A., Mullen, L., & Winograd, C. H. (1990). The natural history of functional morbidity in hospitalized elderly patients. *Journal of the American Geriatrics Society, 38,* 1296–1303.

Horton-Deutsch, S., Farran, C., Loukissa, D., & Fogg, L. (1997). Older adult recipients of home-based mental healthcare services: Who are these patients and what services do they receive? *Home Healthcare Nurse, 15,* 846–854.

Joint International Research Group of the Institute for Bioethics, Maastricht, the Netherlands, and the Hastings Center. (1994). What do we owe the elderly? Allocating social and health care resources. *Hastings Center Report, 24* (suppl.), 1–12.

Kane, R. (1997). *Understanding Health Care Outcomes Research.* Gaithersburg, MD: Aspen Publishers.

Kane, R., & Kane, R. (1981). *Assessing the elderly: A practical guide to measurement.* Lexington, MA: Lexington Books.

Katz, S., & Akpom, C. A. (1976). A measure of primary sociobiological functions. *International Journal of Health Services, 6,* 493–507.

Katz, S., Ford, A. B., Moskowitz, R. W., Jackson, B. A., & Jaffe, M. W. (1963). Studies of illness in the aged: The index of ADL: A standardized measure of biological and psychosocial function. *Journal of the American Medical Society, 185,* 915–919.

Kirsher, B., & Guyatt, G. (1985). A methodological framework for assessing health and disease. *Journal of Chronic Disease, 38,* 27–36.

Kleinpell, R. (1997). Whose outcomes? Patients, providers, or payers. *Nursing Clinics of North American, 32,* 513–520.

Kleinpell, R. (2000). Implementation strategies: Assessing outcomes in the elderly in acute care. *AACN Clinical Issues.*

Kleinpell, R., & Weiner, T. (1999). Assessing outcomes in advanced practice nursing. *AACN Clinical Issues, 10,* 356–368.

Law, M., & Letts, L. (1989). A critical review of scales of activities of daily living. *American Journal of Occupational Therapy, 43,* 522–528.

Le Gall, J., Brun-Buisson, C., Trunet, P., Latournerie, J., Chantereau, S., & Rapin, M. (1982). Influence of age, previous health status and severity of acute illness on outcome from intensive care. *Critical Care Medicine, 10,* 575–577.

Lohr, K. (1988). Outcomes measurement: Concepts and questions. *Inquire, 25,* 37–50.

Loewy, E. (1996). *Textbook of healthcare ethics.* New York: Plenum Press.

Ludwigs, U., & Hulting, J. (1995). Acute physiology and chronic health evaluation II scoring system in acute myocardial infarction: A prospective validation study. *Critical Care Medicine, 23,* 854–859.

Marks, B., Salyer, J., & Geddes, N. (1997). Outcomes research. *Nursing Clinics of North America, 32,* 589–602.

Mayer-Oakes, S. A., Oye, R. K., & Leake, B. (1991). Predictors of mortality in older patients following medical intensive care: The importance of functional status. *Journal of the American Geriatrics Society, 39,* 862–868.

MERLIN Online Public Access Catalog [On-line]. Available: http://laurel.lso.missouri.edu/

McDowell, I., & Newell, C. (1996). *Measuring health: A guide to rating scales and questionnaires.* New York: Oxford University Press.

Mick, D., & Ackerman, M. (1997). Neutralizing ageism in critical care via outcomes research. *AACN Clinical Issues, 8,* 597–608.

Mick, D. J. (in press). Physiological senescence: Effect on care of the traumatically injured and critically ill elderly patient. *Critical Care Nurse.*

Morishita, L., Siu, A., Wang, R., Oken, C., Cadogan, M., & Schwartzman, L. (1989). Comprehensive geriatric care in a day hospital: A demonstration of the British model in the united states. *Gerontologist, 29,* 336–340.

Murray, A. M., Levkoff, S. E., Wetle, T. T., Beckett, L., Cleary, P. D., Schor, J. D., Lipsitz, L. A., Rose, J. W., & Evans, D. A. (1993). Acute delirium and functional decline in the hospitalized elderly patient. *Journal of Gerontology, 48,* M181–M186.

Naylor, M., Brooten, D., Campbell, R., Jacobsen, B., Mezey, M., Pauly, M., & Schwartz, J. (1999). Comprehensive discharge planning and home follow-up of hospitalized elders: A randomized clinical trial. *Journal of the American Medical Association, 281* (7), 613–620.

Naylor, M., Brooten, D., Jones, R., Lavisso-Mourey, R., Mezey, M., & Pauly, M. (1994). Comprehensive discharge planning for the hospitalized elderly: A randomized clinical trial. *Annals of Internal Medicine, 120* (12), 999–1006.

Niskanen, M., & Niskanen, L. (1994). Is the acute physiology and chronic health evaluation (APACHE) scale ageist? *Drugs & Aging, 5* (3), 153–155.

Oye, R. K., & Bellamy, P. E. (1986). Assessing illness severity and outcome in critically ill patients. *Emergency Medical Clinics of North America, 4,* 623–633.

Padilla, G., & Frank-Stromborg, M. (1997). Single instruments for measuring quality of life. In M. Frank-Stromborg & S. J. Olsen (Eds.), *Instruments for health care research* (2nd ed., pp. 114–134). Boston: Jones and Bartlett Publishers.

Parkerson, G., Gehlback, S., Wagner, E., James, S., Clapp, N., & Muhlbaier, L. (1981). The Duke-UNC Health Profile. *Medical Care, 19* (8), 806–828.

Rasin, J. (1997). Measurement issues with the elderly. In M. Frank-Stromborg & S. J. Olsen (Eds.), *Instruments for clinical health-care research* (2nd ed., pp. 44–53). Boston: Jones and Bartlett.

Rauckhorst, L. (1989). Impact of a physician/nurse practitioner team primary care delivery model on selected geriatric long-term care outcomes. *Journal of Nursing Quality Assurance, 4* (1), 62–72.

Resnick, B. (1998). The critically ill older patient. In C. M. Hudak, B. M. Gallo, & P. G. Morton (Eds.)., *Critical care nursing: A holistic approach* (pp. 66–86). Philadelphia: Lippincott.

Richmond, T., McCorkle, R., Tulman, L., & Fawcett, J. (1997). Measuring function. In M. Frank-Stromborg & S. J. Olsen (Eds.)., *Instruments for health care research.* (2nd ed., pp 75–85). Boston: Jones and Bartlett.

Rubenstein, A., Schairer, C., Wieland, D., & Kane, R. (1984). Systemic bias in functional status assessment of elderly adults: Effects of different data sources. *Journal of Gerontology, 39,* 686–690.

Sage, W., Hurst, C., Silverman, J., & Bortz, W. (1987). Intensive care for the elderly: Outcome of elective and nonelective admissions. *Journal of American Geriatrics Society, 35,* 312–317.

St. Pierre, J. (1998). Functional decline in hospitalized elders: Preventive nursing measures. *AACN Clinical Issues, 9* (1), 109–118.

Tinetti, M. E., Inouye, S. K., Gill, T. M., & Doucette, J. T. (1995). Shared risk factors for falls, incontinence, and functional dependence: Unifying the approach to geriatric syndromes. *Journal of the American Medical Association, 273,* 1348–1353.

Titler, M. G., & Reiter, R. C. (1994). Outcomes measurement in clinical practice. *MedSurg Nursing, 3,* 395–420.

Wetle, T. (1987). Age as a risk factor for inadequate treatment [Editorial]. *Journal of the American Medical Association, 258,* 516.

13

Discharge Planning: Design and Implementation

Mary Naylor, Kathryn Bowles,
Roberta L. Campbell, and
Kathleen M. McCauley

The treatment of elders hospitalized for an acute, often critical, condition is frequently complicated by the coexistence of multiple chronic diseases as well as numerous psychosocial, environmental, and financial problems. Elders with such complex issues are posing a significant challenge to health care providers. First, health care professionals must address the immediate health care needs of these individuals whose hospitalizations are generally the result of an exacerbation of one or more chronic illnesses. Second, providers must maximize the limited time they have to position these patients and their families to more effectively manage the patient's health problems and prevent or minimize the need for future hospitalizations. This chapter is designed to assist nurses and other health care professionals in addressing this later challenge. We will present a number of strategies to assist health care professionals in their efforts to improve the quality of care, promote access to services and information, and reduce the use of costly and inappropriate health care resources. We will emphasize strategies and innovative models of care that promote accurate identification of patients in need of postdischarge referrals and facilitate overcoming barriers to continuity of care.

PATIENT FACTORS CONTRIBUTING TO POOR OUTCOMES

Clinical Factors

In their study involving elders hospitalized for a common medical or surgical condition, Naylor and colleagues found that patients had, on average, five active medical diagnoses (Naylor, Brooten, Campbell, et al., 1999). Similarly, Rich and colleagues learned that more than two thirds of the hospitalized elders who participated in their heart failure management study had hypertension and one third suffered from diabetes (Rich, Beckham, Wittenberg, et al., 1995). The coexistence of several health problems increases the risk of hospitalization in the population of older adults. One group of investigators found that 42% of elders discharged from the hospital with seven or more chronic conditions were readmitted within 2 months (Holloway, Thomas, & Shapiro, 1988).

Somewhat related to the presence of multiple comorbid conditions is the increased tendency of elders to develop complications that result in longer hospital stays. Elders, age 70 and older who underwent coronary artery bypass surgery had longer lengths of stay than younger patients did. Although elders had significantly more serious preoperative health problems such as heart failure or cerebrovascular disease, the main causative factor was an increased tendency to develop atrial fibrillation (Paone, Higgins, Havstad, & Silverman, 1998).

Specific diagnostic or clinical variables found to be predictive of rehospitalization within 90 days include heart failure, diabetes mellitus, hypertension, chronic obstructive pulmonary disease, systolic blood pressure below 115 mm Hg, a white blood cell count equal to or greater than 12,000/mm^3, serum sodium >139 mmol/L, and a blood urea nitrogen >30 mg/dL (Ashton, Kuykendall, Johnson, Wray, & Wu, 1995; Burns & Nichols, 1991; Hennen, Krumholz, Radford, & Meehan, 1995; Rich et al., 1995; Smith, Katz, Huster, et al., 1996).

Other Health Factors

In addition to clinical factors, empirical evidence links emotional status, cognitive status, self-reported health, functional status, and perceived quality of life to poor outcomes among hospitalized elders (Happ, Naylor, & Roe-Prior, 1997). Emotional conditions such as anxiety and depression and cognitive impairments such as dementia and delirium have been associated with significantly longer lengths of stay for older patients (Fulop, Strain, Fahs, Schmeidler, & Snyder, 1998). In this study, cognitive impairment was the variable most predictive of prolonged hospitalization.

Elders who rate their overall health as fair or poor were found to be twice as likely to be readmitted to a hospital (Holloway, Thomas, & Shapiro, 1988; Naylor et al., 1999). A poor self-health rating was significantly correlated with the presence of multiple chronic diseases and perceived functional status impairment in a large sample of Medicare beneficiaries (Holloway, Thomas, & Shapiro, 1988).

At 2 weeks post discharge, Naylor and colleagues found a potential link between a decline in patients' functional status and an increase in hospital readmissions (Naylor, Brooten, Jones, et al., 1994). Depression was predictive of rehospitalizations among older patients with heart disease (Levine, Covino, Slack, et al., 1996). Konstram and colleagues found that participants in the Left Ventricular Dysfunction clinical trials who reported poorer quality of life had a greater number of hospital readmissions and increased mortality rates compared with those who reported a higher quality of life (Konstam, Salem, Pouleur, et al., 1996). Similarly, Rosswurm and Lanham (1998) found that impaired functional ability and a greater number of unresolved health problems at hospital discharge, notably pain and activity and exercise limitations, were predictive of emergency department visits and rehospitalizations.

Similar to Holloway's team (1988), who demonstrated that a combination of factors were linked to readmission, Naylor and colleagues (1994) demonstrated that one or more of the following factors contributed to poor outcomes among a group of elders hospitalized for medical or surgical cardiac conditions: age 80 or older, moderate to severe functional impairment, history of depression, inadequate or inaccessible social support, chronic problems requiring multiple medications or other therapies, fair to poor self-health rating, history of nonadherence to therapies, and history of recent hospitalizations.

PATIENT CHARACTERISTICS AND REFERRALS FOR POSTDISCHARGE FOLLOW-UP

There is little understanding of the patient characteristics that should be considered in guiding discharge referral decisions (Arenth & Marmon, 1995; Pohl, Collins, & Given, 1995; Prescott, Soeken, & Briggs, 1995). Prescott and colleagues found that although the decision not to refer for home care was appropriate in 93% of cases studied, clinicians failed to refer 26% of the sample for whom home care was needed. The findings of several studies focusing on sociodemographic differences associated with referrals for follow-up following hospital discharge serve to highlight this point.

Diwan, Berger, and Manns (1997) found that patients living with a spouse or caregiver were less than half as likely to be referred for skilled nursing or home health than were those with nonspouse caregivers. After controlling for a number of factors, Black elders were found to receive significantly fewer hours of formal home care services after hospital discharge compared with a comparable sample of white elders (Chadiha, Proctor, Morrow-Howell, Darkwa, & Dore, 1995). Women with the same activities of daily living (ADL) limitations as men were much less likely to be referred for home health follow-up (Pohl, Collins, & Given, 1995). These investigators argue that the referral process is guided by a medical model and thus fails to consider the larger context of patients and families. Findings of these studies suggest that even this model is inconsistently applied.

A number of studies have attempted to facilitate identification of patients in need of follow-up after discharge either by identifying patient characteristics most associated with this need (Evans & Hendricks, 1993; Rosswurm & Lanhan, 1998; Solomon et al., 1993) or by developing instruments to predict such needs (Garrard, Bryan, Dowd, Dorsey, & Shapiro, 1987; Pacala, Boult, Reed, & Alberti, 1997). Solomon and colleagues (1993), for example, described four independent predictors of the need for home care, including education < 12 years, less accessible social support, impairment in at least one instrumental ADL, and prior home care use. Bull (1994a) revealed that predischarge functional ability and age predicted home care use 2 weeks after discharge. Unfortunately, there is little consistency in the variables examined, and thus many questions about the cluster of characteristics that are predictive of need remain unanswered. Even when key characteristics are identified, nurses and other health care professionals often fail to appropriately refer patients for home care services (Rosswurm & Lanham, 1998).

The unique needs of hospitalized elders were highlighted in a qualitative study conducted by Ekman, Lundman, and Norberg (1999). These investigators found that although these patients were confident in the ability of health care professionals to manage their illnesses, the hospitalization experience was distressing because of its unpredictability and the inability of these elders to comprehend what was happening. All patients reported experiencing rejection by health care providers at times when they needed help. The focus on the disease during the hospitalization diminished the attention providers paid to the patient's illness experience. A critical component of effective inpatient care and discharge planning must be active attention to the elder as an individual.

HEALTH CARE SYSTEM FACTORS CONTRIBUTING TO POOR OUTCOMES

Continuity of care, recognized as essential to positive outcomes for hospitalized elders, has been defined as the "coordination of the delivery of ongoing health care services over time and across a variety of setting and providers" (Anderson & Helms, 1998, p. 386). Studies have demonstrated that a lack of continuous care contributes to poor outcomes. For example, in their study of more than 1000 patients discharged with a primary diagnosis of heart failure, Martens and Mellor (1997) found that those receiving home care nursing services following hospital discharge had significantly fewer readmissions within 90 days of hospital discharge.

Communication, a critical component of patient care coordination, has been found to be both inefficient and inadequate (Trella, 1994; Worth, Tierney, & Lockerbie, 1994). A number of factors have been linked to problems with communication including poor documentation (Howse & Bailey, 1992; Trella, 1994; Worth et al., 1994), limited use of available technology (Patterson, Blehm, Foster, Fuglee, & Moore, 1995), and conflicts over control of patient information and lack of administrative support (Christiansen, Warrick, Netting, et al., 1991). The findings of a study conducted to describe the influence of selected organizational and medical factors on communication between hospitals and extended care facilities (ECFs) in the referral of elderly patients following discharge revealed that hospitals transferred about three fourths of the patient care data recommended in the literature (Anderson & Helms, 1998). Referrals were more complete if generated from large hospitals and specialty care units and if sent to proprietary ECFs.

Adequate discharge planning is essential to ensure continuity of care. Potthoff, Kane, and Franco (1995) described discharge planning as a complex process of decision making focused on assessment and need identification, selection of agencies, and implementation and evaluation of the plan. Inadequate discharge planning for hospitalized elders can result in what Estes and Swan (1993) describe as the "no-care zone." Care of patients with complex needs is rapidly transferred to informal caregivers who are often unprepared to address these needs.

Bull and Kane (1996) found that gaps in communication were a fundamental source of inadequate discharge planning. Additionally, problems in the identification of patients' needs; role confusion; fragmentation; and lack of knowledge, time, and other resources have been identified as significant barriers to adequate discharge planning for hospitalized elders (Anderson & Helms, 1994; Bull & Kane, 1996; McWilliam & Sangster, 1994; Pottoff, Franco, & Kane, 1995). The absence of standardized assessment criteria and discharge planning guidelines has been defined as contributing factors to the lack of coordinated care (Clemens & Hayes, 1997; Oktay, Steinwachs, Mamon, Done, & Fahey, 1992).

The ability to address the needs of elders across a continuum of healthcare settings is certainly influenced by Medicare's reimbursement for services. For example, Medicare requires that home care services following hospital discharge must be reasonable, necessary, and intermittent based on an assessment of individual needs. Eligible patients must be homebound, under the care of a physician, and in need of skilled nursing care or physical, speech, or occupational therapy. A serendipitous finding in a study conducted by Naylor and colleagues (1999) was that 56% of a group of hospitalized elders who met at least one of the criteria associated with poor outcomes were discharged without formal home follow-up. Some of these "high risk" patients were ineligible for such services because they were not "homebound."

CURRENT AND EMERGING STRATEGIES
TO IMPROVE PATIENT OUTCOMES

The difficulty of managing the care of hospitalized elders at high risk for poor postdischarge outcomes has prompted the development of alternative management systems that address the unique needs of these patients. Among the strategies tested have been geriatric interdisciplinary teams, clinical guidelines, clinical pathways, disease management, case management, discharge planning, and transitional care.

Geriatric Interdisciplinary Teams or Units

In their review of research studies published in 1988, Schmitt and colleagues described the challenging conceptual and methodological problems faced by researchers who attempted to examine the effects of interdisciplinary teams. These problems ranged from research designs that did not adequately control for threats to internal validity to the selection of appropriate outcomes to assess the effects of the team's interventions. Many of these same problems are evident in more recent work. For example, the value of a geriatric consultative team in improving outcomes for elders may have been affected by contamination in a recent study (Slaets, Kaufmann, Duivenvooden, Pelemans, & Schudel, 1997).

Positive outcomes have been demonstrated by some geriatric team interventions. Consultation by a geriatric inpatient team resulted in significant reductions in hospital admissions and lower death rates at 6 months post discharge (Thomas, Brahan, & Heywood, 1993). A team intervention that included a geriatrician with geropsychiatric training resulted in improved independence of patients at discharge, shorter lengths of hospital stay on both index admissions and readmissions within 6 months, and fewer readmissions to nursing homes within the first year after discharge (Slaets et al., 1997). A cost savings of approximately $3000 per patient was demonstrated in the intervention group. The testing of a geriatric team intervention involving telephone follow-up resulted in beneficial effects for caregivers (Silliman, McGarvey, Raymond, & Fretwell, 1990). These investigators concluded that the intervention may have given caregivers a greater sense of mastery and self-confidence, resulting in improved health ratings. A few studies have focused on the testing of team interventions for specific patient groups. For example, using a preintervention, postintervention design, Gold and Bergman (1997) found that a geriatric consultation team was helpful in selecting appropriate sites for admission of elderly emergency department patients and in making recommendations for appropriate outpatient and community follow-up for nonadmitted patients.

Clinical Guidelines

Guidelines to assist in the evaluation and management of patients with complex health needs are increasingly available to providers. In 1989, the Agency for Healthcare Research and Quality (AHRQ) began the development of guidelines to health care providers to make appropriate care decisions. Clinicians can access information online at the National Guideline Clearinghouse (NGC) site at http://www.guideline.gov or link to it from the AHRQ site at http://www.ahrq.gov. The NGC allows the clinician to compare two or more guidelines side-by-side, to view syntheses of guidelines that indicate similarities and differences, and to link to full-text guidelines, where available. Guidelines have been developed for common health problems, such as unstable angina, heart failure, acute pain management, and so on. Some guidelines have been designed to facilitate treatment and stabilization of patients during the acute phase of illness; others provide recommendations for the care of such patients in both inpatient and outpatient settings. To date, there is little empirical evidence of the extent to which these guidelines influence the practice of physicians responsible for the care of older adults over an acute episode of illness, nor have published studies examined the adherence of nurses to clinical practice guidelines.

Clinical Pathways

Many clinical settings are now using pathways to guide clinical practice and promote quality care. Typically, pathways are developed by staff in a given hospital or other health care setting for a specific population and a given length of stay. Content areas include type and frequency of monitoring, treatments, diet, medications, activity and patient and family education. Most often, pathways guide care in only one setting (i.e., hospital admission through discharge). For example, clinical pathways to "fast track recovery" have been implemented for elderly coronary artery bypass patients. Despite a higher incidence of preoperative comorbid conditions, longer intubation times, and a greater incidence of postoperative atrial fibrillation in patients age 70 and older, Lee and colleagues demonstrated that the use of a pathway led to no differences in operative mortality rates when compared with younger patients (Lee, Swain, Andrey, Murrell, & Geha, 1999). Most elders were discharged from the intensive care unit on the day after the surgery; 35% were discharged before the 5th operative day. The report of this study failed to describe the adjustment and recovery period, although readmission rates of older patients were similar to those of younger patients.

Managed care has influenced the development of paths that span multiple settings over an extended time period. For example, a 12-month pathway has been developed to link the acute, recovery, rehabilitation, and maintenance phases of care for patients receiving interventional cardiology procedures (Doran, Sampson, Staus, Ahern, & Schiro, 1997). A clinical pathway was used to identify health-care patterns and problems for a group of cardiac surgical patients. Patients were found to have knowledge deficits in the areas of substance use (i.e., smoking cessation), nutrition, physical activity, and pain (Sampson & Doran, 1998). Although the authors suggested educational strategies to resolve these deficits, the study was not designed to evaluate the effectiveness of the pathway. In general, there is limited empirical evidence available regarding the actual use of clinical pathways or their effects on patient outcomes.

Disease Management

Disease management has been defined as the "systematic, population-based approach to identify persons at risk, intervene with specific programs of care, and measure clinical and other outcomes" (Epstein & Sherwood, 1996, p. 836). Disease management programs are generally designed for multidisciplinary use and targeted at patient populations with specific, common health conditions such as diabetes, asthma, congestive heart failure, and so on.

Evidence related to the effectiveness of disease management is just beginning to emerge. In a randomized clinical trial targeting elderly heart failure patients, Rich and colleagues (1995) tested the effects of conventional care supplemented by a nurse-directed interdisciplinary team with those achieved by conventional, physician-directed care alone. The intervention consisted of intensive patient education, dietary consultation, social service evaluation, medication review, and close follow-up after discharge by a home health specialist and study nurse. At 90 days post hospital discharge, the intervention group demonstrated the following outcomes compared with the control group: all cause readmissions were reduced by 56% ($p = 0.04$) and the number of patients experiencing multiple readmission was reduced by 61% ($p = 0.01$). Patients in the intervention group also experienced an improved quality of life and greater compliance with medications and diet than usual care patients. The cost analysis revealed a net per patient savings of $460.

Much more common are reports of preintervention or postintervention designs to evaluate the effects of disease management, particularly on health resource usage (Roglieri, Futtermahn, McDonough, et al., 1997). These efforts have consistently demonstrated reductions in costly hospitalizations compared with the preintervention phase, suggesting the potential of disease management in improving outcomes. Rigorous testing is the next logical step.

Case Management

Case management by nurses or others specially trained to coordinate the delivery of care to patients across settings may be an effective method to reduce fragmentation and improve patient and cost outcomes (Robinson, Mead, & Boswell, 1995; Zelle, 1995). Generally, case management describes a care coordination function, although the term has also been used to include the provision of direct care. Case managers may be nurses, social workers, therapists, or other health professionals.

The benefits of case management systems implemented by nurses for patients with chronic conditions such as hyperlipidemia (Becker, Raqueno, & Yook, 1998), hypertension (Pheley et al., 1995), and diabetes mellitus (Aubert, Herman, Waters, et al., 1998; Weinberger, Kirkman, Samson, et al., 1995) have been demonstrated. Nurse case management systems have also achieved positive effects on risk behaviors that contribute to exacerbations of chronic illnesses such as smoking and exercise (DeBusk, Miller, Superko, et al., 1994).

A successful model of case management by nurses was developed at Carondolet St. Mary's Hospital and Health Center to assist high-risk elders in accessing services in a timely manner (Lamb, 1992). The nurse case manager is at the center of the Nursing Network, an integrated system of nursing care. Network components include acute inpatient care, extended and long-term care, home care, hospice, and ambulatory care. An evaluation of the effects of this model revealed that elders cared for by case managers had greater confidence in self-care, improved symptom management and less frequent use of hospital and emergency services (Lamb, 1992).

The evidence in support of nurse-led case management systems, particularly for high-risk elders, is not all positive. Gagnon and colleagues conducted a randomized clinical trial (RCT) to examine the effects of a nurse case management intervention compared with usual care in a sample of frail, older adults living in Canada who were discharged from the emergency department (Gagnon, Schein, McVey, & Bergman, 1999). Study findings revealed that the intervention group was more likely to use emergency health services without a concomitant increase in health benefits such as improved quality of life, functional status, or even satisfaction with care.

There is tremendous variation in the design and services provided by case management systems. Many do not offer the comprehensive services required by elders (Fox, Wicks, & Newacheck, 1993; Harrington, Lynch, & Newcomer, 1993). Recommendations of case managers are sometimes not implemented by patients' physicians (Harrington et al., 1993). Many authors have recommended a multidisciplinary, case management model to ensure successful outcomes for patients requiring extended follow-up (Katz, 1993; Landefeld, Palmer, Kresevic, Fortinsky, & Kowal, 1995). Clearly, additional study of the effects of case management systems is warranted.

Discharge Planning

Effective discharge planning, which includes the design and implementation of an individualized plan to guide the transition from hospital to home or an extended care facility, has been demonstrated to be an effective method in promoting timely discharge and preventing poor postdischarge outcomes. Bull (1994b) conducted a qualitative study to obtain information on patients' and professionals' perspectives on quality. Study findings revealed that communication, a process that consisted of asking questions, getting answers, and questioning inconsistencies, was identified by both patients and professionals as a key component of successful discharge planning. Additionally, Bull, Hansen, and Gross (2000) reported that continuity of care and the extent to which older patients and family caregivers felt prepared to manage care following hospitalization were the best predictors of their satisfaction with discharge planning.

Despite the recognized importance of discharge planning, few studies have examined the ability of nurses to anticipate patients' postdischarge needs. Reiley and colleagues conducted an exploratory study to determine how well primary nurses predict the functional status of their patients 2 months after discharge and to assess whether patients and nurses agree about patients' understanding of the postdischarge treatment plan (Reiley, Iezzoni, Phillips, et al., 1996). Study findings revealed that nurses consistently underestimated the functional ability of their patients and overestimated patients' knowledge regarding their treatment plans. Cockram and colleagues found that the lack of referrals was due to the general nursing staff's limited expertise in disability assessment and in expediting patients' discharge (Cockram, Gibb, & Kalra, 1997). Nurses working on specialized care units had greater expertise in these areas, most likely because of interactions with specialized geriatric team members.

Care outcomes may be influenced by the hospital's model of discharge planning. Kelly and McClelland (1985), as cited in Anderson and Helms (1993), described a typology of discharge of five discharge planning models including primary nurse, discharge planner, liaison nurse, bedside staff, and multiprofessional collaboration. Anderson and Helms (1993) examined whether the hospital's discharge planning model affected the quantity and quality of communication about patients referred for home health care. Study results revealed that about half of the patient data recommended in the literature was actually transferred and most of the data were background in nature. Additionally, the discharge planning model used was found to make a difference in both the amount and the nature of data shared with liaison nurses providing the greatest amount of data. The researchers were careful to point out that although the models describe areas of responsibility, they are not operational in the traditional sense.

A number of studies have tested discharge planning innovations designed to improve patient outcomes. The findings of an RCT conducted by Evans and Hendricks (1993) revealed that a discharge planning intervention targeting high-risk patients increased the likelihood of a successful transition to home and decreased the likelihood of unscheduled readmissions through the 9-month study period. Similarly, an RCT conducted by Naylor and colleagues (1994) demonstrated the potential of a comprehensive discharge plan designed specifically for older adults and implemented by advanced practice nurses (APNs) in decreasing readmissions and associated costs for medical cardiac patients through 6 weeks post discharge. Findings from this study also demonstrated the potential of a more intensive, longer-term intervention for elders at high risk for poor outcomes.

Transitional Care

Transitional care generally refers to care and services that promote the safe and timely transfer of patients from one level of care to another (e.g., acute to subacute) or from one type of setting to another (e.g., hospital to home) (Happ, Naylor, & Roe-Prior, 1997). Unfortunately, there are few examples of empirically based models of transitional care.

In 1981, an interdisciplinary model of transitional care (comprehensive discharge planning and home follow-up) implemented by APNs was developed (Brooten, Brown, Munro, et al., 1988; Brooten, Munro, Roncoli, et al., 1989). This health care innovation was originally designed to enable earlier hospital discharge of vulnerable patients by substituting a portion of hospital care with transitional home follow-up by APNs. The model now focuses on improving postdischarge outcomes for vulnerable groups that are discharged following shortened lengths of hospital stays.

In contrast to most health care delivery systems, the use of the transitional care model with hospitalized elders uses state of the art interventions, relies on the professional judgment of clinical experts, and attempts to promote a strong patient-provider relationship and continuity of care from the hospital to patients' homes. To date, this model of care with hospitalized elders has been the focus of two completed RCTs and one ongoing National Institute of Nursing Research–funded RCT.

Recently, the findings of the second RCT were published (Naylor et al., 1999). This clinical trial examined the effectiveness of an APN-centered discharge planning and home follow-up intervention for elders at high risk for poor outcomes on patient and cost outcomes. The sample consisted of 363 elders hospitalized for a common medical or surgical condition who met at least one of the criteria found to be associated with poor outcomes in an earlier study. At 24 weeks after the index hospital discharge, control group patients were more likely to be readmitted at least once ($p < 0.001$). Fewer intervention patients had multiple readmissions ($p = 0.01$), and time to first readmission was increased in this group ($p < 0.001$). The intervention resulted in estimated per patient savings in postdischarge Medicare reimbursements of almost \$3000.

Findings from this study revealed that the protocol used by APNs was not sufficiently targeted to help elders with heart failure manage the multiple, disabling symptoms and difficult treatment regimens associated with this illness. The presence of poor general health behaviors and other comorbid conditions only added to the complex care needs of these elders. The testing of a comprehensive intervention targeted at this challenging patient group and implemented by APNs who are experienced in the care of elders with heart failure and who have the support of a multidisciplinary team is the focus of an ongoing RCT.

SUMMARY

In this chapter we have discussed clinical and other health factors that contribute to the complexity of care management for hospitalized elders. Studies have found that multiple, comorbid conditions, as well as specific diseases or biochemical alterations, can increase the risk of hospital readmission. Patients with physical, functional, or psychological impairments may also experience poor outcomes.

One important, and often underused, resource for positive patient outcomes is skilled home care. Continuity of care across settings is enhanced through a comprehensive needs assessment, timely discharge planning, individualized patient and family-focused care, and multidisciplinary communication and collaboration.

Nurses and other health care professionals can employ various strategies to improve the quality of care older patients and their families receive. Evidence-based practice may be promoted through the use of clinical guidelines or pathways, geriatric interdisciplinary teams, disease management, discharge planning, or case management. There is, however, limited empirical evidence about the effectiveness of these strategies to guide clinical decision making.

On the other hand, there is growing evidence that models of transitional care reduce fragmentation and improve patient and cost outcomes. Discharge planning and home follow-up implemented by APNs aimed at high-risk patients extended the time to first readmission, decreased multiple readmissions, and generated savings in Medicare reimbursements. Further testing of this model is needed with other populations of elders.

REFERENCES

Anderson, M. A., & Helms, L. B. (1993). An assessment of discharge planning models: Communication in referrals to home care. *Orthopedic Nursing, 12* (4), 41–49.

Anderson, M. A., & Helms, L. B. (1994). Quality improvement in discharge planning: An evaluation of factors in communication between health care providers. *Journal of Nursing Care Quality, 8* (2), 62–72.

Anderson, M. A., & Helms, L. B. (1998). Extended care referral after hospital discharge. *Research in Nursing and Health Care, 21,* 385–394.

Arenth, L. M., & Mamon, J. (1985). Determining patient needs after discharge. *Nursing Management, 16* (9), 20–24.

Ashton, C. M., Kuykendall, D. H., Johnson, M. L., Wray, N. P., & Wu, L. (1995). The association between the quality of inpatient care and early readmission. *Annals of Internal Medicine, 122,* 415–422.

Aubert, R. E., Herman, W. H., Waters, J., Moore, W., Sutton, D., Peterson, B. L., Bailey, C. M., & Koplan, J. P. (1998). Nurse case management to improve glycemic control in diabetic patients in a health maintenance organization: A randomized controlled trial. *Annals of Internal Medicine, 129,* 605–612.

Becker, D. M., Raqueno, J. V., & Yook, R. M. (1998). Nurse-mediated cholesterol management compared with enhanced primary care in siblings of individuals with premature coronary disease. *Archives of Internal Medicine, 158,* 1533–1539.

Brooten, D., Brown, L. P., Munro, B. H., York, R., Cohen, S. M., Roncoli, M. & Hollingsworth, A. (1988). Early discharge and specialist transitional care. *Image: Journal of Nursing Scholarship, 20,* 64–68.

Brooten, D., Munro, B. H., Roncoli, M., Arnold, L., Brown, L. P., York, R., Hollingsworth, A., Cohen, S., & Rubin, M. (1989). Developing a program grant for use in model testing. *Nursing and Health Care, 10,* 314–318.

Bull, M. J. (1994a). Use of formal community services by elders and their family caregivers two weeks following hospital discharge. *Journal of Advanced Nursing, 19,* 503–508.

Bull, M. J. (1994b). Patients' and professionals' perceptions of quality in discharge planning. *Journal of Nursing Care Quality, 8* (2), 47–61.

Bull, M. J., Hansen, H. E., & Gross, C. R. (2000). Predictors of Satisfaction with Discharge Planning for Elders with Heart Failure and Their Family Caregivers. *Journal of Cardiovascular Nursing, 14* (3), 76–87.

Bull, M., & Kane, R. L. (1996). Gaps in discharge planning. *Journal of Applied Gerontology, 15,* 486–500.

Burns, R., & Nichols, L. O. (1991). Factors predicting readmission of older general medicine patients. *Journal of General Internal Medicine, 6,* 389–393.

Chadiha, L. A., Proctor, E. K., Morrow-Howell, N., Darkwa, O. K., & Dore, P. (1995). Post-hospital home care for African-American and White elderly. *Gerontologist, 35,* 233–239.

Christianson, J. B., Warrick, L. H., Netting, F. E., Williams, F. G., Read, W., & Murphy, J. (1991). Hospital case management: Bridging acute and long-term care. *Health Affairs, 10,* 173–184.

Clemens, E. L., & Hayes, H. E. (1997). Assessing and balancing elder risk, safety and autonomy: Decision-making practices of health care professionals. *Home Health Care Services Quarterly, 16* (3), 3–21.

Cockram, A., Gibb, R., & Kalra, L. (1997). The role of a specialist team in implementing continuing health care guidelines in hospitalized patients. *Age & Aging, 26,* 211–216.

DeBusk, R. F., Miller, N. H., Superko, H. R., Dennis, C. A., Thomas, R. J., Lew, H. T., Berger, W. E., Heller, R. S., Rompf, J., Gee, D., Kraemer, H. C., Bandura, A., Ghandour, G., Clark, M., Shah, R. V., Fisher, L., & Taylor, C. B. (1994). A case management system for coronary risk factor modification following acute myocardial infarction. *Annals of Internal Medicine, 120,* 721–729.

Diwan, S., Berger, C., & Manns, E. K. (1997). Composition of the home care service package—predictors of type, volume, and mix of services provided to poor and frail older people. *Gerontologist, 37,* 169–181.

Doran, K., Sampson, B., Staus, R., Ahern, C., & Schiro, D. (1997). Clinical pathway across tertiary and community care after an interventional cardiology procedure. *Journal of Cardiovascular Nursing, 11* (2), 1–14.

Ekman, I., Lundman, B., & Norberg, A. (1999). The meaning of hospital care, as narrated by elderly patients with chronic heart failure. *Heart & Lung, 28,* 203–209.

Epstein, R. S., & Sherwood, L. M. (1996). From outcomes research to disease management: A guide for the perplexed. *Annals of Internal Medicine, 124,* 832–837.

Estes, C. L., & Swan, J. H. (1993). *Long-term care crisis: Elders trapped in the no-care zone.* Newbury Park, CA: Sage.

Evans, R. L., & Hendricks, R. D. (1993). Evaluating hospital discharge planning: A randomized clinical trial. *Medical Care, 31,* 358–370.

Fox, H. B., Wicks, L. B., & Newacheck, P. W. (1993). Health maintenance organizations and children with special needs. A suitable match? *American Journal of the Disabled Child, 147,* 546–552.

Fulop, G., Strain, J. J., Fahs, M. C., Schneider, J., & Snyder, S. (1998). A prospective study of the impact of psychiatric comorbidity on length of hospital stays of elderly medical–surgical inpatients. *Psychosomatics, 39,* 273–280.

Gagnon, A. J., Schein, C., McVey, L., & Bergman, H. (1999). Randomized controlled trial of nurse case management of frail older people. *Journal of the American Geriatric Society, 47,* 1118–1124.

Garrard, J., Dowd, B. E., Dorsey, B., & Shapiro, J. (1987). A checklist to assess the need for home health care: Instrument development and validation. *Public Health Nursing, 4,* 212–218.

Gold, S., & Bergman, H. (1997). A geriatric consultation team in the emergency department. *Journal of the American Geriatrics Society, 45,* 764–767.

Happ, M. B., Naylor, M. D. & Roe-Prior, P. (1997). Factors contributing to rehospitilization of elderly patients with heart failure. *Journal of Cardiovascular Nursing, 11* (4), 75–84.

Harrington, C., Lynch, M., & Newcomer, R. J. (1993). Medical services in social health maintenance organizations. *Gerontologist, 33,* 790–800.

Hennen, J., Krumkolz, H. M., Radford, M. J., & Meehan, T. P. (1995). Readmission rates, 30 days and 365 days postdischarge, among the 20 most frequent DRG groups, Medicare inpatients age 65 or older in Connecticut hospitals, fiscal years 1991, 1992, and 1993. *Connecticut Medicine, 59,* 263–270.

Holloway, J. J., Thomas, J. W., & Shapiro, L. (1988). Clinical and sociodemographic risk factors for readmission of Medicare beneficiaries. *Health Care Financing Review, 10* (1), 27–35.

Howse, E., & Bailey, J. (1992). Resistance to documentation: A nursing research issue. *International Journal of Nursing Studies, 29,* 371–380.

Katz, K. S. (1993). Project headed home: Intervention in the pediatric intensive care unit for infants and their families. *Infants & Young Children, 5* (3), 67–75.

Konstam, V., Salem, D., Pouleur, H., Kostis, J., Gorkin, L., Shumaker, S., Mottard, I., Woods, P., Konstam, M. A., & Yusuf, S. (1996). Baseline quality of life as a predictor of mortality and hospitalization in 5,025 patients with congestive heart failure. *American Journal of Cardiology, 78,* 890–895.

Lamb, G. (1992). *Conceptual and methodological issues in nurse case management research.* Washington, DC: American Nurses.

Landefeld, C. S., Palmer R. M., Kresevic, R., Fortinsky, R., & Kowal, J. (1995). A randomized trial of care in hospital medical units especially designed to improve the functional outcomes of acutely ill older patients. *New England Journal of Medicine, 32,* 1333–1338.

Lee, J. H., Swain, B., Andrey, J., Murrell, H. K., & Geha, A. S. (1999). Fast track recovery of elderly coronary bypass surgery patients. *Annuals of Thoracic Surgery, 68,* 437–441.

Levine, J. B., Covino, N. A., Slack, W. V., Safran, C., Safran, D. B., Boro, J. E., Davis, R. B., Buchanan, G. M., & Gervino, E. V. (1996). Psychological predictors of subsequent medical care among patients hospitalized with cardiac disease. *Journal of Cardiopulmonary Rehabilitation, 16,* 109–116.

Martens, K. H., & Mellor, S. D. (1997). A study of the relationship between home care services and hospital readmission of patients with congestive heart failure. *Home Healthcare Nurse, 15,* 123–129.

McWilliam, C. L., & Sangster, J. F. (1994). Managing patient discharge to home: The challenges of achieving quality of care. *International Journal for Quality in Health Care, 6,* 147–161.

Naylor, M. D., Brooten, D., Campbell, R., Jacobsen, B. S., Mezey, M. D., Pauly, M. V., & Schwartz, J. S. (1999). Comprehensive discharge planning and home follow-up of hospitalized elders—A randomized clinical trial. *Journal of the American Medical Association, 281,* 613–620.

Naylor, M. D., Brooten, D., Jones, R., Lavizzo-Mourey, R., Mezey, M., & Pauly, M. (1994). Comprehensive discharge planning for the hospitalized elderly—A randomized clinical trial. *Annals of Internal Medicine, 120,* 999–1006.

Oktay, J. S., Steinwachs, D. M., Mamon, J., Done, L. R., & Fahey, M. (1992). Evaluating social work discharge planning services for elderly people: Access, complexity, and outcome. *Health and Social Work, 17,* 290–298.

Pacala, J. T., Boult, C., Reed, R. L., & Aliberti, E. (1997). Predictive validity of the PRA Instrument among older recipients of managed care. *Journal of the American Geriatrics Society, 45,* 614–617.

Paone, G., Higgins, R. S., Havstad, S. L., & Silverman, N. A. (1998). Does age limit the effectiveness of clinical pathways after coronary artery bypass graft surgery. *Circulation, 98,* 98.

Patterson, P. K., Blehm, R., Foster, J., Fuglee, K., & Moore, J. (1995). Nurse information needs for efficient care continuity across patient units. *Journal of Nursing Administration, 25* (10), 28–36.

Pheley, A. M., Terry, P., Pietz, L., Fowles, J., McCoy, C. E., & Smith, H. (1995). Evaluation of a nurse-based hypertension management program: Screening, management, and outcomes. *Journal of Cardiovascular Nursing, 9,* 54–61.

Pohl, J. M., Collins, C., & Given, C. W. (1995). Beyond patient dependency: Family characteristics and access of elderly patients to home care services following hospital discharge. *Home Health Care Services Quarterly, 15* (4), 33–47.

Potthoff, S. J., Kane, R. L., & Franco, S. J. (1995). *Hospital discharge planning for elderly patients: Improving decisions, aligning incentives* (Master Contract 500-92-0048). Minnesota: University of Minnesota Institute for Health Services Research.

Prescott, P. A., Soeken, K. L., & Briggs, M. (1995). Identification and referral of hospitalized patients in need of home care. *Research in Nursing and Health, 18,* 85–95.

Reiley, P., Iezzoni, L. I., Phillips, R., Davis, R. B., Tuchin, L. I., & Calkins, D. (1996). Discharge planning: Comparison of patients and nurses' perceptions of patients following hospital discharge. *Image: Journal of Nursing Scholarship, 28,* 143–147.

Rich, M. W., Beckham, V., Wittenberg, C., Leven, C. L., Freedland, K. E., & Carney, R. M. (1995). A multidisciplinary intervention to prevent the readmission of elderly patients with congestive heart failure. *New England Journal of Medicine, 333,* 1190–1195.

Rich, M. W., Gray, D. B., Beckham, V., Wittenberg, C., & Luther, P. (1996). Effect of a multidisciplinary intervention on medication compliance in elderly patients with congestive heart failure. *American Journal of Medicine, 101,* 270–276.

Robinson, D. K., Mead, M. J., & Boswell, C. R. (1995). Inside looking out: Innovations in community health nursing. *Clinical Nurse Specialist, 9,* 227–229, 235.

Roglieri, J. L., Futterman, R., McDonough, K. L., Malya, G., Karwath, K. R., Bowman, D., Skelly, J., & Warburton, S. (1997). Disease management interventions to improve outcomes in congestive heart failure. *American Journal of Managed Care, 3,* 1831–1839.

Rosswurm, M. A., & Landham, D. M. (1998). Discharge planning for elderly patients. *Journal of Gerontological Nursing, 24* (5), 14–21.

Sampson, B. K., & Doran, K. A. (1998). Health needs of coronary artery bypass graft surgery patients at discharge. *Dimensions of Critical Care Nursing, 17,* 165–168.

Schmitt, M. H., Farrell, M. P., & Heinemann, G. D. (1988). Conceptual and methodological problems in studying the effects of interdisciplinary geriatric teams. *Gerontologist, 28,* 753–764.

Silliman, R. A., McGarvey, S. T., Raymond, P. M., & Fretwell, M. D. (1990). The senior care study. Does inpatient interdisciplinary geriatric assessment help the family caregivers of acutely ill older patients? *Journal of the American Geriatric Society, 38,* 461–466.

Slaets, J. P., Kauffmann, R. H., Duivenvooden, H. J., Pelemans, W., & Schudel, W. J. (1997). A randomized trial of geriatric liaison intervention in elderly medical inpatients. *Psychosomatic Medicine, 59,* 585–591.

Smith, D. M., Katz, B. P., Huster, G. A., Fitzgerald, J. F., Martin, D. K., & Freedman, J. A. (1996). Risk factors for nonelective hospital readmissions. *Journal of General Internal Medicine, 11,* 762–764.

Solomon, D. H., Wagner, D. R., Marenberg, M. E., Acampora, D., Cooney, L. M., & Inouye, S. K. (1993). Predictors of formal home health care use in elderly patients after hospitalization. *Journal of American Geriatrics Society, 41,* 961–966.

Trella, R. (1994). From hospital to home: Bridging the gaps in care. *Geriatric Nursing, 15,* 313–316.

Weinberger, M., Kirkman, M. I., Samsa, G. P., Shortliffe, E. A., Landsman, P. B., Cowper, P. A., Simel, D. L., & Feussner, J. R. (1995). A nurse-coordinated intervention for primary care patients with non-insulin-dependent diabetes mellitus: Impact on glycemic control and health related quality of life. *Journal of General Internal Medicine, 10,* 59–66.

Worth, A., Tierney, A., & Lockerbie, L. (1994). Community nurses and discharge planning. *Nursing Standard, 8* (21), 25–30.

Zelle, R. S. (1995). Follow-up of at-risk infants in the home setting: Consultation model. *Journal of Obstetrical, Gynecological, and Neonatal Nursing, 24* (1), 51–55.

14

Family Responses to Critical Care

Jane S. Leske and Susan M. Heidrich

A major assumption of family-centered critical care is that family members, as well as patients, are affected by critical illness and in need of care. What if the patient is elderly? What family stresses are produced by a critical illness? Who are family to critically ill elderly patients? What is the impact of critical care on the family? What are the unique characteristics of the aged population that need to be considered in providing nursing care? What are effects of discharge and subsequent caregiving on family members? The family can function as a source of support for the patient and as a resource for the nursing staff. The elderly spouse, adult children, siblings, grandchildren, great-grandchildren, and other family members and friends all play unique roles during a critical illness and ultimately in the treatment, rehabilitation, and discharge of the elderly patient.

Although continuing knowledge is being obtained about the biology of aging and treatment modalities in advanced age, little research has been conducted in the area of family members of elderly patients who are critically ill. Little is known about how middle-aged or aged family members interpret the critical care experience. However, nurses need to understand the family system of a critically ill geriatric patient in order to provide optimal and holistic care.

Hospitalization for a critical illness can disrupt even the most highly organized and functional family. Assessment and interventions with family members of aged patients require consideration of the earlier questions. The contents of this chapter will focus on ways to identify and organize the contribution of family members to optimal outcomes for geriatric patients, as well as ways to limit family stress and foster family functioning.

STRESS AND THE FAMILY IN CRITICAL CARE

Since critical illness often occurs without warning, there is little time for family members to prepare for this experience. Most families usually report feeling powerless, vulnerable, and helpless (Schlump-Urquhart, 1990; Solursh, 1990). They have no clear knowledge of what to expect from health professionals caring for their family member or what to expect in regard to the illness and expected outcome. Families can act as buffers for patient stress and serve as valuable patient care resources. However, when families have high levels of stress, they may be unable to support the patient and, in fact, may transfer their stress to the patient. Unmitigated family stress may manifest itself in distrust of hospital staff, noncompliance with the treatment regimen, and even lawsuits. It is advantageous for everyone that care is provided so that optimal levels of family functioning are supported.

Any illness severe enough to necessitate admission to the intensive care unit (ICU) is life threatening and can precipitate severe stress within any family system. Stresses produced by critical illness vary in intensity and duration but certainly have the potential to create a heavy burden for families. Fear of death, uncertain outcome, emotional turmoil, financial concerns, fatigue, role changes, disruption of routines, and unfamiliar hospital environments are a few of the sources of stress for family members (Kleiber et al., 1994; Titler, Cohen, & Craft, 1991). In contrast to the family of younger persons, however, family members of elderly patients most likely have had prior experiences with critical care. Whether these experiences were positive or negative may determine their response to the stress of another critical care situation (Leske & Heidrich, 1996). In addition, some family members may view critical illness of an elderly person as a normal part of aging (Peirce, Wright, & Fulmer, 1992). In fact, critical illness may trigger some anticipatory grieving. Some families may feel more prepared for death as an outcome with older family members than with younger family members and so begin to grieve before death.

Stress also may interfere with the ability of any family to use effective coping skills and maintain patterns of family functioning (McCubbin & McCubbin, 1991). Basic coping techniques do not seem to change with age, and it is important to remember that emotional coping styles are determined more by the personality characteristics of the person than by their age (Andres, Bierman, & Hazzard, 1985). However, because elderly persons may anticipate serious illness in old age, they may use different coping resources for dealing with critical illness in the family. They may also show less overt emotional distress in a critical situation.

Even though older persons may exhibit less outward distress during a crisis, have had previous experience with critical illness situations, or consider such an experience normative or expected in old age, this should not be interpreted to mean that they need less support or attention from health care providers. Attention to how elderly family members are coping with the stress of the situation is essential because, in the critical care setting, most families appear to have a profound positive impact on the critically ill patient's response to treatment (Simpson & Shaver, 1990). Families can serve as valuable patient care resources. Most aged patients will return home rather than to another institution. Furthermore, family members provide most noninstitutional care for the elderly. The family care provider and the elderly patient form a dyad that is not always apparent in the ICU. The interruption in family ties during critical illness has important implications for nursing care and discharge planning. Because families' responses to stress have implications for the family, patient, and nursing staff, it is advantageous for everyone that nurses direct care so that optimal levels of family functioning are supported.

FAMILY THEORIES AND CONCEPTS USEFUL IN CRITICAL CARE

The American population is aging in two important ways. First, the number of people who are old is increasing and, with the aging of the baby-boomers, the proportion of the population that is old will increase dramatically. Second, life expectancy has increased, while disability has decreased. This means that people are living longer and are healthy for more years of life than ever before (Manton, Stallard, & Corder, 1995). For the critical care nurse, these changes mean that a greater proportion of their patients can be expected to be "geriatric" patients and, more importantly for this discussion, these patients can be expected to have other family members involved in their care.

Critical care interventions have been shown to provide significant benefits to older persons, including the very old (Rush, 1997). Mortality rates for older ICU patients are similar to those for all age ranges (Kass, Castriotta, & Malakoff, 1992; Wu, Rubin, & Rosen, 1990). However, elderly persons admitted to ICUs fall into two very distinct groups: those who are functionally independent but struck by an acute serious illness such as myocardial infarction and those who are frail and have multiple degenerative illnesses whose condition becomes unstable (Kaufman, 1998). It is the second group that composes 70 to 80% of hospital admissions and that poses the most dilemmas for families and health professionals.

The introduction of the concept of "family-centered care" has led to important changes in the nursing care of childbearing and childrearing families, particularly in the care of critically ill infants and children. This concept can also be applied to families of critically ill geriatric patients. Two concepts are central to the notion of family-centered care: enabling and empowerment. Enabling involves providing the means for family members to use or acquire competencies needed to care for their loved one. Empowerment is the interaction between the nurse and family members that maintains or gives a sense of control to the family member. Although the relationship between a parent and a young child differs substantially from that of an adult child and elderly parent or between elderly spouses, these two concepts can still be used to ensure comprehensive and compassionate care of the geriatric patient in critical care.

A second theory useful in understanding family and health provider interactions in the ICU is family systems theory. A key concept in family systems theory is that a change in one part of the system (for example, the hospitalization of a critically ill parent) affects the entire family system, resulting in a strain on coping resources and possibly family distress. One way that systems, such as families, attempt to maintain or restore equilibrium and thereby reduce distress is by controlling "inputs and outputs"; for example, controlling what is allowed to enter or leave the system. A major input and output that is very relevant to ICU nurses is the two-way communication of information.

In family systems theory, families have been described as "open" or "closed" systems according to how much communication and support is allowed to enter or leave the family system. Some families are "closed" systems. For these, information sharing or use of outside resources is not trusted and is perceived as disruptive and causing stress to the family. Such families may neither offer nor be receptive to teaching or information gathering by the nurse. These families are sometimes labeled as being "in denial" or "uncooperative," but these families are acting in ways that they perceive are in the best interest of the family. Other families are "open" systems and perceive the exchange of information or resources as adding energy and stability to the system. Open families can be very receptive and cooperative in receiving and giving information or support, or they can be viewed as "demanding" or "controlling" because of their insistence on getting the answers that they need. Again, these families are acting in ways that, in their view, are best for the family. The key to effective communication with both types of families is developing trust.

In addition to systems theory, an understanding of family developmental issues can assist the nurse in dealing effectively with families of elderly patients. Family development is a powerful paradigm that has been greatly overlooked as a therapeutic framework. A family crisis may occur when a critical illness does occur. The degree of disruption to the family system is affected by the timing of the illness in the family life cycle, the nature of the illness, the openness of the family system, and the role of the ill person (Carter & McGoldrick, 1980). Therefore, it is important to consider families in the larger time frame of family development.

Spouses of critical care geriatric patients typically are older and perhaps frail. Siblings, who are increasingly important as sources of support in old age, also may be older and frail. Illness is a prominent concern to most older adults. Fears of loss of physical and mental functioning, chronic pain, and degenerating conditions are common concerns even though most elderly do maintain good health. Older individuals in our society are often stereotyped as frail, depressed, lonely, and cognitively slow or impaired. It would be a mistake for nurses working with these family members to hold these attitudes, particularly because the salient transitions of later life hold the potential for transformation and growth. In fact, research on aging shows that older persons are happier and more satisfied with life than young or middle-aged persons are. Further, variability in health, cognitive ability, and emotional well-being is greater in old age than at any other time in life (Ansello, 1988; Gurainik, LaCroix, & Everett, 1988). In addition, there is a myth that older persons are isolated from their families. Although some family members may live in distant communities, most elderly persons have daily or weekly contact with family members.

Adult children of the geriatric patient are often in midlife. In terms of age, this stage usually extends from the mid-40s to the mid-60s. There is currently little terminology to describe this phase of the family life cycle. Some use the term "empty nest," but this has negative connotations. Many demographic changes in adult development have made this a lengthy stage in the family life cycle. Typically, at this time of life, children are teenagers or in college, bringing both emotional and financial stresses; careers are often at their peak; the quality of marital relationships can decline; physically people begin to notice signs of aging or first develop a serious health problem; and often both time and money are devoted to helping care for aging parents. Having aging and ill parents, in and of itself, is a stressor. For the first time, the adult child may be confronted with his or her own mortality, as well as the parent's. A critical illness in the parent often changes the parent-child relationship so that roles reverse, and the adult child is given the responsibility of making decisions, communicating family wishes, or interacting with health care providers.

Understanding developmental issues for a family may be crucial to understanding the impact of the critical illness of the elderly patient. Other family members may be called upon to assume new roles and responsibilities. In addition, prior divorce can negatively affect the parent-child relationship even in the latter part of life, weakening economic ties and reducing informal caregiving (Schone & Pezzin, 1999). Researchers have reported that divorced parents may not be able to count on the economic and personal support of their children. Divorced fathers are particularly vulnerable to receiving less care in later life because of weaker ties with their children. In addition, the ties to children may be further weakened by remarriage. It appears that remarried parents received less informal care from their children and purchase more hours of formal care (Schone & Pezzin, 1999). These results raise concerns about future generations of elderly patients who will have experienced higher rates of divorce and may place greater demands on social and economic programs for assistance.

Gillis and Knafl (1999) describe a third conceptual approach to family care in their review of nursing research on families in non-normative transitions. They suggest that several time-bound processes can be seen among families in response to events such as serious illness. First, the family must formulate an initial response to the illness by defining the threat, impact, and experience. Families may need assistance in defining this threat in a realistic way, or they may need the nurse to help correct the misperceptions about the situation. On the other hand, nurses need to understand the family's perception and definition of the illness. This is the root of many of the dilemmas around decision making for the frail, elderly patient. Stereotypes and lack of information about the health, emotional responses, and family relationships of the older family members can interfere with adequate assessment of the family.

Families also must begin to understand how family life has to adapt and how resources must be garnered to treat the critical illness. Then the family learns how to manage the illness in the context of other ongoing aspects of daily life (such as paying bills, doing the grocery shopping, and, for older persons, getting to their own doctor's appointments). How families manage this process is not well-understood. Yet, critical care nurses can be attuned to these ongoing issues of the family and prepare families for these demands. Understanding how families cope and adapt in response to developmental changes can be used as a guide in identifying major family issues.

IMPACT OF CRITICAL CARE ON THE FAMILY

In many instances, a family member, most often an elderly wife, has cared for the geriatric patient admitted to the ICU. Caregiving can be a chronic and stressful event, with negative effects on the caregiver's emotional well-being and financial well-being. Caregiver distress has been described in numerous ways by caregivers, including feelings of burnout, depression, isolation, fear, frustration, anxiety, low morale, sleeplessness, fatigue, and loneliness (Brody, 1990). Alarmingly, caregivers have reported even higher levels of depression and psychological distress, a more negative affect, and higher use of psychotropic drugs than people in the general population have (Cuellar & Butts, 1999; Neundorfer, 1991).

Caregiving also affects the physical health of the caregiver. One large epidemiological study has shown that elderly caregivers who experience emotional strain are more likely to die than are noncaregiving controls (Shulz & Beach, 1999). Nurses dealing with spouses who have been caregivers of the ICU patient need to be aware that these family members are at greater risk not only for emotional distress and depression but also for serious physical health problems. The added stress of having a spouse admitted to the ICU puts that caregiver in a high-risk situation in relation to his or her own health. Therefore, any ways in which the nurse can intervene to reduce the distress of the family members and to increase health-protective behaviors of that family member should be used. Nursing interventions also need to focus on discharge planning for the caregiver as well as for the patient. Because of shortened length of hospital stays and higher acuity needs in the discharged patient, caregivers often continue to provide care after hospitalization (Clark, 1997). The needs of caregivers, such as support for themselves as well as support services for the patient, should be part of discharge planning if family-centered care is the goal (Fournet, 1992).

Sometimes the needs of the older ICU patient and the needs of the family member, particularly an elderly spouse, conflict. For example, confusion and agitation are common, but distressing, sequelae of acute illness or admission to an ICU, or both, for older patients. Estimates of the incidence of acute confusion range from 24 to 80% of all hospitalized elderly patients (Foremen, 1989). The downward trajectory into acute confusion is often viewed as a normal progression of events, and the patient is allowed to pass without benefit of intervention. Prompt intervention is essential because of the increased morbidity and mortality associated with untreated acute confusional states (Francis & Kapoor, 1992). It is recommended that a history of confusion be sought for all elderly patients. One way to minimize acute confusion is to have familiar persons in the critical care environment. The elderly spouse may be asked or know from experience whether staying with the patient will help reduce these symptoms (Juneau, 1996; Tolley & Prevost, 1997). Yet that same spouse, because of his or her age, may be highly fatigued and sensitive to the same environmental stressors, such as sensory overload, as the patient and in need of rest and time away from the hospital to maintain health.

Communication with health care providers also can be a significant stressor, particularly when decisions about treatment must be made. Family members, particularly those who are elderly, may have a limited understanding of what the information that health care providers give them really means. At times, health care providers assume that family members understand if no questions are asked. Family members also may think they understand what health professionals are saying when in reality they do not. Research has pointed out that physicians and patients, physicians and family members, and patients and family members either do not communicate or, when they do, misunderstand or misperceive the communication. This is especially problematic when the communication is about end-of-life treatment decisions (Kaufman, 1998). For example, family members may inform the nurse that the patient does not want to be on life support, but they do not understand that mechanical ventilation is life support. Research on family decision making during stressful periods or crisis is limited. Most of the nursing research on decision making in the clinical setting focuses on the process and analysis of decisions made by nurses or physicians rather than by families of patients.

Health professionals often assume that older adults prefer quality of life over quantity, but that is not always the case, even for the very old. Many do prefer quality over quantity and would choose less invasive procedures if they were critically ill. Some, however, prefer quantity of life in their current state of health. Unfortunately, as seen in one study, neither health professionals nor family members could accurately predict the patient's preference (Tsevat et al., 1998). In addition, as Kaufman (1998) noted in an ethnographic study of an ICU, when faced with critical decisions in an ICU, families are unsure of "what to want" (p. 722) besides the recovery of their loved one. Often it is the nurse who notes the communication problem or who is in the position of translating and ensuring understanding among family members, patients, and health care providers.

Because of the enormous amount of time that a family spends at the hospital after a critical illness, a series of changes may occur within the family system. These may include reorganization of roles and tasks, changes in communication patterns, and emotional struggles. These changes may even become more complicated in geriatrics, because there are multiple adult family members, representing a couple of generations, with varying levels of responsibility to the elderly patient. These levels of responsibility need to be assessed considering current and past relationships the patient has had with the family; the degree of economic threat the illness poses to the family; trajectory expectations for the illness that the family holds; and the impact of the rehabilitation, discharge, and possible disability on the ability to perform the caregiving role.

The preexisting levels of stress in families may be a predictor of their reaction to the critical care crisis. Because family crises evolve over time, families are seldom dealing with a single crisis. Prior strains contribute to increased family stress (McCubbin & McCubbin, 1991). Most families carry residual strains that result from unresolved hardships from earlier stressors. There is strong support that chronic strains and daily hassles have debilitating effects on family well-being. Experiencing multiple stressors over long periods can lead to enormous strain, a situation that places the family at risk for difficult adaptation to the critical illness (Failla & Jones, 1991; McCubbin & McCubbin, 1991). Prior research suggests that prior strains, rather than the actual stressor event, predict psychosocial family adaptation (LaVee, McCubbin, & Olson, 1987). However, the stress of severe patient illness contributes to increased difficulty with family adaptation. At this time a clear need exists to evaluate factors such as the mental health, physical health, and functional ability of the patient's potential primary caregiver, as well as the caregiver's ability to manage stress.

The obvious role of the critical care nurse is to manage the physiological crisis of the patient. Keeping up with the procedures and technological explosion is one explanation for the lack of nursing intervention with families. Several factors described in the literature may serve to deter nurses from including families in the domain of care. Nurses are often rewarded by others for completing tasks, carrying out the medical regimen, learning new technology, and, in doing so, keeping the unit running smoothly. On the other hand, care that is rendered to the family is not as easily recognizable and thus may not be fostered. Many nurses do not perceive themselves as qualified and knowledgeable to provide family care. However, family assessment and intervention is a key element of complete care. It cannot be emphasized enough that a nurse cannot talk to the family too much.

RESPONSES OF AGED FAMILY MEMBERS

Gerontological research consistently shows that, as people age, they become less and less like others of the same age (Ansello, 1988). This evolving awareness of the increasing heterogeneity of older people suggests that an elderly person's biological, cognitive, and psychological function can vary greatly, from healthy and active to severely debilitated (Guarainick et al., 1989). Elderly family members differ from younger family members in important ways that potentially affect how they cope with the stress of critical illness:

- They have diminished baseline physiological reserve.
- They may have chronic illnesses that can exacerbate or intensify the response.
- They report less emotional distress but develop somatic symptoms indicative of distress.
- They may need longer time to process information.
- They may have family members that live far away.
- They may have friends or neighbors, instead of relatives, that provide a support system.
- They may have different attitudes and expectations towards health care providers.

These age-related changes need to be taken into account when dealing with older family members because they may affect how well the family members can cope with and adapt to the critical illness situation. These changes also need to be addressed when assessing the family, particularly because the patient may return to the care of the aging spouse.

GENERAL NEEDS OF FAMILY MEMBERS
AFTER CRITICAL ILLNESS

Numerous studies have been conducted to identify various needs of families when one member was hospitalized in a critical care unit (Alpen & Halm, 1992; Foss & Tenholder, 1993; Freichels, 1991; Hickey, 1990; Kleinpell & Powers, 1992; Leske, 1991, 1992a; Walters, 1995; Warren, 1993). Most results are based on data obtained from the Critical Care Family Needs Inventory (CCFNI) or a researcher-modified version of this instrument. The CCFNI consists of 45 need statements that are to be rated on a scale of 1 (not important) to 4 (very important) by family members. The needs have been identified in a variety of patient populations, including cardiac surgery, terminal illness, trauma, spinal cord injury, burns, and general critical care patients. Although families have many needs, five main areas of concern repeatedly arise: families place the utmost importance on receiving assurance, remaining near the critically ill person, receiving information, being comfortable, and having support (Leske, 1991, 1992a).

Assurance reflects the family's need to hope for a desired outcome, part of which is based on their confidence and trust in the health care system. Family members' need for personal contact and to remain physically and emotionally close to the critically ill person also is important. Following initial notification of a life-threatening illness, all families need to have consistent and realistic information about the ill member. In addition, personal comforts allow family members to remain near the ill member for extensive periods of time. Support reflects the variety of resources, support systems, or supportive structures that families need after a critical illness. All of these needs appear universal and are not associated with age, gender, relationship to patient, prior ICU experience, or patient medical diagnosis, at least during the first few days of the critical care experience (Leske, 1992b). Research results also show some inconsistencies among perceptions of patients, families, and health-care professionals about the importance of family needs. Family members tend to rate needs as more important than nurses do. Similarly, marked disagreement has been found between family members and nurses about how well needs are met. The obvious conclusion is that the family member's perception of needs has to be assessed for an effective plan of care to be developed. It is the individualizing of interventions to meet these needs that require age-specific considerations.

MEETING FAMILY NEEDS

Patients with good support systems have higher survival rates, better recovery experiences, and fewer postcrisis sequelae (O'Malley & Menke, 1988; Tracey, Fowler, & Magarelli, 1999). To determine appropriate and supportive interventions, nurses must first accurately assess family members. Given prior evidence that meeting family needs can reduce family stress, the question arises: How do nurses intervene to meet family needs to promote optimal family health and coping during critical illness, especially when the patients are elderly?

UNDERSTANDING FAMILY GOALS

Integral to intervening to meet family needs is recognizing the goals of any family during the critical care experience. Families experiencing a critical illness are confronted with several major adaptive tasks related to stage of family life cycle and needs for assurance, visitation, information, comfort, and support (Leske, 1992a). These goals also are important for aged family members. Goals for family life cycle stage include dealing with the critical illness of a parent or spouse. Some family goals for meeting assurance needs include developing confidence and trust in the health-care team, keeping or redefining hope, and managing discouraging or dreadful news. Family goals for visitation needs consist of maintaining familial relationships, networking with the health care team, and participating in patient care planning. Learning what needs to be known and balancing understanding with information overload, making decisions, and understanding the hospital environment are family goals for meeting information needs. An additional family goal is to balance work, home, and hospital activities while taking care of themselves. Family goals for meeting support needs include handling problems that arise, seeking or accepting assistance, and preparing for the role changes with an uncertain future. When the family members are elderly, there may be a tendency to not involve them fully in formulating plans of care or to adequately address their unique goals (Cohen, 1988). This may be due to stereotypes and myths about the abilities and desires of elderly persons. However, standards of practice state that nurses continually evaluate family responses to interventions in order to determine progress toward goal attainment (American Nurses Association, 1987).

AREAS FOR FAMILY ASSESSMENT

Assessment is the act of viewing the family situation from a database in order to identify specific areas for intervention. The focus of the nurses' initial interaction with the family is to assess the initial response to and understanding of the critical illness situation.

Initial Family Contact

Initial contact with family members is very important because it sets the foundation for a trusting relationship between the nurses and family (Bouley et al., 1994; Hickey, 1990). Ideally, nurse-family contact is initiated as soon as possible after the critical event. Most families need immediate and tangible information in order to balance the acute state of uncertainty. Allowing a family to wait without any knowledge about the situation conveys a blatant lack of respect for any family's value and dignity. Early contact has been reported to reduce family stress, anxiety, and uncertainty (Leske & Heidrich, 1996). Acknowledgment of feelings, such as "it is very difficult to wait," communicates support and conveys to the family that their situation is recognized. The knowledge that someone else is empathetic is comforting to most family members.

Nurses should be prepared for a variety of responses, such as crying, anger, hysteria, frustration, impatience, and even withdrawal. However, initial responses from aged family members may be difficult to predict. Today's cohort of elderly were brought up in an era in which displaying emotions or asking for help was considered unacceptable. The nurse may need to anticipate the concerns of elderly persons and not assume that silence or acquiescence means that there are no problems. The nurse focuses on the immediate problems related to the critical care experience and encourages the family members to do likewise. Meeting in an area that provides privacy and is separate from the general waiting room is conducive to a productive initial family meeting (Schlump-Urquhart, 1990).

Gathering the Family Database

Gathering a family database can be facilitated by obtaining information that includes family roles and relationships. The family assessment lays the foundations for future planning. The information helps align family expectations with interventions in order to promote satisfaction with care. Questions to consider for the family database include: What does the family need most? Are there other health care professionals who should be consulted? In the process of gathering such data, families will ask fundamental questions that need to be addressed: What happened? How did it happen? Why? Because the admission to ICU is such a stressful time for the family, the nurse may not be able to gather all the family information during the initial interview. Data can be easily added to the family profile after each subsequent family interview. When gathering information about aged family members, a number of factors need to be considered. These include health of the older person; closeness (physical and emotional) of other family members, particularly siblings and adult children; role of the elderly person in the family, particularly in the case of spouses; and who makes treatment decisions.

Assess Health of Aged Family Member

With aged family members, special attention should be directed to their physical condition. Elderly persons, particularly women, report an average of three chronic health problems. The most common include hypertension, other cardiovascular disease, and arthritis. Often, the older person is taking multiple medications, both prescription and over the counter (Strickland, 1988; VanNostrand, Furner, & Susman, 1993). Older persons typically also experience some deficits in hearing and vision. Each of these factors need to be considered in developing appropriate strategies for aged family members.

Another important consideration is the emotional well-being of the older family member. As noted earlier, many older persons do not report emotional distress, at least to the same extent that younger adults do. This is, in part, because of their socialization to keep feelings private, their need to "keep a stiff upper lip" and not burden others with their problems, and the stigma attached to emotional "problems" (George, 1989). Asking an older person about feelings of anxiety, depression, or signs of emotional distress may elicit a denial of any kind of affective symptoms. When an aged person is experiencing emotional distress, however, he or she is likely to report or seek treatment for somatic symptoms and not attribute these symptoms to stress. Symptoms such as insomnia, early waking, loss of appetite, indigestion, and headaches are common symptoms experienced by older persons (Heidrich, 1993; Heidrich & D'Amico, 1993). These may be due to chronic health problems, common physiological changes associated with aging, or emotional distress. Asking questions about these types of symptoms, their onset and duration, will provide some basis for the nurse to assess the emotional well-being of the aged family member and suggest interventions to reduce the severity of symptoms.

Assess Availability of Other Family Members

Most elderly persons live with a spouse or alone, independently in the community (American Association of Retired Persons, 1993; Bureau of the Census, 1991). Given the geographic mobility in the U.S. population, adult children and siblings may not live close by. However, even when elderly individuals are separated physically from their immediate family, they do maintain frequent contact by telephone. Because of this, family members are an important source of emotional support to the older person, but they may not be available to provide more instrumental types of support (Cutrona, Russell, & Rose, 1986). Necessities such as transportation to the hospital, taking care of household chores, paying the bills, and preparing meals can loom as major problems for an elderly family member during a critical care experience. The nurse needs to identify whether other family members, especially adult children, are available and what kinds of support they can offer.

Friends are particularly important to aged persons as sources of both qualitative and instrumental support (Thompson & Heller, 1990). It is often the support network of friends and neighbors who need to be called upon to fill in gaps when the family member is elderly. In dealing with the aged, the family database should contain information about friends and neighbors who may be the available and essential support persons.

Assess Aged Family Member's Role

Typically, the aged family member of a critically ill older adult is the spouse, although it may be a sibling or a child. Knowledge about generational differences in family roles is necessary to guide nurses in gathering essential information. For instance, many women who are now in their 70s and 80s and still have spouses have no knowledge of their family finances. They may not know about their sources of income or their expenses, how to pay bills, or what kind of life insurance policies their husbands have. They may not have a drivers' license and may never have learned how to drive a car. Younger health professionals may not be aware of these generational differences or may attribute the wife's lack of information or knowledge of how to get things done to some age-related cognitive "decline," rather than to how earlier generations of women were socialized into family roles. The nurse needs to be sensitive to the fact that an older woman may be dealing with issues and making decisions in areas in which she has had no previous experience. This may be an added source of stress for the older family member that may not be present in younger or middle-aged persons.

Assess Family Spokesperson for Treatment Plans

The issue of designating a family spokesperson is of immense importance during a critical care situation, but who takes the telephone calls may be different from who makes treatment decisions with older family members. Critical care nurses need to be prepared for disagreements among family members about treatment options (Kapp, 1991). Even health care professionals may disagree about treatment plans. When the critically ill patient is elderly, there are often family issues about treatment options. Although many family members state they know what the older patient would want, this information may be inaccurate or may not be used appropriately to make treatment decisions (Kapp, 1991; Sonnenblick, Friendlander, & Steinberg, 1993). The nurse needs to be prepared to deal with conflicting family wishes and emotional responses when treatment decisions are being made for elderly family members.

SUGGESTED FAMILY INTERVENTIONS

Interventions with family members begin on orientation to the critical care area and continue throughout the critical care period. Suggested nursing interventions and activities associated with the five need categories serve as a guide for initial implementation.

Orient to Critical Care Environment

Regardless of previous experience with critical care or lack of it, the critical care environment can be very intimidating to family members. The vast array of machines and technology is overwhelming. Family members report that the greater the number of machines involved in patient care, the more serious the illness. They describe the sounds emitted by machines as alarms that signify a crisis; therefore, the more alarms, the greater the crisis. In addition, the "Do Not Enter" signs on the door are obstacles to family visitation.

Families not experienced with critical illness do not know what to expect. Feelings of anxiety are intensified when entering the ICU for the first time. Factors that contribute to family anxiety include unusual sounds and odors, complex equipment, numerous critically ill patients, and the many treatments and procedures that the patient undergoes. Families may perceive the business of the ICU as chaotic and disorganized, and they may feel that they "are in the way." Aged family members are especially concerned about "not bothering anyone." However, educating families about their loved one's illness, treatments, and physical status helps prepare families for what they will encounter when they visit the patient (Cray, 1989).

Providing Assurance and Hope

Providing assurance is especially important for any family experiencing uncertainty in diagnosis, treatment, and outcome of illness, regardless of the age of family members. Establishing a calm and relaxed atmosphere that will support a trusting and empathetic relationship is a necessary part of assurance. Professionals and families need to establish a relationship that is mutually respectful, trusting, and collaborative. The development of any further interventions will depend on the initial rapport established between care providers and family members.

Nursing interventions that provide assurance are difficult to describe, probably because nurses provide assurance by exhibiting genuine concern for family members' welfare while listening, encouraging, and positively responding to them. Exchanging of names is an important but simple introduction that is often overlooked in nurse-family interaction. However, addressing aged family members or patients by their first name unless specifically asked to do so may be inappropriate. Using first names may convey a lack of respect or loss of dignity to the older person. Be cautious about communicating ageist attitudes, even inadvertently, such as referring to someone as a "sweet little old lady."

Results of prior research indicate that to feel hope is a very important need of family members of the critically ill (Leske, 1991). Nurses need to support hope because hope can be associated with positive patient outcomes (Tracey, Fowler, & Magarelli, 1999). Many hope-inspiring strategies focus on relationships with others. These relationships involve nurses, family, friends, and a higher power (Kaye & Heald, 1996). Recalling the joyous times can help families focus on positive aspects of family relationships. Reminiscence with family members may provide the nurse with information on how to personalize patient care (McQuay, Schwartz, Goldblatt, & Gian-grasso, 1995; Westphal, 1995).

Facilitating Visitation

The need for family members to remain near the critically ill patient is important. By seeing the critically ill patient, family members validate the seriousness of the situation (Eichhorn, Meyers, & Guzzetta, 1995). It is reported that most family members desire an unlimited number of visits per day and believe that visiting is important to the recovery of the critically ill patient (Halm & Titler, 1990). Family members feel that their visits affect patients by calming their fears, uplifting their spirits, promoting a positive attitude, and giving some inner strength for recovery. Balancing the needs of family members with the needs of the patient, unit, and health care personnel is no easy task. However, visitation practices should have a scientific base, rather than one governed by institutional or environmental regulations. Visitation contracts appear to be a popular compromise between rigid rules and unlimited policies. By using a visitation contract, visiting frequency, length of visit, and approved visitors are tailored to individual family situations. Family members need unit telephone numbers and who to contact for information on the patient. In addition, beeper systems have offered family members respite from the waiting room vigil (Menkhaus, Turner, Gueldner, & Michele, 1996).

Remember that, for a number of reasons, some older people may have difficulty getting to and from the hospital. Also, their own health problems may interfere with their ability to spend long hours in the ICU waiting room. However, even when the spouse must remain at home, she or he can make important contributions to the patient's recovery. Specific arrangements for telephone call updates and progress reports may be a beneficial intervention.

Managing Information

The need for information is one of the most important needs of any family member after critical illness (Daley, Kleinpell, Lawinger, & Casey, 1994; Henneman, McKenzie, & Dewa, 1992; McGaughey & Harrison, 1994; McGaughey, 1994). Mendonca and Warren (1998) examined the needs of family members of 51 ICU patients (mean age = 62.84 years) and the extent to which family members felt their needs were met. Eight of the top 10 needs were related to obtaining information about the patient. Information giving is an important intervention aimed at preparing or moving the family toward understanding and accepting the critical situation and possible outcomes. Nursing interventions are designed to foster family member's management of the vast amount of information that may be directed to them.

Providing information to elderly family members requires special approaches to accommodate age-related changes that may influence the ability to understand or retain new information. Sensory overload from the strange environment of the hospital or critical care unit and sensory impairments, such as declines in vision and hearing, may interfere with aged family member's ability to process or retain information. Aged family members are just as capable of remembering and understanding as younger family members are. However, under conditions of environmental and memory overload, difficulty can occur with processing of information. For instance, many older persons have some hearing loss. An unfamiliar and stressful environment may exacerbate the problem. Be careful not to misinterpret a hearing loss as a cognitive impairment. When there is a hearing loss, it is helpful to speak in lower tones but no louder than you would with colleagues.

Modifying traditional teaching approaches to address the special needs of elderly family members will enhance the effectiveness of any teaching (Dellasega, Clark, McCreary, Helmuth, & Schan, 1994). Reducing memory "overload" by initially providing only essential information to relieve their immediate concerns will be more effective than providing too much information. Simple terminology without medical jargon will enhance the older family member's ability to understand and remember explanations.

New material is best processed if it is presented in small increments at frequent but manageable intervals. Continual identification of the aged family member's energy level is an important consideration; fatigue can influence processing ability. Complicating the issue of providing information is the fact that the educational level is generally lower in the elderly than it is in younger generations. About 40% of those age 75 years or more are high school graduates; the number is lower for Blacks and Hispanics (American Association of Retired Persons, 1992; Bureau of Census Statistical Brief, 1986). Because of the differences in educational levels, most written materials should be prepared at about the 8th grade level of reading and, because of vision loss with age, in larger print.

Knowledge of age-related differences in information processing can help the critical care nurse use special skills when providing information. Speaking at a slower pace; being visible; making sure the family members have a needed prosthesis, such as a hearing aid; and allowing increased time for responses and additional questions are all measures that can enhance communication.

Facilitating Comfort

Sitting in the waiting room produces changes in eating habits, lack of physical or mental activity, and certainly prevents people from employment

(Bengtson, Karlsson, Wahrborg, Hjalmarson, & Herlitz, 1996). It is well documented, however, that most family members are not worried about physical comfort during the initial critical care experience (Leske, 1992a). However, if family members are to remain an effective source of support for the patient, they must receive adequate rest, nutrition, and personal hygiene. This is especially important now that patients are discharged earlier, and some are discharged directly home from the ICU. Family members need to have high energy levels in order to maintain the hospital "vigil" and care for the discharged patient. They often need to be encouraged to eat and take some time away from their relentless vigil.

These considerations take on added importance when the family member is elderly. Aged family members often have musculoskeletal limitations and decreased mobility. Sitting for hours in the waiting room can be painful. Typical waiting room furniture contributes to problems for the older family member. For instance, no one has identified comfortable chairs for the elderly who may have arthritis, osteoporosis, or pulmonary problems. It is important to assess if waiting will be difficult. In addition, aged family members need to be encouraged to take breaks from sitting and to walk around.

The lights and noise of the waiting room and surrounding areas also may interfere with adequate vision. Because of the normal changes in vision with age, some aged family members may find it difficult to navigate the hospital maze. Glare from lighting and small print on signs and cluttered directional maps may contribute to confusion and anxiety in the older person.

Enhancing Support

Nurses use many mechanisms to provide support to families, but few of these methods have been evaluated. Even the appropriateness of viewing nursing interventions as a supplement to existing family resources has been questioned (Gilliss, Neuhaus, & Hauck, 1990). It is impractical for nurses and possibly unhealthy for families for practitioners to provide all the necessary family support. Therefore, family groups are being used during the critical care experience (Halm, 1990). These groups provide the opportunity for participants to share common experiences, build mutual support, ventilate common concerns, foster a sense of hope, reduce anxiety, and obtain information common to the groups' needs (McQuay, 1995; Sabo et al., 1989).

Within the current cohort of aged people, however, there may be some for whom sharing feelings, personal issues, and private family matters is unacceptable. A support group may not be a beneficial intervention because the idea is foreign to some aged family members and not part of their upbringing or lifestyle. They have not been socialized to participate in these groups. If they would attend, special attention would need to be directed to particular issues of older persons. Support groups also may be more acceptable if the content focuses on information and tasks rather than sharing feelings and concerns. The critical care nurse will need to take direction from the group, rather than have a set agenda.

A commonly used method for assisting with support is to ask the aged family member to identify others who assist with specific tasks. Both friends and family, particularly adult children, may be available to help with day to day tasks and problems. Remember that friends may be more important than family members in providing emotional support and nurture to the older person. Asking the aged family member if he or she has a close friend or confidante is one way of assessing the availability of emotional support. Encouraging the older person to take some time to talk to or be with friends may give them permission to take care of themselves.

ROLE OF NURSE WITH FAMILY MEMBERS

At times, the family of the patient in critical care may replace the patient in the typical nurse-patient relationship so the relationship becomes the nurse-family relationship. This partnership between nurse and family may take a while to develop or may never develop adequately, leaving families and staff working toward different goals for the patient. There are strategies used by families and nurses that help develop this relationship. The strategies used by nurses include demonstrating commitment, persevering, and being involved (Hupcey, 1998). Demonstrating commitment involves responding to the family member as a person, spending time with the family, encouraging family participation, showing empathy, and respecting family rituals. Persevering requires spending time with difficult families and gathering information so you know the family. Being involved includes concepts of patient advocacy and bending bureaucratic rules.

Family strategies for developing the nurse-family relationship in critical care include determining who is the "good" nurse, how to be a "good" visitor, and how to be trustworthy. Families spend time trying to evaluate staff and determining which nurses are the "good" nurses (Hupcey, 1998). They watch care provided and look for signs of kindness and genuine interest on the part of the nurse toward the patient. This critique of nursing staff continues in the waiting room as families discuss who to trust and who provides competent care. Many families also invest a lot of effort into trying to please the nursing staff and be "good" visitors. They try to be friendly, cooperative, and help the nurses out. They may bring gifts and provide positive feedback. As the nurse-family relationship develops, families begin to trust certain nurses and accept the nurse's explanations without constant questioning. They begin to go home and take care of themselves.

SUMMARY

The ultimate goal for any family faced with a critical illness is to reorganize and stabilize its function as the affected member progresses from the acute to the rehabilitative phases of recovery. Stabilization of family function is achieved to the extent that the family can mobilize the necessary resources to cope effectively with the situation.

It is well-documented that families can use some intervention, especially in early stages of the patient's illness and treatment, but it remains unclear as to what specific interventions are the most effective. It is even less clear as to which interventions are effective for aged family members. The majority of families confronted with critical illness may do well, with or without specific interventions (Leske & Heidrich, 1996). On the other hand, the stresses associated with critical illness may increase family vulnerability to a wide range of emotional, behavioral, or adjustment problems. The aged family member may be at increased risk for changes in family roles and routines that alter his or her ability to fully participate in patient care. Research is needed to develop theoretically grounded and empirically based approaches for aged family member interventions. Until then, critical care nurses are encouraged to be creative and innovative in designing and evaluating interventions to meet specific family member needs. The challenges are to identify which interventions are helpful to aged families and how they can best be used in clinical practice.

Hospitalization for a critical illness can disrupt even the most highly organized and functional family. Family-focused care may mitigate family stress by providing support based on the unique needs of each family. Family members may suffer as much distress as the patient. They, too, deserve special attention and consideration. Professionals who are interested in the welfare and functioning of the family must ensure that the family members of the patient receive adequate and appropriate care, no matter what their ages.

REFERENCES

Alpen, M. A., & Halm, M. A. (1992). Family needs: An annotated bibliography. *Critical Care Nurse, 12* (2), 32, 41–50.

American Association of Retired Persons. (1993). *A profile of older Americans.* Long Beach, CA: American Association of Retired Persons.

American Nurses' Association. (1987). *Standards and scope of gerontological nursing practice.* Kansas City, MO: American Nurses Association.

Andres, R., Bierman, E. L., & Hazzard, W. R. (1985). *Principles of geriatric medicine.* New York: McGraw-Hill.

Ansello, E. F. (1988). A view of aging America and some implications. *Caring, 7,* 62–63.

Bengtson, A., Karlsson, T., Wahrborg, P., Hjalmarson, A., & Herlitz, J. (1996). Cardiovascular and psychosomatic symptoms among relatives of patients waiting for possible coronary revascularization. *Heart & Lung, 25,* 438–443.

Bouley, G., von Hofe, K., & Blatt, L. (1994). Holistic care of the critically ill: Meeting both patient and family needs. *Dimensions of Critical Care Nursing, 13,* 218–223.

Brody, E. M. (1990). Social factors in care: The elderly patient's family. In W. R. Hazzard, E. L. Bierman, & J. P. Blass (Eds.), *Principles of geriatric medicine and gerontology* (2nd ed., pp. 232–240). New York: McGraw-Hill.

Bureau of the Census. (1991). *Census of population and housing (1991). Summary population and housing characteristics.* Washington, DC: U.S. Department of Commerce.

Bureau of the Census Statistical Brief. (1986). *Age structure of the U.S. population in the 21st century* (U.S. Department of Commerce, SB-1-86). Washington, DC: U.S. Government Printing Office.

Carter, E. A., & McGoldrick, M. (1980). *The family life cycle: A framework for family therapy.* New York: Gardner Press.

Cohen, E. S. (1988). The elderly mystique: Constraints on the autonomy of the elderly with disabilities. *Gerontologist, 28* (suppl.), 24–31.

Clark, M. C. (1997). A causal functional explanation of maintaining a dependent elder in the community. *Research in Nursing & Health, 20,* 515–526.

Cray, L. (1989). A collaborative project: Initiating a family intervention program in a medical intensive care unit. *Focus on Critical Care, 16,* 212–218.

Cuellar, N., & Butts, J. B. (1999). Caregiver distress: What nurses in rural settings can do to help. *Nursing Forum, 24* (3), 24–30.

Cutrona, C., Russell, D., & Rose, J. (1986). Social support and adaptation to stress by the elderly. *Journal of Psychology and Aging, 1,* 47–54.

Daley, K. M., Kleinpell, R. M., Lawinger, S., & Casey, G. (1994). The effect of two nursing interventions on families of ICU patients. *Clinical Nursing Research, 3,* 414–422.

Dellasega, C., Clark, D., McCreary, D., Helmuth, A., & Schan, P. (1994). Nursing process: Teaching elderly clients. *Journal of Gerontological Nursing, 20* (1), 31–38.

Eichhorn, D. J., Mayers, T. A., & Guzzetta, C. E. (1995). Family presence during resuscitation: It is time to open the door. *Capsules & Comments in Critical Care Nursing, 3* (1), 8–13.

Failla, S., & Jones, L. C. (1991). Families of children with developmental disabilities: An examination of family hardiness. *Research in Nursing and Health, 14,* 41–50.

Foreman, M. (1989). Confusion in the hospitalized elderly: Incidence, onset, and associated factors. *Research in Nursing & Health, 12,* 21–29.

Foss, K. R., & Tenholder, M. F. (1993). Expectations and needs of persons with family members in an intensive care unit as opposed to a general ward. *Southern Medical Journal, 86,* 380–384.

Fournet, C. (1992). Support for significant others of elderly patients. *AACN Clinical Issues in Critical Care Nursing, 3,* 73–78.

Francis, J., & Kapoor, W. (1992). Prognosis after hospital discharge of older medical patients with delirium. *Journal of the American Geriatrics Society, 40,* 601–606.

Freichels, T. A. (1991). Needs of family members of patients in the intensive care unit over time. *Critical Care Nursing Quarterly, 14* (3), 16–29.

George, L. K. (1989). Stress, social support, and depression over the life course. In M. S. Markides & C. L. Cooper (Eds.), *Aging, stress, and health* (pp. 241–267). New York: Wiley.

Gillis, C. L., & Knafl, K. A. (1999). Nursing care of families in non-normative transitions: The state of science and practice. In A. S. Hinshaw, S. L. Feetham, & J. L. Shaver (Eds.), *Handbook of clinical nursing research* (pp. 231–249). Thousand Oaks, CA: Sage.

Gilliss, C. L., Neuhaus, J. M., & Hauck, W. W. (1990). Improved family functioning after cardiac surgery: A randomized trial. *Heart & Lung, 19,* 648–654.

Gurainick, J. M., LaCroix, A. Z., & Everett, D. F. (1989). *Aging in the eighties: Advance data from vital and health statistics, 170.* Hyattsville, MD: National Center for Health Statistics.

Halm, M. A. (1990). Effects of support groups on anxiety of family members during critical illness. *Heart & Lung, 19,* 62–71.

Halm, M. A., & Titler, M. (1990). Appropriateness of critical care visitation: Perceptions of patients, families, nurses, and physicians. *Journal of Nursing Quality Assurance, 5,* 25–37.

Heidrich, S. M. (1993). The relationship between physical health and psychological well being in elderly women: A developmental perspective. *Research in Nursing & Health, 16,* 123–130.

Heidrich, S. M., & D'Amico, D. (1993). Physical and mental health relationships in the very old. *Journal of Community Health Nursing, 10,* 11–21.

Henneman, E. A., McKenzie, J. B., & Dewa, C. S. (1992). An evaluation of interventions for meeting the information needs of families of critically ill patients. *American Journal of Critical Care, 3,* 85–93.

Hickey, M. (1990). What are the needs of families of critically ill patients? A review of the literature since 1976. *Heart & Lung, 19,* 401–415.

Hupcey, J. E. (1998). Establishing the nurse-patient relationship in the intensive care unit. *Western Journal of Nursing Research, 20,* 180–194.

Juneau, B. (1996). Special issues in critical care gerontology. *Critical Care Nursing Quarterly, 19,* 71–75.

Kapp, M. B. (1991). Health care decision making by the elderly: I get by with a little help from my family. *Gerontologist, 31,* 619–623.

Kass, J. E., Castriotta, R. J., & Malakoff, T. (1992). Intensive care unit outcomes in the very elderly. *Critical Care Medicine, 20,* 1666–1671.

Kaye, J., & Heald, G. (1996). Spirituality among family members of critically ill adults. *American Journal of Critical Care, 5,* 242.

Kaufman, S. R. (1998). Intensive care, old age, and problems of death in America. *The Gerontologist, 38,* 715–725.

Kleiber, C., Halm, M., Titler, M., Montgomery, L. A., Johnson, S. K., Nicholson, A., Craft, M., Buckwalter, K., & Megivern, K. (1994). Emotional responses of family members during a critical care hospitalization. *American Journal of Critical Care, 3,* 70–76.

Kleinpell, R. M., & Powers, M. J. (1992). Needs of family members of intensive care unit patients. *Applied Nursing Research, 5,* 2–8.

LaVee, Y., McCubbin, H. I., & Olson, D. H. (1987). The effects of stressful life events and transitions on family functioning and well-being. *Journal of Marriage and the Family, 49,* 857–873.

Leske, J. S. (1991). Overview of family needs after critical illness: From assessment to intervention. *AACN Clinical Issues in Critical Care Nursing, 2,* 220–226.

Leske, J. S. (1992a). Needs of adult family members after critical illness— prescriptions for interventions. *Critical Care Nursing Clinics of North America, 4,* 587–596.

Leske, J. S. (1992b). Comparison ratings of needs importance after critical illness from family members with varied demographic characteristics. *Critical Care Nursing Clinics of North America, 4,* 607–613.

Leske, J. S., & Heidrich, S. M. (1996). Interventions for aged family members. *Critical Care Nursing Clinics of North America, 8,* 91–102.

Manton, K. G., Stallard, E., & Corder, L. (1995). Changes in morbidity and chronic disability in the U.S. elderly population: Evidence from 1982, 1984, and 1989 National Long Term Care Surveys. *Journal of Gerontology: Social Sciences, 50B,* S194–S204.

McCubbin, M. A., & McCubbin, H. I. (1991). Family stress theory and assessment: The resiliency model of family stress, adjustment, and adaptation. In H. I. McCubbin & A. Thompson (Eds.), *Family assessment inventories for assessment and research* (pp. 3–32). Madison, WI: University of Wisconsin Press.

McGaughey, J., & Harrison, S. (1994). Developing an information booklet to meet the needs of intensive care patients and relatives. *Intensive and Critical Care Nursing, 10,* 271–277.

McGaughey, J. (1994). Understanding the information needs of patients and their relatives in intensive care units. *Intensive and Critical Care Nursing, 10,* 186–194.

McQuay, J. E. (1995). Support of families who had a loved one suffer a sudden injury, illness, or death. *Critical Care Nursing Clinics of North America, 7,* 541–547.

McQuay, J. E., Schwartz, R., Goldblatt, P. C., & Giangrasso, V. M. (1995). "Death-telling" research project. *Critical Care Nursing Clinics of North America, 7,* 549–555.

Mendonca, D., & Warren, N. A. (1998). Perceived and unmet needs of critical care family members. *Critical Care Nursing Quarterly, 21,* 58–67.

Menkhaus, S., Turner, N., Gueldner, S., & Michele, Y. (1996). Effectiveness of the family beeper program (FBP) in the critical care unit. *American Journal of Critical Care, 5,* 236.

Neundorfer, M. (1991). Family caregivers of the frail elderly: Impact of caregiving on their health and implications for interventions. *Family & Community Health, 14,* 48–58.

O'Malley, P., & Menke, E. (1988). Relationship of hope and stress after myocardial infarction. *Heart & Lung, 17,* 184–190.

Peirce, A. G., Wright, F., & Fulmer, T. T. (1992). Needs of the family during critical illness of elderly patient. *Critical Care Nursing Clinics of North America, 4,* 497–606.

Rush, P. (1997). Guidelines for critical care and the elderly: The search continues. *Critical Care Medicine, 25,* 1619–1620.

Sabo, K., Kraay, C., Rudy, E., Abraham, T., Bender, M., Lewandowski, W., Lombardo, B., Turk, M., & Dawson, D. (1989). ICU family support group sessions: Family members' perceived benefits. *Applied Nursing Research, 2,* 82–89.

Schlump-Urquhart, S. R. (1990). Families experiencing a traumatic accident: Implications and nursing management. *AACN Clinical Issues in Critical Care Nursing, 1,* 522–534.

Schone, B., & Pezzin, L. (1999). Parental marital disruption and intergenerational transfers: An analysis of lone elderly parents and their children. *Demography, 36* (3), 287–297.

Schulz, R., & Beach, S. R. (1999). Caregiving as a risk factor for mortality. *Journal of the American Medical Association, 282,* 2215–2219.

Simpson, T., & Shaver, J. (1990). Cardiovascular responses to family visits in coronary care unit patients. *Heart & Lung, 19,* 344–351.

Solursh, D. S. (1990). The family of the trauma victim. *Nursing Clinics of North America, 25,* 155–162.

Sonnenblick, M., Friendlander, Y., & Steinberg, A. (1993). Dissociation between the wishes of terminally ill parents and decisions by their offspring. *Journal of the American Geriatrics Society, 41,* 599–604.

Strickland, B. R. (1988). Sex-related differences in health and illness. *Psychology of Women Quarterly, 12,* 381–399.

Thompson, M. G., & Heller, K. (1990). Facets of support related to well being: Quantitative social isolation and perceived family support in a sample of elderly women. *Psychology & Aging, 5,* 535–544.

Titler, M. G., Cohen, M. Z., & Craft, M. J. (1991). Impact of adult critical care hospitalization: Perceptions of patients, spouses, children, and nurses. *Heart & Lung, 20,* 174–182.

Tolley, G., & Prevost, S. (1997). Case management of critically ill elders: A case study. *AACN Clinical Issues in Critical Care Nursing, 8,* 635–642.

Tracy, J., Fowler, S., & Magarelli, K. (1999). Hope and anxiety of individual family members of critically ill adults. *Applied Nursing Research, 12,* 121–127.

Tsevat, J., Dawson, N. V., Wu, A. W., Lynn, J., Soukup, J. R., Cook, E. F., Vidaillet, H., & Phillips, R. (1998). Health values of hospitalized patients 80 years or older. *Journal of the American Medical Association, 279,* 371–375.

VanNostrand, J. F., Furner, S. E., & Susman, R. (Eds). (1993). Health data of older Americans: United States, 1992. *National Center for Health Statistics: Vital Health Stat 3, 27.*

Walters, A. J. (1995). A hermeneutic study of the experiences of relatives of critically ill patients. *Journal of Advanced Nursing, 22,* 998–1005.

Warren, N. A. (1993). Perceived needs of the family members in the critical care waiting room. *Critical Care Nursing Quarterly, 16* (3), 56–63.

Westphal, C. G. (1995). Storyboards: A teaching strategy for families in critical care. *Dimensions of Critical Care Nursing, 14,* 214–221.

Wu, A. W., Rubin, H. R., & Rosen, M. J. (1990). Are elderly people less responsive to intensive care? *Journal of the American Geriatrics Society, 38,* 621.

PART III

Specialized Practice in Critical Care Nursing

15

Trauma Care

Karen L. Johnson and Steven B. Johnson

Trauma is a disease that affects people of all ages. It is the most frequent cause of death in persons less than 44 years of age and is considered by some to be exclusively a young person's disease. However, the elderly patient population is not exempt from trauma. Independent of age, injury is the leading cause of all physician contacts and the fifth most common cause of death in people older than 65 years (Young, Cephas, & Blow, 1998). As older adults experience good health and maintain an active life style, they continue to engage in activities they have enjoyed throughout their lives, but they are at greater risk for injury related to these activities (Robbins & Courts, 1997). Reports have shown the rate of elderly involved in trauma to be as high as 29% (Marciani, 1999).

The elderly are predisposed to traumatic injuries because of the inevitable consequences of aging. Age-related deterioration of the senses and changes in postural stability, motor strength, balance, and coordination reduce the ability to react to or avoid environmental hazards (Santora, Schinco, & Trooskin, 1994). These limitations are further exacerbated by conditions such as dementia, arthritis, and postural hypotension. Osteoporosis, a common disease process in elderly women, has been implicated as a major contributing factor to the high incidence of fractures seen in elderly trauma patients. Research also suggests that elderly patients incur more physiological compromise as a result of less severe anatomic injury (DeKeyser, Carolan, & Trask, 1995).

Once injured, the elderly have a more prolonged hospitalization and rehabilitation than younger patients with similar injuries have, and they consume a greater portion of the cost of trauma care. Considerable debate exists about the proper expenditure of resources for the care of the elderly, especially in situations in which the long-term outlook for meaningful survival and functional recovery appears bleak (Carrillo, Richardson, Malias, Cryer, & Miller, 1993).

DISTINGUISHING FEATURES OF TRAUMA
IN THE ELDERLY

The elderly may experience similar types of injuries as younger people experience; however, there are distinct differences in injury pattern, effect, postinjury course, and outcome that occur with advancing age (Schwab & Kauder, 1992). The principles of trauma resuscitation and management generally remain the same for trauma patients of all ages. However, it is essential that critical care clinicians understand and appreciate age-related physiological changes and the age-dependent physiological reactions that occur in response to injury and therapy. Detailed histories must be obtained in an effort to get a complete picture of events surrounding the injury. Trauma patients over age 65 have a higher mortality rate, longer hospital stays, more complications, a common mechanism of injury, and poorer outcomes than their younger counterparts do. These unique aspects of geriatric trauma must be considered when planning care for this subset of elderly trauma patients (Rauen, 1992).

Mechanism of Injury and Injury Patterns

Mechanisms of injury tend to be different in the elderly than they are in the young. Falls predominate, followed by motor vehicle crashes, and pedestrians hit by motor vehicles (Champion et al., 1990).

The elderly experience the majority of all falls that result in injuries (DeKeyser et al., 1995). These falls are less likely to be from great heights, as they are in younger patients. They most commonly occur from level surfaces or from steps. Most of the injuries occur in the winter months, in or about the home. Because many of the falls by the elderly can be caused by an underlying medical problem, management of the elderly fall victim must include an evaluation of events and conditions immediately preceding the fall. A sudden decrease in cerebral blood flow (due to cardiac dysrhythmias, venous pooling, autonomic insufficiency) or a metabolic derangement (hypoglycemia, hypoxia, anemia) is often the cause (Schwab & Kauder, 1992). For these reasons, patients who present with a fall-related injury should receive a thorough search for an inciting event. A concentrated effort to delineate any underlying problems (environmental or medical) should be taken.

The exposure of the elderly to motor vehicle trauma is a consequence of the increasing growth of the elderly population and the growing number of elderly drivers and occupants of motor vehicles. Elderly drivers appear to have low crash rates compared with younger drivers, in large part because they drive much less often. When the groups are normalized for the number of miles driven, the 65 and older group has the second highest crash rate after new drivers (Santora et al., 1994). Motor vehicle crashes are the leading cause of trauma-related death in the group aged 65 to 75 (Schwab & Kauder, 1992). Most deaths occur from side impact crashes and are the result of driver error. These crashes may occur as a result of a combination of factors (Table 15.1). A thorough history of the injury must be obtained from the patient, family, and prehospital personnel. If the patient is responsive, it is important to determine if any particular events precipitated the crash. For example, a patient may have experienced chest pain or shortness of breath before losing control of the vehicle. This history can provide valuable information and can alter the treatment plan.

A moving vehicle is one of the most devastating mechanisms of injury. The elderly are involved in crashes as pedestrians more commonly than any other age group, including children (National Safety Council, 1992). Half of all deaths that occur at crosswalks occur in individuals over age 65 (Robbins & Courts, 1997). Physiological diminution of cerebral and motor skills and alterations in visual and auditory acuity may cause elder pedestrians to walk directly into the path of oncoming vehicles. In addition, many older adults are unable to quickly cross the intersection before traffic signals change. Elderly pedestrians struck by motor vehicles most commonly have head, chest, and leg injuries.

Although falls and vehicular trauma account for the most serious injuries seen in the intensive care unit in the geriatric population, older adults are increasingly becoming victims of violent crime and abuse. There is an increased incidence of assaults with blunt objects and penetrating trauma to this population. Traumatic abuse of elders includes physical violence and neglect. A high index of suspicion must be maintained when an elderly individual appears bruised, battered, poorly nourished, or unkempt or has an inconsistent pattern of injury (McMahon, Schwab, & Kauder, 1996).

Outcome

Mortality after trauma is usually the result of direct injury to organs and tissues or from indirect injury from the myriad physiological and biochemical derangements that accompany trauma (Perdue, Watts, Kaufman, &

TABLE 15.1   Factors That Predispose the Elderly to Motor Vehicle Crashes

Exacerbation of acute or chronic medical conditions
Physiological diminution of cerebral skills
Physiological diminution of motor skills
Cognitive deficits in memory and judgment
Alterations in visual and auditory acuity
Medications that interfere with safe driving
Deterioration in strength and slower reaction times
Increased exposure by continued use of the car as a primary source of transportation

Trask, 1998). Trauma in the elderly has been shown to be associated with a higher mortality in spite of less severe injuries. The increased mortality is related to both the cause and the severity of injuries, as well as the number of resultant complications. The results from the Major Trauma Outcome Study (Champion et al., 1990) showed that mortality increases directly with age greater than 55 years, regardless of injury mechanism, severity, or body region injured. The higher elderly mortality has been attributed to the effects of preexisting diseases such as ischemic heart disease, obstructive lung disease, cirrhosis and diabetes (Perdue et al., 1998). Complications that occur following trauma can have an impact on mortality. Elderly patients suffer a greater number of complications post injury than do younger trauma patients (Champion et al., 1990).

Relatively minor trauma can be the event that changes an elderly person with a relatively independent lifestyle to one who requires prolonged rehabilitation or skilled nursing care. This necessitates discharge planning early in the course of admission. Although mortality rates are the most visible means of measuring outcome, functional status at the time of discharge and over the long term is of far greater importance to the elderly survivors of severe injury and their families (Schwab & Kauder, 1992).

A few studies have addressed the functional outcome of the elderly, but the results are contradictory. Studies have used widely different approaches to the measurement of disability, which has resulted in wide variety in both the rate and degree of reported dysfunction after serious injury (Holbrook, Anderson, Seiber, Browner, & Hoyt, 1999). As a consequence, it is not clear whether intensive treatments lead to comparable outcome results in young and elderly trauma patients with multiple injuries. Such data might have consequences on therapeutic strategies, health care planning, and the allocation of resources (Van der Sluis, Klasen, Eisma, & ten Duis, 1996).

The adverse effect of trauma on survival in elderly patients is not isolated to the immediate postinjury period but can last for years after the trauma episode. The reason for this persistent negative effect on survival is unknown. One reason may be that once injured, elderly patients never regain their level of preinjury health, perhaps as a direct result of loss of function secondary to injury, complications of injury, or a depletion of body energy stores (Gubler et al., 1997).

Impacts of Limited Physiological Reserve on Resuscitation Phase

The concept of "limited physiological reserve" in the elderly trauma patient highlights the key difference between the average younger trauma patient with normal physiological reserve and the elderly patient with underlying physiological derangements (Schwab & Kauder, 1992). The concept is consistent with age-related physiological alterations that occur in virtually every organ system. The extent of abnormal underlying physiological characteristics differs greatly between individuals. These age-related physiological changes produce widely variable responses to injury, particularly after age 55. In a young person, a predictable normal physiological response to trauma can be assumed. These same assumptions cannot be made in the severely injured geriatric patient. It is important to remember that resting organ function may be preserved in the elderly, but the ability to augment function in response to traumatic stress may be greatly compromised.

Elderly patients typically have limited physiological reserve in many organ systems. Diminished physiological function in the elderly may be identified by a decrease in cardiac index, pulmonary compliance, and renal function. In the elderly, marginal cardiac reserve is usually associated with coronary artery disease, and marginal respiratory reserve is related to loss of pulmonary elasticity. The decreased ability of the kidneys to handle fluid challenges during resuscitation may also add to the propensity for early cardiopulmonary complications.

Fluid resuscitation is an integral intervention in the trauma resuscitation phase. The amount of fluid to be administered may have to be corrected for the lesser lean body mass of the elderly (Demarest, Osler, & Clevenger, 1990). Chronic volume depletion and total body potassium depletion may occur in the elderly as a result of chronic diuretic therapy. This may necessitate more volume and potassium supplementation. Isotonic electrolyte solutions, used for the initial resuscitation of trauma patients of all ages, provide intravascular volume expansion. Ringer's lactate is the fluid of choice. Although normal saline is a satisfactory replacement for many conditions, it has the potential for producing hyperchloremic acidosis when used in volumes commonly administered during a trauma resuscitation. This potential is more critical in the elderly patient with impaired renal reserve.

The assessment and management of hypovolemic shock is more complex in the elderly trauma patient. Loss of physiological reserve and presence of preexisting conditions are likely to produce conflicting hemodynamic data. The older adult may appear to be hemodynamically stable in the face of inadequate perfusion. This can occur for several reasons. Elderly patients may be taking drugs to induce beta blockade and calcium channel blockade for the management of hypertension and angina. These drugs interfere with conduction through the atrial ventricular node and produce bradycardia. An absence of tachycardia in patients who take these drugs may be misconstrued as adequate stroke volume and cardiac output. Increased circulating catecholamines in the young heart increase heart rate in the face of increased oxygen demand. However, with advancing age, sensitivity to exogenous and endogenous catecholamines decreases. For this reason, the expected compensatory tachycardia produced by shock states may not occur and a diminished heart rate may be observed (Robbins & Courts, 1997). Age-related changes in the heart include a stiffening of the myocardium, resulting in decreased left ventricular compliance. This impairs pump function and cardiac reserve. Therefore, cardiac output can be significantly less than in younger patients.

All of the previous factors exacerbate the difficulties in resuscitating the elderly trauma patient. The elderly are as intolerant of overresuscitation as they are of hypovolemia (Demarest et al., 1990). Resuscitation of the elderly should proceed along the guidelines of the *Advanced Trauma Life Support Manual of the Committee on Trauma of the American College of Surgeons* (American College of Surgeons, 1997). The use of invasive hemodynamic monitoring, including the early insertion of pulmonary and peripheral arterial catheters, can facilitate the determination of adequacy of perfusion. Studies have found that, in spite of normal vital signs, cardiac output and mixed venous oxygen saturation can be low in elderly patients (Scalea et al., 1990).

Normal age-related changes make cervical spine clearance (radiographic visualization of C1 through C7) more difficult (Robbins & Courts, 1997). Additional radiography, including magnetic resonance imaging, may be required to clearly view the cervical spine. Kyphosis can make cervical spine immobilization difficult and uncomfortable for geriatric patients.

Monitoring of body temperature is particularly important in the elderly because hypothermia increases postinjury complications. Advancing age impairs the ability to regulate body heat production and heat loss related to hypothyroidism, decreased muscle mass, decreased metabolic rate, and peripheral vascular changes. Hypothermia should be prevented through the use of warm intravenous fluids, warm blankets, and heat lamps.

The need for nutritional support appears to be greater in elderly trauma patients than it is in well-nourished younger patients. Physiological changes associated with aging influence glucose tolerance, renal clearance, and serum growth hormone. The older patient's lack of physiological reserve makes it imperative that early nutritional support be initiated. However, glucose tolerance decreases with normal aging and enteral or parenteral feeding may result in marked hyperglycemia, particularly when it is associated with the insulin resistance that accompanies trauma and critical illness (Marciani, 1999). Nutritional consults are imperative to ensure optimal nutritional support. Enteral feeding is the clear choice as the most effective physiological route for providing nutrition. A feeding tube should be positioned past the pylorus and the enteral formula product administered should be individualized to meet the unique needs of the geriatric patient with traumatic injuries.

Preexisting Conditions

Response to injury depends on the extent of individual physiological reserve and presence of preexisting conditions. Preexisting conditions complicate the treatment response and recovery and increase the risk of death in older patients with trauma (Robbins & Courts, 1997). The mortality rate varies according to the type of medical condition and the number of conditions. Although cardiovascular disease and hypertension are common among elderly trauma patients, the presence of renal disease or malignancy is associated with the highest mortality (Milzman, Boulanger, & Rodriquez, 1992).

Preexisting cardiac disease can greatly complicate the management of patients with severe trauma. There are higher complication and mortality rates in patients with cardiac disease, but early recognition, accurate monitoring, and aggressive correction of abnormalities as they arise can substantially improve prognosis (Wilson, 1994).

Chronic pulmonary disease is one of the most prevalent preexisting medical disorders and has been associated with high mortality rates (O'Brien & Criner, 1994). The high mortality presumably is due to the respiratory complications of trauma, coupled with reduced pulmonary reserve and the increased prevalence of pulmonary complications.

Trauma patients of all ages are at risk for acute renal failure through a variety of mechanisms (direct injury, renal hypoperfusion, hypoxia, direct cellular toxicity), but this risk is intensified for patients with chronic renal insufficiency. Patients with chronic renal insufficiency have little tolerance for further nephron loss from trauma, sepsis, hypovolemia, or drug toxicity. Therefore, it is imperative to protect the kidney by maintaining adequate perfusion and avoiding nephrotoxic insults. Special attention must be given to fluid resuscitation in patients with preexisting renal disease because of their limited or absent ability to excrete solutes and fluids. Invasive hemodynamic monitoring is helpful in guiding resuscitation efforts because urine output and acid-base balance are unreliable markers as end points of resuscitation.

Normal endocrine system functioning is necessary for immediate survival posttraumatic injury. The endocrine system regulates fluid, electrolyte, and substrate balance during the early and late stresses associated with multisystem trauma. Preexisting endocrine system dysfunction may inhibit the elderly trauma patient's ability to respond to severe stress. In addition, chronic endocrine disease, such as diabetes mellitus, can impair widespread organ function. These may occur on a clinical or subclinical basis. Endocrine deficiencies may present insidiously and may be recognized only during severe stress. Therefore, critical care clinicians must have a high index of suspicion for possible endocrine disorders in all trauma patients, but especially in those with sudden clinical deterioration or unexplained fluid and electrolyte imbalance (Boulanger & Gann, 1994).

MANAGEMENT CONSIDERATIONS FOR SPECIFIC INJURIES IN THE ELDERLY

Traditional trauma protocols have been well-established for the treatment of young trauma patients. As clinicians have come to recognize how older trauma patients differ from younger trauma patients, they have recognized the need to tailor management plans to meet these patients' special needs.

In the milieu of limited physiological reserve and preexisting conditions, even a minor injury can compromise the elderly trauma patient. The best outcomes have been achieved through immediate invasive monitoring and mechanical ventilation, aggressive volume resuscitation, special vigilance against complications and early mobilization of the patient (Stamatos, Sorensen, & Tefler, 1996).

Head Injuries

Falls are the most common mechanism of head injury in the elderly. There is a higher incidence of subdural and intraparenchymal hematomas. As the brain undergoes a progressive loss of volume with age, the space around the brain becomes larger. Because of these age-related anatomic changes, the incidence of subdural hematomas is three times higher in the elderly (Demarest et al., 1990). This is an important consideration because gradual neurological decline may be the only symptom of a subdural hematoma.

Medical management of acute head injuries in the elderly is the same as for younger patients. Computerized tomography (CT) is indicated for decreasing level of consciousness, declining Glascow Coma Scale scores, and changes in pupillary reactivity. Management should include strategies to promote optimal cerebral perfusion pressure through interventions to augment mean arterial pressure and reduce intracranial pressure. Prompt surgical evacuation may be required for mass lesions.

Neurological recovery after severe head injury may be prolonged, and chances of mental reconstitution are less at advancing ages. Severity of head trauma is generally greater in the elderly and has been attributed to preexisting brain injury and underlying brain disease. The chronic use of some medications, particularly anticoagulants, can worsen head injury.

Early involvement of the family in the decision for aggressive management is extremely important in the management of the elderly with severe head injury. This is particularly so for patients remaining in a coma for more than 5 days and those showing signs of increased intracranial pressure (Santora et al., 1994). Previously stated patient desires and advanced directives should be discussed with the family when decisions about withholding aggressive support need to be made.

Spinal Cord Injuries

Most spinal cord injuries occur in men between the ages of 18 and 25, but when these injuries occur in the older adult, the results can be devastating. The age at the time of injury affects long-term rehabilitation. It has been reported that only 59% of spinal cord injury patients ages 61 to 86 years old survive more than 2 years, compared with 95% of patients ages 16 to

30 (Stamatos et al., 1996). Besides having a higher mortality rate, older adults experience more complications post injury and are hospitalized longer than are younger patients with spinal cord injuries.

Injury to the vertebrae is uncommon until the fifth and sixth decades of life, at which time the incidence of injury increases significantly. As ligaments and joints become less elastic with advancing age, overstretching occurs more easily. Degenerative joint disease and osteoporosis contribute to reduced anatomic strength and spinal stability. As a result, minimal trauma can cause dislocations or fractures in the spinal column.

Patients who sustain spinal cord injuries have a high risk of developing complications post injury. These include gastrointestinal bleeding, deep vein thrombosis, pulmonary emboli, pneumonia, infection, skin breakdown, contractures, and emotional distress. Older patients are at an even greater danger of developing these complications and therefore require vigilant monitoring and meticulous care to prevent them (Stamotos et al., 1996).

Chest Trauma

Chest trauma in the elderly is commonly the result of motor vehicle crashes. Common injuries include rib fractures and hemothoraces. The slowness with which these fractures heal in combination with impaired pulmonary and immunologic reserve in elderly patients makes rib fractures a particularly treacherous injury. For these patients a small contusion or a few rib fractures may necessitate mechanical ventilation, and only a few days on the ventilator may result in pneumonia that can ultimately prove fatal. Elderly patients with chest trauma have a higher incidence of cardiac arrest than younger patients do because of limited cardiopulmonary reserve (Shorr, Rodriquez, & Indeck, 1989).

Various age-related physiological changes can impair respiratory function and hinder recovery. These include calcification of costal cartilage, which stiffens the rib cage; increased rigidity and decreased recoil in the lungs; weaker respiratory muscles; and fewer, less functional alveoli. All of these result in decreased vital capacity and functional residual capacity. Pain associated with rib fractures can be intense and can impair effective coughing and deep breathing. This can lead to atelectasis, mucous plugging, and pneumonia, which all further impair ventilation and oxygenation. Aggressive pulmonary toilet can be achieved through effective pain management regimes. Analgesics must be used with caution to avoid any respiratory depression. Regional anesthetic therapy (epidural anesthesia) is often effective. Early mechanical ventilation should be considered in patients who have failed more conservative means of pulmonary support.

Management of the geriatric trauma patient with chest injury should include careful fluid management, aggressive chest physiotherapy, effective pain management, prevention of deep vein thrombosis and pulmonary emboli, cardiac rhythm monitoring, and measurement of cardiac output.

Abdominal Trauma

Prompt and accurate diagnosis of intra-abdominal trauma is imperative because the elderly are intolerant of shock and unnecessary laparotomy (Demarest et al., 1990). Determination of intra-abdominal injury is made using physical examination, diagnostic peritoneal lavage, or abdominal CT, or a combination of these. However, diagnostic peritoneal lavage may be contraindicated however in elderly persons who have undergone previous major abdominal operative procedures (Schwab & Kauder, 1992). Splenic rupture is an uncommon injury in the elderly because of the relative atrophy of this organ (McMahon, Schwab, & Kauder, 1996).

Fractures

The high incidence of osteoporosis in the elderly leads to an increased incidence of fractures. Hip fractures remain the most frequent cause of hospital admission for trauma in the elderly (Santora et al., 1994). Responsible for this epidemic is the combination of loss of bone density, increased bone fragility, and the propensity for the elderly to fall.

Efficient and effective management of hip fractures in the elderly involves following general guidelines employed in the management of the multiply injured trauma patient. These protocols involve early fracture fixation and early patient mobilization. These strategies can be effective in decreasing pulmonary complications post fracture.

Wound Healing

All aspects of wound healing appear to be influenced by the aging process. The inflammatory and proliferative phase are decreased with delayed angiogenesis, delayed epithelialization, and delayed remodeling (Marciani, 1999). Fibroblast function diminishes and impairs collagen synthesis necessary for wound repair. Wound repair and healing is also affected by age-associated changes in immunologic function. T-cell production and function decline with age. Progressive atrophic changes in the lymphoid system are manifested by a decrease in lymphoid cells that results in a decrease in cell-mediated and humoral responses to antigenic stimuli. These age-related changes in immunologic function compromise wound healing and affect the elderly patient's ability to resist infection. Principles of wound management in the elderly have been recommended by Marciani (1999) and are summarized in Table 15.2.

Mortality from tetanus in developed countries is largely limited to the elderly. Some elderly people may not have been fully immunized against tetanus, making them vulnerable when they have tetanus prone wounds (McMahon et al., 1996). Both immunization and prophylaxis should be considered after potential exposure in the elderly.

REHABILITATION

The aim of rehabilitation is to restore the patient to former functional status and to maintain or maximize the remaining function. Special rehabilitation treatment efforts may be required in the geriatric patient. Unlike the younger trauma patient population in which rehabilitation outcomes can be dramatic, the geriatric patient is likely to realize more subtle progress (Santora et al., 1994).

The time interval between injury and restoration of ambulation is crucial. During this time the patient is susceptible to the hazards of immobility, including compromised cardiopulmonary function, muscle atrophy and contractures, skin breakdown, development of deep vein thrombosis and pulmonary emboli. Therefore, efforts to promote mobility are essential and should include passive and active range of motion exercises while on bedrest and then progression to assisted transfers and eventually ambulation. However, these rehabilitation efforts can present special challenges in the geriatric patient. Passive range of motion is essential to the patient with arthritis. Arthritis with resultant ligament and joint capsule ossification decreases baseline flexibility and increases pain and disability. Ambulation is not always possible because of other injuries, fatigue, previous stroke, or incoordination.

PREVENTION

Given the high risk of trauma to the elderly in terms of mortality, change in lifestyle, and financial cost, primary preventive measures are of the utmost importance. Three injury prevention strategies have been proposed: (1) preevent, which focuses on increasing public awareness through educa-

TABLE 15.2　Wound Management in the Elderly

Excision of ragged wound edges (vascularity is reduced)
Prophylactic use of antibiotics (when potential for infection is increased)
Longer maintenance of sutures (wound healing is delayed)

tional promotion and programs that may influence legislation; (2) event, which centers on efforts to reduce the energy transfer during the injury process; and (3) postevent, which deals with efforts to improve resuscitation (Santora et al., 1994). Educational programs should be offered to geriatric groups to prevent injury. These programs should promote safety in the home and may include such interventions as a home safety inspection to assess heights of beds and toilets, use of throw rugs, and lighting of indoor hallways and outdoor walkways. Motor vehicle crashes may potentially be reduced by identification of impaired drivers, including those with hearing or visual impairments, disabling musculoskeletal disorders, dementia, or medications that decrease these skills. In an effort to refresh skills and update traffic knowledge, driver education programs for adults greater than age 55 have been established by the American Association of Retired Persons. Pedestrian prevention programs have been shown to reduce fatal and serious injury in the elderly. Prolongation of stop light times to accommodate the decreased rate of walking of the elderly, modifications of road and crosswalk signs, tighter speed limit enforcement, and safety education presentations at senior centers have been effective in decreasing the incidence of pedestrian-vehicular crashes in the elderly.

SUMMARY

The critically ill elderly trauma patient poses a unique and complex picture that requires an understanding of age-related physiological changes, concomitant effects of acquired diseases, and the interaction of these processes on recovery after a traumatic insult. These processes vary from person to person. This increases the need for individualized management of the critically ill traumatically injured geriatric patient.

REFERENCES

American College of Surgeons, Subcommittee on Advanced Trauma Life Support. (1997). *Advanced trauma life support course for physicians.* Chicago: American College of Surgeons.

Boulanger, B. R., & Gann, D. S. (1994). Management of the trauma victim with pre-existing endocrine disease. *Critical Care Clinics, 10,* 537–566.

Carrillo, E. H., Richardson, J. D., Malias, M. A., Cryer, H. M., & Miller, F. B. (1993). Long term outcome of blunt trauma care in the elderly. *Surgery, Gynecology & Obstetrics, 176,* 559–564.

Champion, H. R., Copes, W. S., Sacco, W. J., Lawnick, M. M., Keast, S. L., Bain, L. W., Flannagan, M. E., & Frey, C. F. (1990). The Major Trauma Outcome Study: Establishing national norms for trauma care. *Journal of Trauma, 30,* 1356–1365.

DeKeyser, F., Carolan, D., & Trask, A. (1995). Suburban geriatric trauma: The experiences of a level I trauma center. *American Journal of Critical Care, 4,* 379–382.

Demarest, G. B., Osler, T. M., & Clevenger, F. W. (1990). Injuries in the elderly: Evaluation and initial response. *Geriatrics, 45,* 36–42.

Gubler, K. D., Davis, R., Koepsell, T., Soderberg, R., Maler, R. V., & Rivara, F. P. (1997). Long term survival of elderly trauma patients. *Archives of Surgery, 132,* 1010–1014.

Holbrook, T. L., Anderson, J. P., Sieber, W. J., Browner, D., & Hoyt, D. B. (1999). Outcome after major trauma: 12 month and 18 month follow-up results from the trauma recovery project. *Journal of Trauma, 46,* 765–773.

Marciani, R. D. (1999). Critical systemic and psychosocial considerations in the management of trauma in the elderly. *Oral Surgery, Oral Medicine, & Oral Pathology, 87,* 272–280.

McMahon, D. J., Schwab, C. W., & Kauder, D. (1996). Comorbidity and the elderly patient. *World Journal of Surgery, 20,* 113–120.

Milzman, D. P., Boulanger, B. R., Rodriguez, Z., Soderstrom, C. A., Mitchell, K. A., & Magnant, C. M. (1992). Pre-existing disease in trauma patients: A predictor of fate independent of age and injury severity score. *Journal of Trauma, 32,* 236–243.

National Safety Council. (1992). Accident facts. Chicago: National Safety Council.

O'Brien, G. M., & Criner, G. J. (1994). Chronic pulmonary disease. *Critical Care Clinics, 10,* 507–522.

Perdue, P. W., Watts, D. D., Kaufman, C. R., & Trask, A. L. (1998). Differences in mortality between elderly and younger adult trauma patients: Geriatric status increases risk of delayed death. *Journal of Trauma, 45,* 805–810.

Rauen, C. A. (1992). Trauma and the elderly: The impact on critical care. *AACN Clinical Issues in Critical Care Nursing, 3,* 149–154.

Robbins, L. M., & Courts, N. F. (1997). Care of the traumatized older adult. *Geriatric Nursing, 18,* 209–215.

Santora, T. A., Schinco, M. A., & Trooskin, S. Z. (1994). Management of trauma in the elderly patient. *Surgical Clinics of North America, 74,* 163–186.

Scalea, T. M., Simon, H. W., Duncan, A. O., Atweh, N. A., Sclafani, S. J. A., & Phillips, T. F. (1990). Geriatric blunt trauma: Improved survival with early invasive monitoring. *Journal of Trauma, 30,* 129–136.

Schwab, C. W., & Kauder, D. R. (1992). Trauma in the geriatric patient. *Archives in Surgery, 127,* 701–706.

Shorr, R. M., Rodriquez, A., & Indeck, M. C. (1989). Blunt chest trauma in the elderly. *Journal of Trauma, 29,* 234–237.

Stamatos, C. A., Sorensen, P. A., & Tefler, K. M. (1996). The older trauma patient. *American Journal of Nursing, 96,* 192–200.

Van der Sluis, C. K., Klasen, H. J., Eisma, W. H., & ten Duis, H. J. (1996). Major trauma in young and old: What is the difference? *Journal of Trauma, 40,* 78–82.

Wilson, R. F. (1994). Trauma patients with pre-existing cardiac disease. *Critical Care Clinics, 10,* 461–506.

Young, J. S., Cephas, G. A., & Blow, O. (1998). Outcome and cost of trauma among the elderly: A real life model of a single payer reimbursement system. *Journal of Trauma, 45,* 800–804.

16

Medical Intensive Care

Marquis D. Foreman and Ruth M. Kleinpell

Patients aged 65 years to 84 years currently constitute 58% of the adult critical care population with the highest rates of admission to the intensive care unit (ICU) occurring among those aged 70 years to 79 years (Castilo-Lorente, Rivera-Fernandez, & Vazqauex-Mata, 1997; Tullman & Dracup, 2000). Although the outcome of critical illness is in part affected by age, age is not the most important determinant of prognosis following ICU treatment (Chelluri, Grenvik, & Silverman, 1995; Kleinpell & Ferrans, 1998). Intensivists agree that severity of illness and concurrent health status have a significantly greater impact on the use of intensive care resources and outcomes of critical care than age has (Chelluri et al., 1995; Jacobs, van der Vliet, van Roozendale, & van der Linder, 1988; McLish, Powell, Montenegro, & Nochonovitz, 1987; Nicholas, Le Gall, Alperovitch, Loirat, & Villers, 1987; Scheffler, Knaus, Wagner, & Zimmerman, 1982). However, great debate continues about the appropriateness of ICU treatment for the elderly, and rationing of ICU technologies on the basis of age has been proposed (Callahan, 1996, 1998).

The dilemma regarding the appropriateness of intensive care for the elderly is extraordinarily complex and confounded by conflicting evidence about the benefits of intensive care for the elderly. The elderly are more vulnerable to less than desirable outcomes of intensive care in part because of the lack of clarity about what the desirable outcomes of care for the elderly are, as well as because of the presence of multiple chronic illnesses and their complex treatments and the environment in which the intensive care is provided. Psychosocial, cognitive, and physiological factors also contribute to the risk of poorer outcomes of intensive care; many of these issues are presented elsewhere in this text and by Tullman and Dracup (2000). Additional facets of this dilemma are presented in this chapter. Physiological alterations associated with aging contribute to an elder's vulnerability to poorer outcomes of care; these are reviewed in this chapter. Because elderly patients with chronic illness often experience exacerbations in their condition, hospitalization is often required. Specialized treatment in special care units for chronically critically ill patients has been explored as a viable treatment option. Appropriate use of ICU therapies is recognized as a necessary component of ICU treatment of the critically ill elderly. The use of invasive therapies during critical illness continues to be debated, and the impact of age on the outcome of critical illness with the use of invasive treatments is being called into question. Lastly, quality of life, which is increasingly being addressed in the medical and lay literature, remains an important consideration in the treatment of the critically ill elderly. These issues will be discussed relative to care of the critically ill elderly.

AGE-RELATED CHANGES AND IMPACT ON CRITICAL ILLNESS

Physiological decline in virtually every body system in the elderly places them at even greater risk when they experience any critical illness. Changes in the cardiovascular system include myocardial hypertrophy and hemodynamic changes that lead to decreased cardiac reserve. Conduction system changes result in a decreased number of pacemaker cells in the sinoatrial node, contraction time is slowed, and a slowed ventricular filing rate and increased vessel stiffness result (Forrest, 2000; Ribera-Casado, 1999). Although blood pressure rises with age, hypertension is not a normal age-related physiological event. Yet, hypertension is a prevalent cardiovascular disease commonly found in the elderly because of age-related changes in vascular compliance.

Aging results in a gradual decline in renal blood flow, glomerular filtration rate, renal tubular resorptive capacity, and sodium excretion (Forrest, 2000; Muhlberg & Platt, 1999). Changes in bladder capacity occur as bladder muscles weaken, and incomplete emptying may occur. Incontinence can also occur and may result from bladder outlet changes, stress incontinence, or central nervous system disorders. Changes in renal functioning with age can alter the renal excretion of drugs, resulting in decreased excretion rates (Muhlberg & Platt, 1999) (see also chapter 10).

Immune system changes that occur with aging include a decline in the humoral and cell-mediated immune responses. With a decrease in normal immunological functions, the elderly patient is more susceptible to infections and malignancy (Forrest, 2000).

Changes associated with aging that affect pulmonary functioning include a decrease in vital capacity and respiratory excursion, increased residual volume, and a decrease in ventilatory response to hypoxia and hypercapnia and in alveolar-capillary gas-diffusing capacity (Forrest, 2000). Respiratory function is further compromised in the elderly because of decreased lung compliance and weakened respiratory musculature.

Gastrointestinal system changes that occur with aging include a decrease in gastric motility, gastric mucosa atrophy, and diminished absorption capacity (Forrest, 2000). The elderly are more likely than younger persons are to have deficient levels of serum albumin, protein, vitamins, and hemoglobin because of malabsorptive and gastrointestinal disorders such as gastritis, peptic ulcer disease, vascular ischemia, and pancreatic disease (Forrest, 2000). The elderly also may experience xerostoma, or dry mouth, difficulties swallowing, and problems with dentition that can alter their nutritional intake.

The aging process also affects the integument system, resulting in degenerative changes in elastic and collagen tissues, decreased vascularity, and increased capillary fragility. These factors contribute to increased skin fragility, loss of body hair, increased healing time, and increased susceptibility to pressure sores (Forrest, 2000). Additionally, loss of subcutaneous tissue and a decrease in sweat glands contribute to the diminished ability of the skin to maintain body temperature (Forrest, 2000).

Age-related changes that occur in the nervous system include neuronal cell loss, changes in synaptic transmissions, slowed conduction of the nerve impulses, and loss of peripheral nerve functions (Forrest, 2000). Sensory and motor disorders and mental status changes can result.

An understanding of the physiological changes that occur with aging are important in assessing the needs of the elderly patient who is critically ill. Because aging occurs differently in different individuals, it is requisite that nursing care goals be individualized. Nursing care of elderly ICU patients is concerned with all body systems.

CHRONICALLY CRITICALLY ILL

The length of stay in intensive care units is typically short, on the average of 3–4 days. However, since the late 1980s there has been a growing patient population with protracted stays of up to months. These patients have been labeled "the chronically critically ill." Although this patient population is not exclusively elderly, it is predominately elderly. The chronically critically ill create great conflict and burden: Their care is costly to institutions, the benefits and outcomes of intensive care are unclear, and recovery for these patients is slow and difficult. As a consequence, these patients and their families and care providers are greatly dissatisfied and frustrated with the current models of care. Moreover, in this era of scare resources (limited intensive care nurses and beds) the chronically critically ill place even greater demands on ICU resources (Daly, Rudy, Thompson, & Happ, 1991).

The chronically critically ill are those patients who are physiologically stable but continue to require intensive medical and nursing care and various forms of life support as a result of complications or underlying chronic health conditions exacerbated by a protracted critical illness (Daly et al., 1991; Rudy et al., 1995). Although these patients have survived the most acute phase of a life-threatening illness and continue to require sustained ventilatory and nutritional support (Rudy et al., 1995), the impact of treatment and prognosis may appear uncertain or less favorable (Rockwood et al., 1993).

One alternative approach to the care of these chronically critically ill patients that has proven successful is the special care unit. These units have been designed specifically to meet the unique needs and challenges of this patient population. The goal of these special care units is to improve the outcomes of care while improving the satisfaction of patients, families, and care providers and decreasing the costs of care.

The special care environment as originally conceived (Daly et al., 1991) targets physiologically stable patients, and as a result physiological monitor technology monitoring is limited. Care is provided to patients by experienced critical care nurses in private rooms; care actively involves the patient and their families, promotes rehabilitation, and focuses on the long-term management of specific patient care problems. Initial testing of this model of care has demonstrated great success in minimizing costs while maximizing outcomes and satisfaction with care (Douglas et al., 1996; Rudy et al., 1995)

USE OF INVASIVE THERAPIES

ICUs first appeared in the 1940s as outgrowths of postoperative recovery rooms, and by 1980 almost every hospital had at least one ICU (Draper, 1983). The ICU serves as a place for monitoring and care of patients with actual or potentially severe physiological instability requiring technical or artificial life support (Task Force of the American College of Critical Care Medicine, Society of Critical Care Medicine, 1999).

ICUs were originally expected to decrease mortality and decrease overall costs of medical care (Hilberman, 1975). However, the cost of intensive care treatment has escalated as a result of the expensive equipment, supplies, and therapies rendered in ICU settings. ICU treatment currently accounts for 15 to 20% of costs for total hospital care, with the average cost of an ICU stay ranging from $12,000 to $22,000 (Fakhry, Kercher, & Rutledge, 1996; Friedman, Steiner, & Scott, 1998). Appropriate use of ICU resources is important; data remain lacking on the use and outcome of life-sustaining technologies in the elderly. Some surgical and invasive procedures are now routinely performed in elderly patients who have good outcomes; however, the cost of invasive technologies has raised the question of the appropriate use of costly ICU care.

Two principle roles of ICUs are life support of organ-system failure in critically ill patients and monitoring of stable, noncritically ill patients who may require intensive care treatment or life support (Knaus, Draper, & Wagner, 1983). ICU treatment should be reserved for patients with treatable medical conditions with reasonable prospect of recovery (Task Force, 1999).

Guidelines have been developed for admission of patients to the ICU based on expert opinion and the relevant literature, which outline that life-threatening or critical conditions require ICU treatment, regardless of age (Task Force, 1999).

Decisions about admission and treatment of patients in the ICU, however, are often clinical judgments based on diagnosis and instability. Prognostic scoring systems that classify a patient's prognosis of surviving a critical illness episode exist (Cullen, Civetta, & Briggs, 1974; Knaus et al., 1995; Teres & Lemeshow, 1987). However, they are often used as an additional parameter to guide treatment and not as the sole determinant of whether a patient should received invasive treatments in the ICU. The decision to aggressively treat a critically ill elderly patient is a complex one, and several issues need to be considered.

Factors that have an impact on response to invasive treatments and outcome from critical illness for the elderly include physiological changes that occur with the aging process and comorbidities. Studies of the influence of age and surgical mortality have found that underlying disease processes and timing of surgical intervention influenced risk, not simply age (Lubin, 1993). Additional research has shown that functional measures, including physical functioning and severity of illness were important predictors of hospital outcomes for patients aged 70 and older (Broslawski, Elkins, & Algus, 1995; Inouye et al., 1998).

Although many therapies rendered in the ICU are invasive, many are medically indicated. The use of emergent resuscitative treatments such as cardiopulmonary resuscitation and defibrillation are indicated for life-threatening conditions and are recognized as warranted therapies during critical illness to prevent imminent death in a patient with a prognosis for survival. The use of other invasive treatments, such as the insertion of chest tubes for pleural drainage, lumbar puncture for spinal fluid analysis, and intubation for maintenance of respiratory function depend on the patient condition and medical need.

The use of other invasive therapies is not clearly outlined. For example, the routine use of hemodynamic monitoring has recently been questioned (Pulmonary Artery Catheter Census Conference Participants, 1997). The use of hemodynamic monitoring was once a commonplace invasive treatment in the ICU. Recent analysis of the benefits of hemodynamic monitoring, specifically the use of the pulmonary artery catheter, has raised concern about the risk of iatrogenic infection and the escalating costs (Leibowitz, 1996). Routine use of the pulmonary artery catheter is now not recommended for routine monitoring of low-risk patients in the ICU, regardless of age (Taylor et al., 1997).

The assumption that elderly patients cost more to care for because they present a higher risk has been cited as a reason that invasive treatments or surgical interventions might be limited solely on the basis of age (Del Guerico, 1996). Recent research has found that patients age 75 and older received fewer ICU therapies, despite higher severity of illness and mortality rates (Castillo-Lorente et al., 1997). Pressure to reduce health care cost increases has been suggested as a reason for rationing invasive and life-sustaining ICU treatments in critically ill elderly patients (Mick & Ackerman, 1997).

It is evident that continued research on outcomes of ICU care for the elderly is necessary if ICU resources are to be used efficiently.

QUALITY OF LIFE

Advancing technology has raised concerns about quality of life as an outcome variable of ICU treatment. Quality of life is being increasingly addressed in health care and medical literature yet rarely is a precise definition of the term given. References to and uses of the term quality of life vary widely, and, often, references to quality of life are made without specification to the meaning of quality of life (King, 1998). Terms that have been equated with quality of life include life satisfaction, worth of life, value of life, and self-esteem (Ferrans, 1990, 1996; Padilla & Frank-Stromborg, 1997). Definitions of quality of life suggest that it pertains to well-being, satisfaction of needs, life satisfaction, self-esteem, overall experience and condition of life, general happiness, and health-related quality of life (Dean, 1997; Ferrans, 1990, 1996; George & Bearon, 1980).

Both objective terms, such as physical functioning, and subjective terms, such as attitudes and feelings of well-being, have been used to describe quality of life. A multidimensional perspective of quality of life, incorporating objective and subjective components has been proposed for measuring quality of life in elderly patients (Lawton et al., 1999). The importance of using both objective and subjective dimensions for measuring quality of life in the elderly has also stressed the importance of functional status and health status (George & Bearon, 1980).

Research related to quality of life outcomes for the critically ill elderly has focused predominantly on objective measures such as age, survival, functional activity levels, ability to live at home, and hospital readmissions (Campion, Mulley, Goldstein, Barnett, & Thibault, 1981; Capuzo, Bianconi, Contu, Pavoni, & Gritti, 1996; Chelluri, Pinsky, Donahoe, & Grenvik, 1993; Hurel, Loirat, Saulneir, Nicholas, & Brivet, 1997; Konopad, Noseworthy, Johnston, Shustack, & Grace, 1995; McLean, McIntosh, King, Leung, & Byrick, 1985; Zaren & Hedstrand, 1987). Of those studies that measured quality of life subjectively, only overall measurements of quality of life have been used (McHugh, Havill, Armistead, Ullal, & Fayers, 1997; Patrick, Danis, Southerland, & Hong, 1988; Sage, Hurst, Silverman, & Bortz, 1987). Additionally, small sample sizes and little information on specific aspects of quality of life limit the usefulness of previous research for predicting outcomes for the elderly.

Several studies assessing outcomes after critical illness for elderly patients focusing on functioning or symptoms have also included assessments of quality of life. Responses from elderly cardiac surgery patients revealed favorable quality of life (McHugh et al., 1997), and a 1-year follow-up of elderly patients after ICU treatment found improving quality of life (Chelluri et al., 1993); however, additional research is needed.

Limited data are available regarding the long-term status and quality of life of elderly patients after ICU treatment. Additionally, the vagueness of the concept and failure to adequately define and adequately measure quality of life has limited the usefulness of the current research on quality of life of the critically ill elderly. Research specific to quality of life outcomes for the elderly has not been addressed sufficiently. To determine the impact of ICU treatment on the quality of life of the critically ill elderly patients, more comprehensive assessments of quality of life are needed.

SUMMARY

Although the elderly experience age-related changes that can influence outcome from critical illness, age alone does not influence the course of recovery after ICU treatment. Clinical outcomes of ICU care vary depending on illness severity, concurrent disease, and health status. Certain diseases and conditions are associated with particularly high ICU mortality rates, yet underlying disease has been identified as the most significant predictor of ICU outcome (Berensen, 1984; Oye & Bellamy, 1991; Scheffler et al., 1982; Ryan et al., 1997; Wu, Rubin, & Rosen, 1990). Previous research has shown that although age is related to ICU mortality rates, it is not as important a predictor of outcome as severity of illness, previous health status, and diagnosis (Wu et al., 1990; Beck, Taylor, Millar, & Smith, 1997). Age should never be used as the sole criterion for denying critically ill elderly patients indicated ICU treatment (Lubin, 1993). Until accurate data are available on the costs and use of life-sustaining technologies, the elderly as a group should be afforded ICU treatment (Kleinpell & Ferrans, 1998). Additionally, quality of life and alternative methods of caring for the critically ill elderly need to be explored further to meet the health care needs of this growing population.

REFERENCES

Beck, D. H., Taylor, B. C., Millar, B., & Smith, G. (1997). Prediction of outcome from intensive care: A prospective cohort study comparing Acute Physiology and Chronic Health Evaluation II and III prognostic systems in a United Kingdom intensive care unit. *Critical Care Medicine, 25* (1), 9–15.

Berensen, R. (1984). *Intensive care units (ICUs). Clinical outcomes cost and decision making.* Health Technology Case Study No. 28. Washington, DC: U.S. Government Printing Office.

Broslawski, G., Elkins, M., & Algus, M. (1995). Functional abilities of elderly survivors of intensive care. *Journal of American Occupational Association, 95,* 712–717.

Callahan D. (1996). Controlling the costs of health care for the elderly—fair means and foul. *New England Journal of Medicine, 335,* 744–746.

Callahan, D. (1998). *False hopes.* New York: Simon & Schuster.

Campion, E., Mulley, A., Goldstein, R., Barnett, O. & Thibault, G. (1981). Medical intensive care for the elderly. *JAMA, 246,* 2052–2056.

Capuzzo, M., Bianconi, M., Contu, P., Pavoni, V., & Gritti, G. (1996). Survival and quality of life after intensive care. *Intensive Care Medicine, 22,* 947–953.

Castillo-Lorente, E., Rivera-Fernandez, R., & Vazqauex-Mata, G. (1997). Limitation of therapeutic activity in elderly critically ill patients. *Critical Care Medicine, 25,* 1643–1648.

Chelluri, L., Grenvik, A., & Silverman, M. (1995). Intensive care for critically ill elderly: Mortality, costs, and quality of life: Review of the literature. *Archives of Internal Medicine, 155,* 1013–1022.

Chelluri, L., Pinsky, M., Donahoe, M., & Grenvik, A. (1993). Long-term outcome of critically ill elderly patients requiring intensive care. *Journal of the American Medical Association, 269,* 3119–3123.

Cullen, D., Civetta, J., & Briggs, B. (1974). Therapeutic intervention scoring system: A method for quantitative comparison of patient care. *Critical Care Medicine, 2,* 57–60.

Daly, B. J., Rudy, E. B., Thompson, K. S., & Happ, M. B. (1991). Development of a special care unit for chronically critically ill patients. *Heart & Lung, 20,* 45–51.

Dean, H. (1997). Multiple instruments for measuring quality of life. In M. Frank-Stromborg & S. Olsen (Eds.), *Instruments for clinical health-care research* (2nd ed., pp. 135–148). Boston: Jones and Barlett Publishers.

Del Guerico, L. (1996). Does pulmonary artery catheter use change outcome? Yes. *Critical Care Clinics, 3,* 553–557.

Douglas, S., Daly, B. J., Rudy, E. B., Sereika, S. M., Menzel, L., Song, R., Dyer, M. A., & Montenegro, H. D. (1996). Survival experience of chronically critically ill patients. *Nursing Research, 45,* 73–77.

Draper, E. (1983). Benefits and costs of intensive care. *Image, 15,* 90–94.

Fakhry, S., Kercher, K., & Rutledge, R. (1996). Survival, quality of life, and charges in critically ill surgical patients requiring prolonged ICU stays. *Journal of Trauma: Injury, Infection, and Critical Care, 41,* 999–1007.

Ferrans, C. (1996). Development of a conceptual model of quality of life. *Scholarly Inquiry for Nursing Practice, 10,* 293–304.

Ferrans, C. (1990). Quality of life: Conceptual issues. *Seminars in Oncology Nursing, 6,* 248–254.

Forrest, J. (2000). Gerontological alterations. In L. D. Urden & K. M. Stacy (Eds.), *Priorities in critical care nursing* (3rd ed., pp. 69–83). St. Louis: Mosby.

Friedman, B., Steiner, C., & Scott, J. (1998). Rationing of an expensive technology in the United States: Hospital intensive care units in two states, 1992. In D. Chinitz & J. Cohen (Eds.), *Governments and health systems: Implications of differing involvement* (pp. 483–496). New York: Wiley.

George, L., & Bearon, L. (1980). *Quality of life in older persons.* New York: Human Sciences Press, Inc.

Hilberman, M. (1975). The evolution of intensive care units. *Critical Care Medicine, 3,* 159–165.

Hurel, D., Loirat, P., Saulneir, F., Nicolas, F., & Brivet, F. (1997). Quality of life 6 months after intensive care: Results of a prospective multicenter study using a generic health status scale and a satisfaction scale. *Intensive Care Medicine, 23,* 331–337.

Jacobs, C., van der Vliet, J., van Roozendale, M., & van der Linder, C. (1988). Mortality and quality of life after care for critical illness. *Intensive Care Medicine, 14,* 217–220.

King, C. (1998). Overview of quality of life and controversial issues. In C. R. King & P. S. Hinds (Eds.), *Quality of life from nursing and patient perspectives* (pp. 23–33). Boston: Jones and Bartlett Publishers.

Kleinpell, R., & Ferrans, C. (1998). Factors influencing intensive care unit survival for critically ill elderly patients. *Heart & Lung, 27,* 337–343.

Knaus, W., Draper, D., & Wagner, D. (1983). The use of intensive care: New research initiatives and their implications for national health policy. *Milbank Memorial Quarterly, 61,* 561–583.

Knaus, W. A., Harrell, F. E., Lynn, J., Goldman, L., Phillips, R. S., Connors, A. F., Dawson, N. V., Fulkerson, W. J., Califf, R. M., & Debsiens, N. (1995). The SUP-PORT prognostic model. Objective and subjective estimates of survival for seriously ill hospitalized adults. Study to understand prognoses and preferences for outcomes and risks of treatments. *Annuals of Internal Medicine, 122,* 191–203.

Konopad, E., Noseworthy, T., Johnston, R., Shustack, A., & Grace, M. (1995). Quality of life measures before and one year after admission to an intensive care unit. *Critical Care Medicine, 23,* 1653–1659.

Lawton, M. P., Winter, L., Kleban, M. H., & Ruckdeschel, K. (1999). Affect and quality of life: Objective and subjective. *Journal of Aging and Health, 11,* 169–198.

Leibowitz, A. (1996). Do pulmonary artery catheters improve patient outcome? No. *Critical Care Clinics, 12,* 559–568.

Lubin, M. (1993). Is age a risk factor for surgery? *Medical Clinics of North America, 77,* 327–333.

McHugh, G., Havill, J., Armistead, S., Ullal, R., & Fayers, R. (1997). Follow up of elderly patients after cardiac surgery and intensive care unit admission. *New Zealand Medical Journal, 110,* 432–435.

McLean, A., McIntosh, J., King, G., Leung, D., & Byrick, R. (1985). Outcomes of respiratory intensive care for the elderly. *Critical Care Medicine, 13,* 625–629.

McLish, D., Powell, S., Montenegro, H., & Nochonovitz, M. (1987). The impact of age on utilization of intensive care resources. *Journal of the American Geriatric Society, 11,* 983–988.

Mick, D., & Ackerman, M. (1997). Neutralizing ageism in critical care via outcomes research. *AACN Clinical Issues, 8,* 597–608.

Muhlberg, W., & Platt, D. (1999). Age-dependent changes of the kidneys: Pharmacological implications. *Gerontology, 45,* 243–253.

Nicholas, F., Le Gall, J., Alperovitch, A., Loirat, P., & Villers, D. (1987). Influence of patients' age on survival, level of therapy and length of stay in ICU's. *Intensive Care Medicine, 13,* 9–13.

Oye, R., & Bellamy, P. (1991). Patterns of resource consumption in medical intensive care. *Chest, 99,* 685–689.

Padilla, G., & Frank-Stromborg, M. (1997). Single instruments for measuring quality of life. In M. Frank-Stromborg & S. Olsen (Eds.), *Instruments for clinical healthcare research* (2nd ed., pp. 114–134). Boston: Jones and Barlett.

Patrick, D., Danis, M., Southerland, L. I., & Hong, G. (1988). Quality of life following intensive care. *Journal of General Internal Medicine, 3*, 218–223.

Pulmonary Artery Catheter Consensus Conference Participants. (1997). Pulmonary artery catheter consensus conference: Consensus statement. *Critical Care Medicine, 25*, 910–925.

Ribera-Casado, J. M. (1999). Ageing and the cardiovascular system. *Journal of Gerontology and Geriatrics, 32*, 412–419.

Rockwood, K., Noseworthy, T. W., Gibney, R. T. N., Konopad, E., Shustack, A., Stollery, D., Johnston, R., & Grace, M. (1993). One-year outcome of elderly and young patients admitted to intensive care units. *Critical Care Medicine, 21*, 687–691.

Rudy, E. B., Daly, B. J., Douglas, S., Montenegro, H. D., Song, R., & Dyer, M. A. (1995). Patient outcomes for the chronically critically ill: Special care unit versus intensive care unit. *Nursing Research, 44*, 324–331.

Ryan, T., Rady, M., Bashour, A., Leventhal, M., Lytle, B., & Starr, N. (1997). Predictors of outcome in cardiac surgical patients with prolonged intensive care stay. *Chest, 112*, 1035–1042.

Sage, W., Hurst, C., Silverman, J., & Bortz, W. (1987). Intensive care for the elderly: Outcome of elective and nonelective admissions. *Journal of the American Geriatric Society, 35*, 312–317.

Scheffler, R., Knaus, W., Wagner, D., & Zimmerman, J. (1982). Severity of illness and the relationship between intensive care and survival. *American Journal of Public Health, 72*, 449–454.

Task Force of the American College of Critical Care Medicine, Society of Critical Care Medicine. (1999). Guidelines for intensive care unit admission, discharge, and triage. *Critical Care Medicine, 27*, 633–638.

Taylor, R. W., Calvin, J. E., & Matuschak, G. M. (1997). Pulmonary artery catheter consensus conference: The first step. *Critical Care Medicine, 25*, 2064–2065.

Teres, D., & Lemeshow, S. (1987). Evaluating the severity of illness in critically ill patients. In W. C. Shoemaker & E. Abraham (Eds.), *Diagnostic methods in critical care* (pp. 1–17). New York: Marcel Dekker.

Tullman, D. F., & Dracup, K. (2000). Creating a healing environment for elders. *AACN Clinical Issues, 11* (1), 34–50.

Wu, A., Rubin, H., & Rosen, M. (1990). Are elderly people less responsive to intensive care. *Journal of the American Geriatric Society, 6*, 621–627.

Zaren, B., & Hedstrand, V. (1987). Quality of life among long term survivors of intensive care. *Critical Care Medicine, 15*, 743–747.

17

The Coronary Care Unit

Deborah Chyun, Christine Tocchi, and
Sally Richards

Cardiovascular (CV) diseases, which include stroke, hypertension (HTN), arrhythmias, coronary heart disease (CHD), and heart failure (HF), are major contributors to mortality and morbidity in the elderly, accounting for 40% of all deaths in those age 75 to 85 and 48% of all deaths in those 85 and older (American Heart Association [AHA], 1998). CHD and hypertensive heart disease are responsible for most deaths, and along with valvular heart disease are major contributors to HF, the condition responsible for most hospital admissions in the elderly. Although HF is an important problem in the elderly, most coronary care unit (CCU) admissions are for management of arrhythmias, unstable angina, or myocardial infarction (MI). Coexistent with these, however, are other CV conditions and chronic diseases—stroke, peripheral vascular disease (PVD), diabetes mellitus (DM), and renal and liver disease—that may complicate assessment and management of the underlying arrhythmia or CHD. In addition, assessment and management may be complicated by the presence of systemic physiological changes associated with aging. This chapter will review the CV changes associated with aging and CV disease, CV assessment of the elderly individual, and management of common CV conditions found in this population: MI, HF, and arrhythmias. Cardiac medications used in the management of these CV conditions will be discussed in relation to the elderly.

NORMAL AGE-RELATED CHANGES IN THE CV SYSTEM

The normal aging process is not associated with CV disease; however, characteristic changes do occur in the CV system. These include structural alterations in the myocardium, valves, conduction system, and vasculature, as well as functional changes in myocardial performance. Mild increases in left ventricular (LV) wall thickness and cardiac mass without an increase in the LV cavity are often noted (Lewis & Maron, 1992). Cavity size may actually decrease and septal thickness increase, producing a leftward bulging into the LV outflow tract. Reasons for this are unclear but may be attributed to stiffness of the aorta, causing impedance to LV outflow, LV hypertrophy (LVH), and higher systolic blood pressure (SBP), along with the connective tissue changes in the myocardium.

Cardiac valves increase in size with increasing age. In younger individuals, the mitral and tricuspid valves are larger than the pulmonic and aortic valves are, with the aortic being the smallest. With older age, the aortic valve shows the greatest increase in circumference; however, this does not usually cause dysfunction (Lewis & Maron, 1992). With a decrease in cavity size, however, mitral valve leaflets may protrude or bulge upward into the left atrium during systole and be mistaken for mitral valve prolapse (MVP) (Chakko & Kessler, 1992). A fibrous thickening and calcification of the aortic and mitral leaflets is often observed in the elderly (Lewis & Maron, 1992). In the aortic cusps, in milder form this is considered aortic sclerosis, present in approximately 29% of the elderly; occasionally, in about 9% of the elderly, heavier calcification may lead to critical aortic stenosis (AS). Degenerative calcific changes of the atrioventricular (AV) valves are also common and are the second most common cause of HF. Calcification around the mitral annulus, commonly seen in elderly women, may occasionally result in mitral regurgitation (MR), conduction defects, and atrial fibrillation (AF) (Savage, Garrison, & Castelli, 1983).

An age-associated loss of myocytes occurs in the sinus node, contributing to sick sinus syndrome and atrial arrhythmias. In addition, reduction of parasympathetic activity may also contribute to the higher resting heart rate and loss of normal heart rate variability observed in the elderly. Fibrosis within the conduction system and the increase in ventricular mass may result in electrocardiographic (ECG) abnormalities such as minor increases in P wave and PR interval duration, a decreased QRS amplitude, a leftward QRS axis shift, increased QT interval corrected for heart rate, first-degree AV, and bundle branch block (BBB) (Chakko & Kessler, 1992; Fleg, 1999). Left bundle branch block (LBBB), however, is usually associated with significant CV disease and is not a normal age-related finding, nor is LVH. Nonspecific ST changes such as sagging or straightening of the ST segment and T wave flattening are common; their prognostic importance is difficult to ascertain because they are frequently associated with cardiac medications and underlying CV disease. In calcified AS, the ECG is usually abnormal; a normal ECG is not consistent with significant AS (Lombard & Selzer, 1987). AV and intraventricular conduction defects (IVCD) may be seen with mitral calcification (Kotler, Jacobs, & Ioli, 1992). Although atrial and ventricular ectopic beats, AF, and paroxysmal supraventricular tachycardia are often seen in the elderly with normal hearts, AF is often associated with underlying heart disease. Diminished QRS voltage, loss of septal R waves and Q waves in inferior leads, complex ventricular arrhythmias, AV conduction defects, and sick sinus syndrome are not normal age-related findings and may be associated with infiltrative diseases such as amyloidosis (Chakko & Kessler, 1992). In addition, ECG evidence of MI, without preceding angina or symptomatic MI is commonly found in the elderly.

Changes within the intima and media, a loss of elastin and replacement with collagen, and thickening of the smooth muscle layer of the blood vessels lead to stiffness of arterial walls. With increasing age the aorta enlarges and there is a decrease in compliance. These changes are believed to occur even in the absence of atherosclerosis (Lewis & Maron, 1992). Increased systemic vascular resistance, increased SBP, decreased diastolic blood pressure (DBP), and a widened pulse pressure result (Wei, 1999). The age-associated increase in LV mass is largely attributed to these changes, which place an increased mechanical demand upon the heart. Changes also occur in the coronary arteries. Not only are they less distensible, but also they loose their ability to vasodilate, thereby becoming less capable of increasing blood supply to the myocardium. Blood pressure regulation is often compromised because of increased vascular stiffness. Many elderly are sensitive to changes in preload and afterload and are unable to adapt to small increases or decreases in plasma volume. Compensatory CV mechanisms may be delayed or insufficient and may result in syncope because of postural changes, urination, or defecation; these effects may be exacerbated by low sodium levels (Wei, 1999).

Functional changes in myocardial performance also accompany aging. In the absence of CV disease, however, systolic function remains relatively unchanged, as does the response to exercise. Although there is less of an increase in ejection fraction (EF), values at maximal exercise are rarely decreased from basal levels. Cardiac output (CO), maintained primarily by an increase in LV diastolic volume, and exercise capacity, heart rate (HR), maximum oxygen consumption, and vital capacity all decrease with increasing age, although other factors such as muscle atrophy, osteoarthritis, osteoporosis, and deconditioning secondary to a sedentary lifestyle may also contribute (Chakko & Kessler, 1992; Schulman, 1999). In addition, the aging myocardium is less responsive to chronotropic and inotropic effects of catecholamines (Schulman, 1999). With a decreased responsiveness to beta-adrenergic stimulation, the heart is increasingly dependent on the Frank-Starling mechanism to maintain CO; however early diastolic filling is often impaired and preload becomes increasingly dependent on atrial contraction (Chakko & Kessler, 1992). The primary effect of aging on myocardial function is on diastolic function. Although diastolic dysfunction may be seen with a variety of other diseases (HTN, CHD, hypertrophic cardiomyopathy), it is commonly associated with older age in the absence of disease (Chakko & Kessler, 1992). Prolongation of relaxation and abnormalities of ventricular filling are observed. These abnormalities are exacerbated by a increased HR. Although these changes in diastolic function are not usually not enough to cause failure, diastolic abnormalities caused by HTN, AS, or CHD may contribute to precipitating HF (Chakko & Kessler, 1992).

CHANGES ASSOCIATED WITH CD DISEASE

Although age-related changes in the CV system occur in the absence of disease, a variety CV diseases—pulmonary, hypertensive, and valvular heart disease; cardiomyopathy (CM); and HF—are frequently found in the elderly. These need to be considered in the initial assessment, as well as during ongoing management during the CCU stay. Chronic obstructive pulmonary disease (COPD) contributes to CV disease, particularly right ventricular dysfunction, whereas HF and mitral valve disease may lead to pulmonary HTN (Burrows, Alpert, & Ross, 1987).

Untreated or undertreated HTN usually results in LVH. The presence of LVH increases with increasing with age; 33% of men and 49% of women older than 70 have echocardiographic evidence of LVH (Levy et al., 1988). LVH is an important prognostic factor, correlating with subsequent adverse coronary events even after adjusting for other factors. With HTN, concentric hypertrophy, an increase in wall thickness without dilation, is observed, in contrast to other conditions in which dilatation predominates without an increase in wall thickness (Lavie, Milani, Mehra, & Messerli, 1999). However, conditions such as valvular regurgitation and obesity, commonly seen in the elderly and do cause dilation, can also contribute to LVH. LVH is associated with reductions in coronary flow reserve, complex ventricular arrhythmias, and systolic and diastolic dysfunction, all of which contribute to myocardial ischemia, sudden cardiac death, and HF.

Calcification of the aortic valve is the most common valvular disorder seen in the elderly. With mild degenerative calcification, aortic sclerosis, an audible systolic murmur is present even in the absence of obstruction (Chakko & Kessler, 1992). As the valve becomes more rigid, however, the severity of stenosis increases. Noninvasive assessment with an echocardiogram is necessary to differentiate aortic sclerosis from AS. Severe mitral annular calcification (MAC) is also common, especially among elderly women. It is accelerated by the presence of HTN, AS, DM, and chronic renal failure (Chakko & Kessler, 1992). With severe calcification, a rigid curved bar of calcium encircles the mitral orifice and may cause MR or, on rare occasions, mitral stenosis (MS). MR results from the distortion and elevation of the valve leaflet by the calcific mass, making valvular tissue less available for coaptation because the annulus cannot reduce its circumference during systole (Nestico, Depace, Morganroth, Kotler, & Ross, 1984). Calcific AS and MAC are chronic degenerative processes and often coexist; they are unrelated to rheumatic heart disease (RHD), rheumatoid disease, or any form of cardiac inflammation but are associated with HTN, AS, hypertrophic CM, CHD, MVP, Marfan's or Hurler's syndromes, mitral valve replacement, hypercalcemia, chronic renal failure, and metastatic calcification (Kotler et al., 1992). Although rare, erosion can occur and produce heart block. In addition, embolic phenomena, including thromboembolic cerebral vascular events, can occur, along with infective endocarditis.

Although MR may also be due to organic valvular disease, CM, or CHD, the most common cause of MR is MVP (Kotler et al., 1992). Complications of MVP—severe MR, infective endocarditis, cerebral ischemic events, and rupture of chordae tendinae—increase with advancing age (Kolibash, Kilman, & Bush, 1986). Mitral regurgitation due to MVP is progressive, with symptoms appearing around the age 60 even when prolapse was first noted at younger ages (Kolibash, Kilman, & Bush, 1986). With severe chronic MR the individual usually presents with AF and HF (Kotler et al., 1992). With the decrease in RHD, MS is seen with decreasing frequency in the elderly, with most having MR. Most of those affected usually present with symptoms by middle age (Kotler et al., 1992). Rheumatic MS is frequently associated with AF, HF, or pulmonary HTN, or a combination of these, and thromboembolic complications may occur (Kotler et al., 1992).

Aortic regurgitation (AR) is uncommon in the elderly. When present, it is usually a result of aortic root dilatation secondary to syphilis; connective disorders such as anklylosing spondylitis; rheumatoid arthritis; giant cell arteritis; idiopathic dilatation of the ascending or thoracic aorta; or systemic HTN (Kotler et al., 1992). Most individuals present with chronic AR and may be asymptomatic for years. Acute AR, however, can be seen with aortic dissection or a ruptured cusp secondary to infective endocarditis (Kotler et al., 1992).

Dilated, hypertrophic, and restrictive CMs are important contributors to HF in the elderly. In dilated CM, systolic function is impaired. Acute management includes treatment of any underlying myocarditis; medical management of pulmonary congestion and low CO with digoxin, beta-blockers, vasodilators, and diuretics; use of antiarrhythmics; treatment of conduction system disease; and anticoagulation (Backes & Gersh, 1992). Assessment should be made for digoxin toxicity and interactions with quinidine, amiodarone, verapamil, and vasodilators. Dilated CM is more common in the elderly than previously appreciated, and the elderly appear to have a worse prognosis, with few patients older than 65 undergoing transplantation. In hypertrophic obstructive CM (HOCM) chamber size is normal or small, wall thickness is increased, systolic function is hyperdynamic, and diastolic filling is impaired. Considerable controversy exists as to whether HOCM in the elderly represents a different disease than HOCM in the young does. HOCM in the elderly probably results from different pathophysiological processes, with HTN, loss of aortic compliance, and age-related changes in mean septal to LV free-wall thickness contributing to the condition (Backes & Gersh, 1992). In the elderly, cavity contour is ovoid with a normal septal curvature, and fewer elderly have a family history of the disease, whereas they are more likely to have mild HTN (Luchi, 1997). Beta-blockers, calcium antagonists, and disopyramide are used in management. Conduction disturbances and pulmonary edema are common, and orthostatic hypotension may lead to falls. AF can rapidly lead to deterioration, so that cardioversion should be immediately available. Symptomatic sustained ventricular arrhythmias are common and have been successfully treated with amiodarone (Backes & Gersh, 1992). LV septal myectomy and myotomy are reserved for highly symptomatic patients who do not have maximal response to medical therapy (Backes & Gersh, 1992). Although HOCM is also more common than previously appreciated, prognosis appears to be better than it is in younger individuals. The third type of CM, restrictive CM, is characterized by an increase in LV stiffness and early diastolic dysfunction; eventually, however, systolic function is also affected (Backes & Gersh, 1992). Restrictive CM is commonly caused by infiltrative diseases; however, it may also be idiopathic. For any change in ventricular volume, high filling pressures result in low forward output, pulmonary congestion, and right-sided failure. Arterial vasodilators and digitalis may be harmful, whereas calcium channel and beta-blockers improve LV relaxation.

ASSESSMENT IN THE CCU

Initial nursing assessment upon arrival to the CCU may be limited by hemodynamic instability, resuscitative measures, or aggressive therapy aimed at limiting infarct size. As soon as possible, however, the CCU nurse should obtain a thorough history, from the patient or significant other and perform a baseline physical examination (Table 17.1). These data can then be used in conjunction with information obtained from the medical record and results of laboratory and diagnostic tests in identifying actual and potential problems and establishing a plan of care. Despite the fact that the CCU setting is often not the ideal place or time to be providing education to the patients and their caregivers, shortened hospital stays and the abundance of ancillary care personnel outside of the CCU setting necessitate that the CCU nurse take a leadership role in discharge planning.

Nursing assessment closely parallels the medical history. However, whereas the physician uses this information in order to arrive at a medical diagnosis, the same information serves the nurse in assessing the patient's response to treatment and in assisting the individual in subsequent management of symptoms and the underlying condition, health promotion, disease prevention activities, and chronic disease management. Awareness of the patient's own perception of why he or she sought medical care and a detailed analysis of the symptoms will assist in assessing an individual's ability to identify symptoms, knowledge regarding his or her condition and its prognosis, and general health beliefs, along with prior ability to manage

TABLE 17.1   CCU Nursing History and Physical Exam

Chief complaint and history of present illness
Why did you seek help today? (In own words)
Symptoms: chest, arm, neck, jaw, back, abdominal pain; dyspnea, syncope, vertigo, acute confusion, numbness; onset of problem, duration, frequency, bodily location and radiation, intensity, quality, aggravating and alleviating circumstances, associated symptoms; extent to which symptoms interfered with lifestyle; ability to control symptoms

Past medical history
CV: CHD risk factors (HTN, DM, thyroid disease, LDL >100, HDL < 35 in men and < 45 in women, PVD, renal disease, cerebrovascular disease, family history, obesity, smoking); angina, MI, coronary bypass surgery, and/or angioplasty, rheumatic heart disease, AS, AR, MS, MR, MVP, congenital heart defects, valve replacement, CM, HF, HTN, peripheral vascular disease, stroke
Other: DM, thyroid disease, anemia, renal dysfunction, liver disease, alcohol use, COPD, cancer, psychiatric conditions
Functional status and physical activity
Diet and nutritional status, ETOH use
Current medications, including alternative therapies

Psychosocial history
Typical day
Social supports

Review of systems and physical exam
Skin: Ask about: dryness, itchiness, prior decubiti. Observe: color, warmth, bleeding, bruising, turgor, and presence of edema, xanthomas and xanthelasmus; color changes indicative of pressure and potential breakdown
Heart and peripheral vascular: Ask about: claudication, thrombophlebitis, peripheral edema, chest pain, palpitations. Obtain: heart rate and rhythm, SBP and DBP in both arms, postural changes; palpate and auscultate at 2nd–3rd left and right intercostal spaces, lower left sternal border and apex for thrills, extra heart sounds (S3 and S4), murmurs and rubs; describe according to: Timing—Systolic vs. Diastolic—and Duration (holosystolic, or early, mid, or late systolic or diastolic); Loudness (I–VI); Pitch (high, medium, low); Quality (Blowing, rumble, harsh, musical); Location; Configuration (crescendo, decrescendo); Radiation; and Respiratory maneuvers; Carotid and femoral bruits. Review: cardiac exam in medical record for additional abnormalities, including results of diagnostic testing. Palpate: peripheral pulses: brachial, radial, ulnar, femoral, popliteal, dorsalis pedis, and posterior tibial.
Lungs: Ask about: dyspnea, orthopnea, paroxysmal nocturnal dyspnea, cough, color and quantity of sputum, hemoptysis, wheezing, asthma, bronchitis, emphysema, pneumonia. Obtain: respiratory rate, rhythm and observe shape of chest, respiratory effort, and retraction or bulging of interspaces; auscultate lung fields for breath sounds and presence of crackles, wheezes, and rubs. Review: respiratory exam in medical record for additional abnormalities, including results of chest x-ray.

TABLE 17.1 *(continued)*

Neurological: Ask about: visual, hearing or swallowing impairment, fainting, blackouts, seizures, paralysis, weakness, numbness, tingling, tremors, memory. Obtain: Mini-mental status exam; note ability to move extremities. Review: neurological exam in medical record for additional mental status, cranial nerve, motor, sensory, or reflex abnormalities.

Laboratory and diagnostic tests

Serum electrolytes; glucose, sodium, potassium, blood urea nitrogen, creatinine, TSH

Complete blood count

Cardiac enzymes

ECG: rate, rhythm, PR, QRS and QT intervals, QRS axis, atrial and ventricular hypertrophy, myocardial ischemia and infarction

Echocardiogram, ventricular radionuclide studies, cardiac catheterization: LVH, valvular dysfunction, diastolic function, EF, coronary anatomy

ETOH = alcohol; HDL = high-density lipoproteins; TSH = thyroid stimulating hormone

---

this or other medical conditions. Other conditions that may cause the patient to present with chest pain are listed in Table 17.2.

Angina pectoris, a major manifestation of myocardial ischemia and a common finding on CCU admission, is found in 13.7% of women and 21% of men age 65–69 years (Mittlemark et al., 1993). The prevalence is 19% in women age 70–84 and 24.7% in those 85 and older. In men age 70 and older the prevalence of angina is 27.3%. Thus, angina represents an important problem in the elderly population. Although angina usually indicates the presence of underlying CHD, myocardial ischemia can result from a variety of conditions that lead to an imbalance between oxygen supply and demand, for example, LVH and AS. Myocardial ischemia, however, frequently occurs in the absence of angina or its equivalents (jaw pain, numbness, dyspnea, fatigue, or nonspecific symptoms related to transient left ventricular dysfunction). Although the cause is unknown, many elderly have atypical findings or have totally asymptomatic CHD. Atypical manifestations include nontypical chest, shoulder, or back pain; dyspnea; pulmonary edema; and cardiac arrhythmias. In addition, with low levels of physical activity, effort-induced angina may not be provoked. In persons older than 65 years with known CHD, angina is reported by 25–43%, dyspnea by 8–25%, and both by nearly 50%. Angina, therefore, is neither a reliable nor a sensitive marker of myocardial ischemia. In addition, there are multiple noncardiac etiologies of chest pain, and these should be considered in the differential diagnosis. Atypical symptoms or absence of symptoms may lead not only to underdiagnosis of CHD but also, in the setting of acute MI, to delay in seeking treatment and in diagnosis (Meischke, Eisenberg, & Larsens, 1993; Turi et al., 1986) and a higher

TABLE 17.2   Common Causes of Chest Pain

Cervical pathology
  Osteoarthritis
  Spondylitis
  Disc herniation
  Metastases
Chest Wall
  Herpes Zoster
  Pectoral myositis and spasm
  Costochondritis
  Thrombophlebitis
Pulmonary
  Pulmonary embolism
  Pneumothorax
  Pneumonia
  Pleurisy
GI Related
  Gallbladder disease
  Esophageal spasm
  Reflux
  Pancreatitis
  Gaseous distention
Vasculature
  Dissecting abdominal aneurysm
Psychogenic/Neurologic
  Anxiety
  Depression
  Delirium

morbidity and mortality (Kannel & Abbott, 1984; Uretsy, Farquhar, Berezin, & Hood, 1977).

Individuals with asymptomatic ischemia tend to have a higher incidence of asymptomatic MI, underscoring the importance of detecting ischemia early in its course. Silent episodes outnumber symptomatic episodes in patients with chronic stable angina and unstable angina and in asymptomatic patients following MI (Pepine, 1986). Silent ischemia—present in 50,000 to 100,000 persons following MI and in 3 million persons with angina—along with symptomatic ischemia during daily activities, extent of CHD, the degree of LV dysfunction, and unstable angina is associated with an adverse prognosis (Nadelman et al., 1990). Asymptomatic ischemia may also occur in the absence of known CHD and is frequently found in individuals with lower extremity arterial disease and diabetes (Barzilay & Kronmal, 1998).

Awareness of the past medical history will allow the nurse to anticipate problems related to management of other conditions, as well as the potential adverse effects of any cardiac-related treatments. Although age-related differences exist between younger and elderly individuals regarding cardiac risk factors, levels of physical activity, and control of lipids, HTN, obesity, DM, and smoking need to be determined. In those individuals with CHD, secondary intervention aimed at meeting AHA goals for risk reduction needs to be implemented; in those without demonstrated CHD, primary preventive measures need to be instituted (Table 17.3). Assessment of CV disease is important, as is assessment for other chronic conditions commonly found in the elderly. As discussed earlier, CV conditions—angina, MI, coronary bypass surgery and angioplasty, RHD, valvular heart disease, CM, HF, HTN, PVD, and stroke—may complicate assessment and management of the acute CV condition. In addition, the presence of DM may necessitate monitoring of blood glucose and presence of ketones; renal and liver disease may affect pharmacodynamics; anemia, common in the elderly, may affect oxygenation; and COPD may necessitate special precautions when assessing and managing oxygen therapy and beta-blockers.

Despite the benefits of regular exercise in the elderly—improvements in functional status, anxiety, depression, mobility, and mortality—70% of older adults report having no regular exercise, and 60% have not walked a mile within the past year (Kovar, Fitti, & Chyba, 1992). The elderly have higher levels of function disability. Functional status often deteriorates after hospitalization and has been shown to be an important prognostic factor in the elderly after MI (Mayer-Oakes, Oye, & Leake, 1991; Pernenkil et al., 1997). Functional loss appears to be proceeded by a decline in physical performance, and early functional limitations or mild impairments that are not evident clinically have been shown to predict subsequent functional

TABLE 17.3 Guidelines for Primary and Secondary Prevention of CHD

Risk factor	Primary prevention goal	Secondary prevention goal
Smoking	Complete cessation	Complete cessation
BP	≤ 140/90	≤ 140/90
LDL	< 160 mg/dL if 0–1 risk factor < 130 mg/dL if ≥ 2	< 100 mg/dL
HDL	> 35 mg/dL	> 35 mg/dL
TG	< 200 mg/dL	< 200 mg/dL
Physical activity	Regular exercise 3–4 × per week for 30 minutes	Minimum goal: Regular exercise 3–4 × per week for 30 minutes
Weight	BMI 21–25 kg/m²	BMI 21–25 kg/m²
Estrogens	Consider in all postmenopausal women	Consider in all postmenopausal women

BMI = body mass index; HDL = high-density lipoproteins; TG = triglycerides dependence (Gill, Williams, Mendes de Leon, & Tinetti, 1997). Subjects at risk of functional decline may be identified early, prior to loss of function, so that interventions may be targeted. Functional status, therefore, should be assessed as early as possible in the hospital course. There are several brief, easily administered functional assessment tools that can be used.

Inadequate nutrition is present in 10–51% of community-dwelling elderly, 20–60% of hospitalized elderly, and up to 85% of nursing home residents (Constans, Bacq, & Brechot, 1992). Physiological changes, social conditions, long-term effects of chronic disease and medications, functional limitations, cognitive deficits, and impaired vision and sense of smell and taste contribute to this situation. The results of undernourishment or malnutrition include a fall in cardiac index and loss of cardiac muscle mass; decrease in vital capacity, respiratory rate, and minute volume; deterioration of liver function; decrease in glomerular filtration; impairment of cellular immunity, antibody production and complement, and mucosal immunity; increased susceptibility to infection; delayed wound healing; reduced rate of drug metabolism; and impairment of physical and cognitive impairment (Sullivan & Lipschitz, 1997). Management of diet and exercise may pose special challenges to the elderly. It is vital, therefore, that nutritional deficiencies be identified early and corrected.

Prescription and over-the-counter medications that the patient is currently taking should be assessed, along with any alternative therapies. Many elderly who are eligible for aspirin, beta-blockers and angiotensin-converting enzyme (ACE) inhibitors do not receive these medications, despite their importance in reducing CHD-related morbidity and mortality. Medications to treat HTN and lipid abnormalities may not be well-tolerated, and the potential for side effects and drug interactions is increased in the setting of polypharmacy.

Psychosocial factors, personal beliefs and behaviors, and environmental and cultural influences contribute to management of chronic disease. The importance of depression and social support has been well-documented in the elderly (Berkman & Syme 1979; Seeman, Kaplan, Knudsen, Cohen, & Guralnik, 1987), as well as in individuals with CHD (Berkman, Leo-Summers, & Horowitz, 1992; Frasure-Smith, Lesperance, & Talajic, 1993); therefore, these factors need to be assessed and appropriate interventions should be instituted.

A thorough history and physical exam upon admission enables the CCU nurse to identify patients at high risk for complications, both during hospitalization and following discharge, as well as to better assess the effects of therapy. A subjective review of systems provides patient input regarding symptoms; a focused physical examination provides objective measures of dysfunction. Skin breakdown is a major problem in the elderly. In combination with prolonged bedrest, decreased CO, and nutritional depletion, decubitus ulcers may result. It is vital that the CCU nurse carefully assess the skin on a daily basis, with careful attention given to pressure points, and preventive and restorative measures instituted.

As in younger patients, baseline assessment of cardiac and respiratory function, including heart rate and rhythm, blood pressure, heart and lung sounds, and peripheral perfusion is critical. Neurological assessment is often overlooked. Changes in heart rate and rhythm, a decrease in CO, and side effects of cardiac medications may cause significant changes in mental status. The potential for an intracerebral bleed following thrombolytic or anticoagulant therapy or for thromboembolic stroke with valvular disorders or AF highlight the importance of an accurate neurological assessment as early as possible in the CCU course. In addition, because many patients undergo cardiac catheterization, percutaneous transluminal coronary angioplasty (PTCA), or coronary artery bypass graft (CABG) surgery, and may do so under emergent conditions, it is critical that baseline neurological status be documented.

Review of results of diagnostic tests, performed prior to and during hospitalization, is important. Electrolyte abnormalities are common in the elderly, particularly in individuals on chronic diuretic therapy. Anemia is frequently observed and may contribute to hypoxia and myocardial ischemia. Cardiac enzymes assist not only in determining the presence of acute MI and infarct size but also in verifying MI that may have occurred well before admission. A baseline ECG is vital so that ST and T waves, axis changes, and prolongation in PR, QRS, and QT intervals can be assessed in response to medications and ongoing ischemia. Echocardiographic results provide important information on valvular and diastolic function, as well as LVH. Although mild atrial enlargement, less than a 20% increase, is commonly found in the elderly on echocardiogram, ventricular enlargement is abnormal (Chakko & Kessler, 1992). Doppler echocardiography, which is based on measurements reflecting the velocity of blood flow through the mitral valve during ventricular filling is useful for detecting diastolic dysfunction. The M shape that is produced has an initial peak representing early filling (E) and the second reflecting atrial filling (A). Normally the E wave is larger than the A wave; however, with diastolic dysfunction, the pattern is reversed. The A wave becomes larger, and the E to A ratio becomes reversed (Chakko & Kessler, 1992). Because of the reduced rate of early diastolic filling, the descending slope of the E wave also becomes prolonged. The E/A ratio is reduced in elderly subjects even in the absence of CVD. Radionuclide studies assist in determining left ventricular ejection fraction (LVEF) and myocardial perfusion abnormalities; cardiac catheterization results reveal the extent of CHD and the need for revascularization.

MYOCARDIAL INFARCTION

More than 670,000 persons in the United States are hospitalized annually for an acute MI (Tresch, 1998). Approximately 60% of these are persons older than 65 years of age and 32% are over the age of 75 years. Furthermore, 80% of all deaths attributed to MI occur in patients over the age of 75 (Gillum, 1993; Graves, 1992; Gurwitz & Osganian, 1991). Hospital mortality in patients older than 70 years is at least three times that of younger patients after an acute MI, and the survival in the first 2 years following MI has been reported to be as low as 50% (Tresch, 1998).

The reason for the high mortality rate in older patients with acute MI is unexplained, although it is most likely multifactorial in origin. Factors that unfavorably affect the prognosis include LV damage due to long-standing HTN, DM, and valvular heart disease in combination with MI, LV dysfunction and hypertrophy. These factors contribute to electrical instability and arrhythmias. In addition, residual ischemia as a result of long-standing multivessel CHD and previous non–Q wave MI may contribute to increased mortality (Tesch, 1998). Although short-term prognosis is better with non–Q wave MI than with Q wave MI, long-term prognosis is poorer. Complications in the post-MI period are also seen more frequently in older adults as compared with younger individuals. Cardiac disease, superimposed on physiological changes of aging, such as increased LV mass, reduced diastolic compliance, and increased vascular resistance, predispose the older adult with acute MI to HF and other complications. In addition, many older patients have comorbidities that significantly increase the risk for complications and mortality after acute MI.

Clinical Presentation

The presentation of acute MI in the older adult can be extremely variable. The individual may have classic symptoms of chest pain or dyspnea or be completely asymptomatic, or the symptoms may be so vague that they are unrecognized. Atypical presentation of MI is common in the elderly, the prevalence increasing with increasing age (Appelgate, Graves, Collins, Zwaag, & Akins, 1984; Bayer, Chadha, Farag, & Pathy, 1986; Muller, Gould, Betzu, Vacek, & Pradeep, 1990; Solomon et al., 1989). The presence of chest pain with MI may occur in as few as 19% of the elderly presenting with MI (Pathy, 1967). Differentiation of atypical symptoms from other chronic conditions is difficult, and MI may not even be suspected. Individuals may often present with dyspnea, HF, GI symptoms, syncope, stroke, confusion, faintness, giddiness, weakness, or restlessness (Aronow, 1987; Bayer et al., 1986; Konu, 1977; Lusiani, Perrone, Pesevanto, & Conte, 1994; MacDonald, 1984; Tinker, 1981; Tresch, 1987). The person who had suffered an unrecognized MI days to weeks earlier may present to the hospital in HF or with recurrent angina. MI may also be the result of another primary process causing an increase in myocardial oxygen demand or a decrease in flow, such as intercurrent illness, GI bleed, or HF. Because prompt recognition and treatment of MI is crucial to limiting infarct size and preserving myocardial function, it is vital that atypical presentation be recognized (Dracup & Moser, 1991; Reilly, Dracup, & Dattolo, 1994; Turi et al., 1986) and that the patient be assisted in identification of anginal equivalents. Myocardial ischemia and infarction can also exist in the total absence of signs and symptoms, and unrecognized MI is common in the elderly (Kannel & Abbott, 1984; Nadelman et al., 1990).

The initial assessment of the CCU patient has been reviewed previously in this chapter (see Table 17.1). It is important to note that the cardiac enzyme profile may be atypical in the older adult. Because baseline creatine kinase (CK) in elderly patients may be significantly lower than normal because of decreased muscle mass, older patients with MI may not develop CK levels high enough to be interpreted as abnormal. Serial CK-myocardial band (MB) may be more sensitive, and troponin levels, low to undetectable in the serum of healthy individuals, show a rapid rise (within 1 hour) after myocardial injury, even in the elderly. As a sensitive marker, troponin is especially useful in detecting silent MI. In patients with an atypical presentation and lack of CK, CK-MB, or troponin elevation, lactic dehydrogenase (LDH) or serum glutamic-oxaloacetic transaminase (SGOT) levels may reflect MI prior to hospitalization. These enzymes, however, may be elevated secondary to other conditions found in the elderly.

Management

The early management of elderly patients with acute MI is similar to that of younger patients. Differentiation of unstable angina, non–Q wave MI, and evolving Q wave MI should be made. Initial treatment is designed to limit infarct size, ease discomfort, and treat any hemodynamic disturbances. The American College of Cardiology (ACC) and the AHA have developed practice guidelines for the management of acute MI based on scientific evidence and agreement on the efficacy and usefulness of each intervention (AHA, 1999). These guidelines can be used to guide nursing assessment and management, as well as to anticipate additional interventions while the elderly person is in the CCU. These guidelines serve as the basis for the information discussed later. Although initial MI recognition and management guidelines are directed at the emergency department (ED), these may be relevant to the CCU in admitting patients transferred from outlying sites who bypass the ED or in patients admitted from other units within the hospital. A targeted clinical examination and a 12-lead ECG should ideally be performed and interpreted within 10 minutes of arrival, with a door-to-needle time for administration of thrombolytic therapy of less than 30 minutes as a goal. This is clearly a challenge in the elderly, who often present with asymptomatic or atypical presentation or with nonspecific ECG findings. Although oxygen therapy (2–5 L/min) is indicated in the presence of overt pulmonary congestion or arterial desaturation ($SaO_2 <$ 90%), and use during the first 2–3 hours is felt to be useful in all patients, effectiveness beyond 3–6 hours has not been well-established.

Medications used in MI management, along with special precautions in the elderly, appear later in this chapter. Nitrates have been the cornerstone of therapy for ischemic pain, reducing preload and improving coronary perfusion. Intravenous (IV) nitroglycerin (NTG) has been shown to limit infarct size and reduce pain, complications, and mortality (Yusuf, Collins, MacMahon, & Peto, 1988). It is indicated in the first 24–48 hours in patients with HF, large anterior MI, persistent ischemia, or hypertension and longer with recurrent angina or persistent pulmonary congestion. Intravenous morphine sulfate is also effective for treating chest pain.

Aspirin is of proven benefit in patients with acute MI (ISIS-2, 1988). The initial dose of aspirin should be administered as soon as possible after presentation and chewed rather than swallowed to ensure rapid absorption. It should be continued indefinitely on a daily basis unless contraindicated (Antiplatelet Trialists Collaboration, 1988). The use of other antiplatelet agents (dipyridamole, ticlopidine, and clopidogrel) is less well-established. They may be substituted in cases of aspirin allergy or if the patient is unresponsive to aspirin.

Thrombolytic agents, such as tissue plasminogen activator (t-PA), streptokinase (SK), and anistreplase, administered within 6 to 12 hours of onset of acute MI reduce infarct size and improve survival in patients of all ages, including the elderly. Indications for thrombolysis are based on the existence of chest pain and ECG evidence of ST-segment elevation greater than 0.1 mV in two or more contiguous leads. Although several large prospective trials have confirmed the life-saving effects of thrombolytic therapy in older adults, current data show that the elderly are frequently omitted from this therapy. Reasons for this include delayed presentation, atypical symptoms, nondiagnostic ECG, greater frequency of non–Q wave infarctions, increased likelihood of contraindications to thrombolysis, and concerns of the likelihood of stroke and bleeding. The choice of the best thrombolytic agent in the elderly remains controversial, and use is largely a clinical judgment and physician preference. In the Global Utilization of Streptokinase and t-PA for Occluded Arteries (GUSTO) Trial (GUSTO Angiographic Investigators, 1993) use of t-PA showed a small, but significant, reduction in mortality. However, hemorrhagic strokes occurred more frequently with t-PA than they did with SK, especially in the elderly cohort. Because of the concern for intracerebral hemorrhage primary PTCA is frequently considered an alternative to thrombolytic therapy in the elderly (Grines, Browne, & Marco, 1993).

IV heparin is indicated for patients undergoing PTCA or surgical revascularization and appears useful in patients undergoing reperfusion therapy with alteplase and with nonselective thrombolytic agents (SK, anistreplase, urokinase) who are at high risk for systemic emboli. This includes patients with large or anterior MI, previous embolus, or known LV thrombus. Routine use is not advocated within 6 hours in patients receiving a nonselective fibrinolytic agent who are not at high risk of systemic emboli. Subcutaneous heparin is used for patients with non–ST-elevation MI and in all patients not treated with thrombolytic therapy who do not have a contraindication to heparin in order to reduce the risk of venous thrombosis. Heparin therapy is specifically recommended for elderly patients with large anterior MI, HF, AF, and documented LV thrombus. It is given for 3–5 days, followed by 3 months of warfarin. Although glycoprotein IIb/IIIa inhibitors (abciximab, eptifibatide, tirofiban) have been shown to have beneficial effects when used in the setting of non–Q wave MI or in conjunction with PTCA, their use is not currently recommended except in patients with MI without ST elevation who have some high-risk features or refractory ischemia, provided they do not have a major contraindication due to a bleeding risk.

Beta-blockers have been shown to limit infarct size, decrease chest pain, and improve prognosis. At the present time only metoprolol and atenolol have been approved for IV use in the acute MI setting. Contraindications for the use of beta-blockers include marked bradycardia, systolic blood pressure less than 100 mm Hg, first-degree AV block, moderate or severe HF, active wheezing, or history of significant bronchospastic disease. Chronic lung disease without bronchospasm and mild HF are not contraindications. Beta-blockers should be given to patients without a contraindication who can be treated within 12 hours of onset of infarction, irrespective of administration of thrombolytic therapy or primary PTCA, continuing or recurrent ischemic pain, or tachyarrhythmias (AF with rapid ventricular response). They may even be useful with moderate LV failure (bibasilar rales without evidence of low CO) or other relative contraindications, provided that the patient is closely monitored. However, they should not be used in patients with severe LV failure.

The role of ACE inhibitors after MI in patients with significant LV dysfunction (EF < 40%) and no obvious contraindications has been established (Pfeffer et al., 1992; Acute Infarction Ramipril Efficacy [AIRE] Study Investigators, 1993). ACE inhibitors should be used for patients within the first 24 hours of suspected MI with ST-segment elevation > 2 mm in anterior precordial leads or with clinical HF in the absence of hypotension (SBP < 100 mm Hg) or no known contraindications to use of ACE inhibitors, an LVEF < 40%, or clinical HF, although other patients may also benefit from their use.

Calcium channel blockers have not been shown to be of benefit in the setting of acute MI; however, verapamil or diltiazem may be useful in patients in whom beta-blockers are ineffective or contraindicated for relief of ongoing ischemia or control of a rapid ventricular response in AF in the absence of HF, LV dysfunction, or AV block. Diltiazem and verapamil are contraindicated in patients with MI and associated LV dysfunction or HF. Although less well-established, diltiazem may be added to standard therapy after the first 24 hours and continued for 1 year in patients with non–Q wave MI who do not have LV dysfunction, pulmonary congestion, or HF. Nifedipine (short-acting) is generally contraindicated in the routine treatment of MI because of its negative inotropic effects and the reflex sympathetic activation, tachycardia, and hypotension associated with its use.

The usefulness and scientific evidence for the routine administration of magnesium is not agreed upon; however, it is useful in patients with documented magnesium or potassium deficits, or both. These electrolyte imbalances should be considered in elderly patients receiving diuretics prior to MI. Magnesium may also be useful for episodes of torsades de pointes ventricular tachycardia (VT) associated with a prolonged QT interval, as well as in high-risk patients such as the elderly and those for whom reperfusion therapy is not suitable.

Primary PTCA may be used as an alternative to thrombolytic therapy, particularly in elderly patients with acute MI and ST elevation or new or perceived new LBBB who can undergo PTCA of the infarcted artery within 12 hours of onset of symptoms or beyond 12 hours if ischemia persists. Primary PTCA is also beneficial as a reperfusion strategy when thrombolysis is contraindicated or when ST-segment elevation persists in patients with poor flow in the infarct-related artery. The patient should be carefully assessed for PTCA complications—reocclusion, renal insufficiency, and bleeding—because age and the presence of multivessel disease are strongly related to complications. Prior MI, depressed LVEF, and comorbid conditions such as DM and HTN are associated with poorer outcomes following PTCA (Singh, Thompson, & Holmes, 1999).

Coronary angiography in those not undergoing primary PTCA may be useful with cardiogenic shock or persistent hemodynamic instability or with evolving large or anterior infarcts treated with thrombolytics when there is question of artery patency and PTCA is therefore being considered. Coronary angiography and possible PTCA are indicated in patients with spontaneous episodes of myocardial ischemia or with ischemia provoked by minimal exertion during recovery; prior to definitive therapy for a mechanical complication—acute MR, ventricular septal defect (VSD), pseudoaneurysm, or LV aneurysm; or with persistent hemodynamics. The routine use of angiography and PTCA within 24 hours of administration of thrombolytic agents, however, is not recommended. In patients with non–ST-segment elevation, early coronary angiography and intervention therapy are most useful and indicated only in patients with persistent or stuttering episodes of symptomatic ischemia, with or without associated ECG changes, and in the presence of shock, severe pulmonary congestion, or continuing hypotension. Angiography is not recommended within days after receiving thrombolytic therapy, and routine coronary angiography and PTCA are not deemed necessary after successful thrombolytic therapy. CABG is a management option when PTCA fails. It is also considered for persistent or recurrent ischemia refractory to medical therapy, cardiogenic shock, surgical repair of VSD, or mitral valve insufficiency. Of note, emergency PTCA or CABG in elderly patients presenting with cardiogenic shock or heart failure is associated with high morbidity and mortality.

Assessment and Management of Complications

Currently, 30-day mortality following MI in the elderly is estimated at 21% (Normand, Glickman, Sharma, & McNeil, 1996). Advanced age is known to be associated with an increased risk of in-hospital death following MI (Goldberg et al., 1989; Marcus et al., 1990; Rich, Bosner, Chung, Shen, & McKenzie, 1992). Prognostic factors for short-term mortality in the elderly include age; prior HF and PVD; poorer mental and functional status; lower body mass index; HR; SBP; presence of HF; conduction disturbances; shock or cardiac arrest; lower serum albumin levels; higher CK, potassium, blood urea nitrogen, and creatinine levels; lower sodium levels; lower EF; and presence of anterior or Q waves (Normand et al., 1996; Chyun, 1998).

Medical and nursing management during acute MI includes ECG monitoring based on infarct location and the underlying rhythm; bed rest with bedside commode privileges for the initial 12 hours in hemodynamically stable patients free of ischemic-type chest discomfort; avoidance of Valsalva maneuver; careful attention to maximum pain relief; and use of anxiolytics. Evidence is not available that bed rest for more than 12–24 hours in stable patients without complications is beneficial. Prolonged immobility in the elderly may be especially detrimental. In addition to limiting infarct size and preventing ventricular remodeling through medications, goals specific to the elderly include enhancing or maintaining independence and functional ability, early recognition and treatment of delirium and agitation, prevention of pressure ulcers, and ongoing assessment and management of complications.

Delirium, an acute confusional state, is a common, serious, and potentially preventable source of mortality and morbidity for the hospitalized older adult. Features of delirium include acute onset, inattention, fluctuating course, and disorganized thinking (Inouye, Viscoli, Horowitz, Hurst, & Tinetti, 1993). The cause is multifactorial and usually involves a complex interrelationship between a vulnerable patient and noxious insults or predisposing factors (preexisting cognitive impairment or dementia, severe underlying illness and comorbidity, functional impairment, advanced age, chronic renal insufficiency, dehydration, malnutrition, and vision or hearing impairment). Medications, immobilization, use of indwelling catheters, physical restraints, dehydration, malnutrition, medical illness, infections, metabolic imbalances, environmental influences, and psychosocial factors may precipitate delirium. Acute MI or HF superimposed on underlying comorbidities, advanced age, the CCU environment, and technological interventions all place the individual at higher risk of delirium.

Management and prevention of delirium includes treatment of the underlying condition, along with symptomatic and supportive care. Nonpharmacological approaches stress reorientation strategies, techniques to promote sleep and decrease anxiety, maintaining mobility and functional ability, reducing environmental insults, and preventing dehydration. Pharmacological approaches encourage the reduction of multiple medications and treating only those individuals with severe agitation. In the setting of acute MI, limiting medications may interfere with optimal CV management; therefore, ongoing ischemia, HF, and arrhythmias should be assessed for carefully.

Differences have been observed among studies comparing complications in younger and older patients with MI. It has been suggested that reinfarction, HF, hypotension, cardiogenic shock, AF, AV block, and stroke occur more frequently in the elderly, as does rupture of the free wall, septum, and papillary muscle (Chung, Bosner, McKenzie, Shen, & Rich, 1995; Rich et al., 1992). Although specific risk factors for most of these complications have not been identified in the elderly, risk factors for ventricular rupture include the presence of HTN and female gender. Although recurrent chest pain, ventricular arrhythmias, and pericarditis do not appear to be associated with older age, these complications still need to be monitored for in the post-MI period.

Management of recurrent chest pain depends on cause of pain. In the elderly, who may exhibit atypical symptoms, active assessment for ongoing ischemia and reinfarction—ST and other ECG changes and cardiac enzyme elevations—must be made. The nurse must assist in distinguishing among ischemia, pericarditis, and noncardiac causes, be prepared to (re)administer thrombolytics, beta-blockers, and IV NTG, and prepare the patient for possible cardiac catheterization.

HF is found in the elderly with both Q wave and non–Q wave MI. Management usually includes diuretics, nitrates, and oxygen. Although inotropic therapy should be avoided, use of dobutamine and dopamine may be used with severe HF and hypotension (Aronow, 1999). Careful fluid administration can be used to treat hypotension when HF is absent (Aronow, 1999). Hemodynamic monitoring is used for severe or progressive HF or pulmonary edema, cardiogenic shock or progressive hypotension, or suspected mechanical complications (VSD, papillary muscle rupture, or pericardial tamponade) or to manage hypotension that does not respond promptly to fluid administration. Intra-arterial monitoring is useful when treating severe hypotension (SBP < 80 mm Hg) and cardiogenic shock and in patients receiving vasopressors, sodium nitroprusside, or other potent vasodilators and in hemodynamically stable patients receiving NTG for ischemia or IV inotropic agents. Pulmonary artery and intra-arterial monitoring are associated with significant complications—infection, pulmonary infarction, ventricular arrhythmias, heart block, and blood loss—and are not used in the absence of cardiac or pulmonary complications or in patients who are hemodynamically stable. Intra-aortic balloon counterpulsation (IABP) is indicated in cardiogenic shock not quickly reversed with pharmacological therapy, as a stabilizing measure for angiography and prompt revascularization, and in managing acute MR or VSD, recurrent intractable ventricular arrhythmias with hemodynamic instability or refractory post-MI angina.

The elderly should be assessed carefully for complications associated with use of the IABP, particularly in the presence of renal or peripheral vascular disease. In addition, the presence of these invasive interventions may necessitate the use of restraints or sedation. These must be used with caution in the elderly.

AF in the peri-MI period is common in the elderly population. It is best treated with electrical cardioversion and heparin when accompanied by severe hemodynamic compromise or intractable ischemia, although rapid digitalization can slow a rapid ventricular rate and improve LV function. Beta-blockers can also be used in patients without clinical LV dysfunction, bronchospastic disease, or AV block. Diltiazem or verapamil IV can be used if beta-blockers are contraindicated or ineffective; however, these should be used with caution.

Although treatment of isolated frequent premature ventricular contractions (PVCs), couplets, runs of accelerated idioventricular rhythm (AIVR), and nonsustained VT or the prophylactic use of antiarrhythmic therapy when using thrombolytic agents have not been well-established, lidocaine, procainamide, amiodarone, and synchronized cardioversion can be used. Antiarrhythmics should be continued 6–24 hours and then the need for continuation reassessed. Ventricular arrhythmias are common in the elderly in the absence of MI and it may be difficult to determine when treatment should be instituted. VT or ventricular fibrillation (VF) should be promptly treated, however, according to whether the VT is monomorphic or polymorphic. VF and sustained polymorphic VT (> 30 seconds or causing hemodynamic collapse) should be treated with unsynchronized shock starting at 200 joules; if this is unsuccessful a second shock of 200–300 joules should be used; and if necessary, there should be a third at 360 joules. In sustained monomorphic VT associated with angina, pulmonary edema, or hypotension (SBP < 90 mm Hg) a synchronized shock should be delivered at 100 joules with increasing energy levels if not successful. The presence of a pacemaker should be noted prior to cardioversion or defibrillation attempts, as should serum digoxin levels. Careful skin assessment of paddle placement sites should be conducted following resuscitative procedures and appropriate treatment for burns or skin breakdown instituted early. Electrolyte and acid-base disturbances should be corrected. Aggressive attempts to reduce myocardial ischemia with beta-blockers, IABP, and emergency PTCA or CABG may be required for drug-refractory polymorphic VT.

Bradyarrhythmias may be treated with atropine or in severe cases with temporary transcutaneous or transvenous pacing or permanent pacing. Atropine is indicated for sinus bradycardia (SB) with evidence of low CO, peripheral hypoperfusion, or PVCs at onset of symptoms. It may also be used in inferior wall MI with type 1 second-degree or third-degree AV block with symptoms of hypotension, ischemic discomfort, or ventricular arrhythmias; sustained bradycardia and hypotension after administration of NTG; nausea and vomiting associated with morphine; and ventricular asystole. Atropine is not indicated for infranodal AV block that is usually associated with an anterior MI with a wide-complex escape rhythm or asymptomatic SB.

Stroke may result from hemorrhage (15%) or thrombotic or embolic occlusion causing ischemia (85%) in the cerebral circulation (Weinberger, Silvers, & Adam, 1999). Ischemic stroke may result from atherosclerosis, emboli from a cardiac source, or small vessel disease related to HTN and DM. Stroke and CHD share many of the same risk factors. HTN is the major risk factor for stroke, and DM and cigarette smoking also have a role. Although the anatomic location of the stroke determines signs and symptoms, strokes most frequently occur in the cerebral hemispheres, with hemiparesis, sensory loss, loss of vision on the contralateral side, and behavioral and speech disturbances (Weinberger et al., 1999). Neurological examination and computerized axial tomography are performed to determine stroke etiology, so that appropriate medical intervention can be promptly instituted.

Discharge Planning

Individualized teaching post MI needs to begin in the CCU. Once the patient is stable, basic definitions of CHD, angina, and MI should be given to both the patient and the caregiver. Instruction should include the healing process following an MI, when an individual can expect to return to work, normal daily activities, and sexual activity. Fear of loss of independence after an MI is often a major concern of the older adult, especially if the MI was severe. For those with other chronic illnesses, further decline can be devastating. These individuals are at high risk for depression; the social and emotional impact of an MI and the risk of functional disability should be addressed with the patient and the caregiver. The patient and the caregiver should also be provided with information on community resources such as the AHA and support groups. Present living arrangements and whether there is the need of home services should also be reviewed.

Preparation for discharge may include submaximal stress or vasodilator (dipyridamole, dobutamie, or adenosine) ECG or nuclear scintigraphy or exercise stress echocardiography for prognostic assessment or functional capacity. Routine assessment of ventricular arrhythmias is not recommended; however, ambulatory (Holter) monitoring, signal-average ECG, heart rate variability, baroreflex sensitivity monitoring, alone or in conjunction with these or other tests, including functional tests (EF, treadmill tests), may be used for risk assessment after MI. The patient and his or her family should be adequately prepared for these tests.

Older age has consistently been associated with poorer long-term outcomes—death and recurrent MI and HF—following MI (Chyun, 1998; Chyun, Vaccarino, Young, & Krumholz, 1999; Narain et al., 1988). Prognostic factors for development of death, recurrent MI, and HF in the elderly include increasing age; prior HF, MI, PVD, stroke, renal insufficiency, DM, and CABG; poorer mental status, presence of HF, lower SBP, and higher HR and serum potassium levels on arrival; poorer EF, Q wave MI, and HF during hospitalization; myocardial function requiring use of nitrates and diuretics at discharge. Patients and caregivers need to understand the warning signs of HF and recurrent MI such as chest pain, pressure, shortness of breath, indigestion, nausea, dizziness, palpitations, confusion, weakness, and weight gain. A clear plan for obtaining immediate medical attention should be developed. This is especially important if the elderly person lives alone; some type of "medical alert" system may be needed. Understanding and ability to follow the medication regimen are paramount. A thorough assessment of the patient and the caregivers is therefore vital. The elderly individual may be on multiple medications, and the schedule may be confusing. The need to maintain cardiac medications must be stressed, and the risk of the patient abruptly discontinuing beta-blocker, nitrates, and antiarrhythmics must be assessed. All medications should be reviewed with the patient and the caregivers, stressing desired effects, common side effects, and possible interactions with over-the-counter medications. The nurse should also review what to do if medications are accidentally omitted or become too costly to maintain.

Secondary prevention should include initiation of an AHA Step II diet (7% total calories as saturated fat and < 200 mg/dL cholesterol) and, if necessary, medication to reduce low-density lipoprotein (LDL) levels to < 100 mg/dL. Physical activity, weight, blood pressure, and smoking cessation need to be assessed and a plan developed to manage these risk factors (AHA, 1995). Long-term beta blockade should be given to all patients other than low-risk patients without a clear contraindication. Anticoagulants should be given to patients unable to take daily aspirin, post-MI patients in persistent AF, and patients with an LV thrombus and may be useful in patients with LV dysfunction. There is no general agreement on estrogen replacement; however, hormone replacement therapy (HRT) with estrogen plus progestin can be continued in postmenopausal women who were using HRT prior to MI.

Hospitalization for acute MI may provide the only opportunity to maximize CHD management, as well as link the individual to a cardiac rehabilitation program following discharge. The nurse should work with the patient and caregivers to establish goals to foster health promotion and reduce cardiac risk. Although physical activity is central to management of CHD and it is recommended that elderly men and women be strongly encouraged to participate in exercise-based cardiac rehabilitation and that special efforts be made to overcome obstacles to entry and participation (U.S. Department of Health and Human Services [U.S. DHHS], 1995), the elderly, particularly elderly women, are referred to and enroll less frequently in exercise-based cardiac rehabilitation than younger individuals (Ades, Waldmann, Polk, & Coflesky, 1992; Lavie & Milani, 1995; Lavie, Milani, & Littman, 1993).

Strategies for assisting the patient to attend a rehabilitation program, including enlisting the physician in encouraging the patient to attend, are important (Ades, Waldmann, McCann, & Weaver, 1992).

HEART FAILURE

HF is a major public health problem, affecting more than 4 million Americans (AHA, 1998). The prevalence of HF increases with increasing age, and more than 75% of those affected are older than 65 years (U.S. DHHS, 1994). Both the incidence and the prevalence of HF will continue to rise as our population ages and advances are made that decrease mortality in these patients.

HF is associated with a decrease in quality of life and in functional capacity. Multidisciplinary teams have focused on the coordination of inpatient, outpatient, and home care for those with HF and have demonstrated positive outcomes in terms of functional capacity, length of hospital stay, readmission rates, self-care knowledge, patient satisfaction, and quality of life (Naylor et al., 1994; Rich et al., 1995; Venner & Solitro-Seelbinder, 1996). However, HF remains the leading cause of hospitalization in the elderly population (AHA, 1998).

Risk Factors and Precipitating Causes of HF

Although age-related changes in diastolic function are usually not enough to cause overt HF, the presence of other illnesses and conditions may contribute to its development. Those who are older, male, and obese and have HTN, valvular heart disease; a cardiomyopathy, or diabetes are at increased risk for developing HF (Chen et al., 1999; Ho, Pinsky, Kannel, & Levy, 1993). Other factors that may precipitate HF in older adults are depicted in Table 17.4. In the hospital setting, the most common precipitating cause of HF is the aggressive administration of IV fluids (Luchi, Taffet, & Teasdale, 1991).

Clinical Presentation

The clinical presentation of congestive heart failure may include a variety of signs and symptoms reflective of pulmonary congestion and decreased CO. These may include

- difficulty in breathing
  shortness of breath
  dyspnea on exertion

TABLE 17.4   Common Precipitants of Heart Failure in Older Adults

- Uncontrolled hypertension
- Myocardial ischemia or infarction
- Arrhythmias
- Cardiac tamponade & restrictive pericarditis
- Congenital abnormalities/Coarctation of the aorta
- Aortic or Ventricular Aneurysms
- Dietary sodium excess & excess fluid intake
- Aggressive IV fluid replacement & blood transfusions
- Renal insufficiency/decrease in glomerular filtration rate
- Anemia
- Infection/fever
- Hyperthyroidism/hypothyroidism/thyrotoxicosis
- Hypoxemia/Pulmonary embolism/mechanical ventilation with use of positive end expiratory pressure (PEEP)
- Thiamine deficiency/Beriberi & Paget's disease
- Drugs/Medications
  - Alcohol
  - Negative Inotropes (Beta blockers, Calcium channel blockers, Antiarrhythmic agents)
  - Nonsteroidal anti-inflammatory agents
  - Corticosteroids
  - Antineoplastics
  - Estrogen preparations
  - Antihypertensives (clonidine, minoxodil)
  - Excessive licorice (glycyrrhizic acid)
  - Osmotic agents (Albumin, Mannitol)
  - Cardiac toxins (Daunomycin, Doxorubicin, Cyclophosphamide)
- Medication non-compliance

*Adapted from Rich, M. W. (1997). Epidemiology, pathophysiology, and etiology of congestive heart failure in older adults. *Journal of the American Geriatrics Society, 45*, 968–974.

tachypnea
orthopnea or paroxysmal nocturnal dyspnea and disrupted sleep
- fatigue, weakness, and a decrease in exercise tolerance

Physical exam findings may include

- hepatomegaly or splenomegaly
- jugular venous distention (JVD)
- hepatojugular reflux
- basilar crackles, bronchospasm, and wheezing
- presence of S3 heart sound
- displaced posterior MI
- lower extremity edema, ascities, weight gain

- pulses alterans
- cool extremities

The clinical presentation of HF may be atypical in the elderly, and often the differential diagnosis is difficult. With a low CO and decrease in perfusion to the periphery and other organs, the patient may present with a gangrenous extremity, confusion, or worsening dementia. In addition, dyspnea may be absent (Wei, 1994). Although the presence of peripheral edema and basilar rales are common findings in the patient with HF, they are unreliable diagnostic signs, especially in the elderly.

Evaluation

The normal age-related changes in the structure of the heart affect diastolic, rather than systolic, function (Lernfelt, Wikstrand, & Svanborg, 1991). In fact, diastolic dysfunction accounts for up to 50% of the cases of HF in those older than 65 years (Soufer et al., 1985). In the patient with diastolic HF, there is an increased resistance to passive filling of the ventricles during early diastole or relaxation. This is in contrast to systolic failure, where there is a decrease in the contractility of the heart. Both the high ventricular filling pressure and the poor pumping ability of the heart can lead to pulmonary congestion and diminished CO. For this reason, the presentation of diastolic and systolic failure can be similar. However, it is important to distinguish diastolic from systolic failure, because management is influenced by the type of dysfunction present.

Differentiating between systolic and diastolic HF can be accomplished by the use of either an echocardiogram or a radionuclide ventriculogram. Other common diagnostic tests used in the evaluation of patients with HF include chest x-ray, ECG, pulmonary artery catheter readings, and arterial and venous blood sampling (Table 17.5).

Management

Initial goals in the management of the CCU patient with HF are to alleviate symptoms, improve oxygenation and circulation, and correct the underlying causes of the patient's failure. Longer-term goals in the management of HF are to improve exercise tolerance and functional capacity, reduce readmission rates, and decrease mortality. Both pharmacological and non-pharmacological interventions are used to meet these objectives.

Pharmacological Therapy in HF

Pharmacological therapy may include the use of diuretics, vasodilators, ACE inhibitors, digoxin and other positive inotropic agents, or beta-blockers or

TABLE 17.5 Diagnostic Tests in the Patient with Heart Failure

Test	Purpose	Findings
Chest X-ray	Assesses for cardiomegaly, abnormal pattern of pulmonary vasculature, or extracardiac causes to HF	Cardiac enlargement seen with HF except in pericarditis or restrictive disease. May see interstitial, perivascular, or alveolar edema, Kerley's B lines, peribronchial cuffing, pleural effusions, atelectasis. In acute HF, lower pulmonary vessels constrict and upper vessels become better perfused.
Echocardiogram	Measures ventricular wall motion, chamber size, wall thickness, contractile function, and valve function	Distinguishes between diastolic and systolic failure. In systolic dysfunction will see a decreased EF ($< 40\%$). In diastolic dysfunction will see stiffness of ventricular wall and an E/A reversal (normally E wave is greater than A wave). May find an aneurysm, intracardiac shunting, pericardial effusion, or thrombi.
ECG	Determination of precipitating factors: ST-T wave changes, arrhythmias	Myocardial ischemia and infarction, bradyarrhythmias, atrial fibrillation/tachyarrhythmia. Voltage criteria in LVH or low voltage with pericardial effusion.
Pulmonary artery catheter	Measures hemodynamic indices: preload, cardiac output	Normal pulmonary capillary wedge pressure (PCWP) < 12. Will have elevated PCWP > 12 in those with congestion. Helpful in guiding management and success of treatment.

(continued)

TABLE 17.5   *(continued)*

Test	Purpose	Findings
Arterial blood gas/pulse oximetry	Evaluates oxygenation and effect of therapeutic interventions	May see an increase in $PaCO_2$ and a decrease in the PaO_2 caused by tachypnea and poor gas exchange. May see O_2 sat < 90% without supplemental oxygen.
Venous blood testing	Helps determine precipitating cause/monitors side effects and therapeutic effects of treatment: CBC, U/A, BUN/Cr, T4/TSH, Liver enzymes, Electrolytes, PT/PTT, CK, MB	Monitor for anemia, proteinuria, renal insufficiency, thyroid disease, hepatomegaly, hypokalemia/hyperkalemia, therapeutic INR, myocardial infarction

BUN, blood urea nitrogen; CBC, complete blood count; $PaCO_2$, partial pressure of arterial carbon dioxide; PCWP, pulmonary capillary wedge pressure; PT/PTT, prothrombin time/partial thromboplastin time; T4, thyroxine; TSH, thyrotropin stimulating hormone; U/A, urinalysis

a combination of these. These medications are usually used in combination, depending on the patient's symptoms, the severity of HF, and the type of dysfunction present. They are discussed in further detail later in this chapter (Table 17.6). Diuretics are used in both systolic and diastolic HF to relieve congestive symptoms. They decrease preload by promoting the excretion of sodium and water and decrease cardiac filling pressures. They should be used cautiously in patients with diastolic dysfunction, who rely more heavily on preload to maintain an adequate CO.

Vasodilators are also useful in the treatment of systolic and diastolic failure. They decrease preload by increasing venous capacitance and decreasing central venous blood volume. As with diuretics, they should be used cautiously in those with diastolic HF. Hydralazine and isosorbide are useful in combination form. By reducing both preload and afterload, they relieve symptoms and improve exercise tolerance. More importantly, these agents may have a beneficial effect on mortality. Morphine sulfate also has a peripheral vasodilating effect and is useful with pulmonary edema.

ACE inhibitors are important in the management of systolic HF because they improve symptoms and exercise tolerance and decrease mortality. They may also be helpful in diastolic failure because they may regress hypertrophy and reduce wall thickness.

Digoxin increases contractility and decreases HR. It is not used routinely with diastolic failure because it can increase ventricular stiffness and delay

TABLE 17.6   Common Medications Used in Patients with CVD

Medication	Side Effects/Considerations in the Elderly
ACE inhibitors	Hypotension (may need to decrease or withdraw diuretic to avoid); cough; hyperkalemia; azotemia Follow BUN and creatinine Avoid volume depletion may cause hypotension and renal insufficiency; need to correct hyponatremia or volume depletion prior to initiation. Lisinopril advantageous due to QD dosage, useful for compliance Avoid K-sparing diuretics or K supplements May cause hypotension with Etoh
Antiarrhythmics	Increase in ventricular ectopy; risk of sudden death Amiodarone: pulmonary toxicity Disopyramide: severe LV dysfunction; GI hypomotility, presbyopia; caution with obstructive uropathy and glaucoma; caution with decreased renal function; carefully monitor bowel and bladder function; bradycardia with calcium blockers Lidocaine: decreased clearance with HF, beta-blockers, and cimetidine; toxicity more common in elderly; monitor for: confusion, parasthesias, respiratory depression, hypotension, seizures Procainamide: Orthostatic hypotension; toxicity with renal disease; bradycardia with diltiazem and verapamil Quinidine: Orthostatic hypotension; toxicity with liver or renal disease, diltiazem or verapamil; increased reabsoprtion with HCTZ, antacids and carbonic anhydrase inhibitors used to treat glaucoma, and chronic UTIs; barbiturates and rifampin decrease antiarrhythmic effect Magnesium: QT interval, Mg and K levels
Anticoagulants	Bleeding, particularly intracerebral Risk increased with malignant lesions, HTN, cerebrovascular disease, frail, gait disturbances Anticoagulant response increased to warfarin at older ages Chronic disease and increased vascular and capillary fragility may also increase risk Potentiate risk with heparin: ASA, cephalosporins, penicillins Potentiate with warfarin: Etoh; allopurinol, amiodarnoe, ASA, cimetidine, ciprofloxacin, clofibrate, indomethacin, metronidazole, phenylbutazone, quinidine, sulfonanides, thyroxine, plus many others Barbiturates, carbamazepine, glutethimide, rifampin, and Vitamin K decrease anticoagulant effect
Antiplatelet agents	Bleeding GI intolerance with ASA
Atropine	Delirium, urinary retention, constipation

(continued)

TABLE 17.6   *(continued)*

Medication	Side Effects/Considerations in the Elderly
Beta blockers	Increase in HF, hypotension, bradycardia, decrease CO, bronchospasm, SA and AV block; CNS toxicity
	Bradycardia may result with propranolol and cimetidine; bradycardia and hypotension with propranolol and diltiazem or verapamil
	Initiated at low doses due to their negative inotropic effects
Calcium channel	HF, LV dysfunction, AV block, tachycardia, hypotension, postural hypotension (verapamil); lower limb edema, headache, dyspepsia
	Diltiazem: SA dysfunction
	Verapamil: SA and AV block; LV dysfunction with beta-blockers
Digoxin	Toxicity: confusion, nausea, anorexia, hazy vision, arrhythmias (VF)
	Need to monitor elderly closely for toxicity, especially with decreased renal function and lean body mass.
	Increased levels with: quinidine, calcium blockers, amiodarone, triamterene, spironolactone, erythromycin, flecainide, amiodarone, propafenone
	Toxicity with normal levels in presence of: hypokalemia, hypomagnesemia, hypercalcemia, hypoxia, acidosis, acute and chronic lung disease, hypothyroidism
	May cause visual disturbances, depression, and confusion with therapeutic levels
	Decreased absorption with sucralfate
Diuretics	Volume depletion and dehydration, hypokalemia (hyperkalemia with potassium sparing diuretics), hyponatremia, hypomagnesia, prerenal azotemia, incontinence, orthostatic hypotension and falls
	Thiazides: Hyperglycemia; hyperuricemia; hypercalcemia; ineffective with glomerular filtration rate <30 ml/min
	Potassium sparing: Hypomagnesemia; ototoxicity
	Thiazides and K-sparing; are not the drug of choice in elderly with concomitant renal dysfunction.
	Use of K-sparing diuretics with ACE inhibitor therapy may cause hyperkalemia
	NSAIDS may decrease effects of furosemide
Inotropic agents	Increases oxygen consumption and may cause ventricular arrhythmias
Morphine	Respiratory depression, nausea and vomiting, hypotension, sedation, constipation, impaction

TABLE 17.6   *(continued)*

Medication	Side Effects/Considerations in the Elderly
Nitrates	Resting and postural hypotension (especially in patients with an inferior MI complicated by right ventricular involvement); bradycardia; headache; vertigo; weakness; palpitations; medication tolerance; syncope, falls May shunt blood in lungs causing decreased oxygenation, especially with COPD; Hydralazine + isosorbide: Headache; hypotension; flushing With other anti-HTN agents: hypotension, sedation May cause hypotension with Etoh

ACE = angiotensin-converting enzyme; ASA = aspirin; AV = atrioventricular; BUN = blood urea nitrogen; CNS = central nervous system; CO = cardiac output; Etoh = alcohol; GI = gastrointestinal; HCTZ = hydrochlorothiazide; HF = heart failure; HTN = hypertension; K = potassium; LV = left ventricular; Mg = magnesium; MI = myocardial infarction; NSAID = non-steroidal anti-inflammatory; QD = daily; SA = sinoatrial; UTI = urinary tract infection

relaxation. However, digoxin may be useful in those patients with persistent symptoms despite diuretic and ACE inhibitor therapy and in those patients with concomitant AF. Other medications that have a positive inotropic effect are dopamine and dobutamine. Both of these drugs can improve contractility and subsequent CO; however, they also increase myocardial oxygen demand. Amrinone and milrinone are phosphodiesterase inhibitors that have been shown to be beneficial in the management of the hospitalized patient with HF, providing a positive inotropic effect as well as a vasodilation.

Beta-blockers are useful in the management of diastolic HF because of their negative chronotropic effect. By decreasing HR, they lengthen the diastolic filling phase of the cardiac cycle. More recently, beta-blockers have been shown to be beneficial in the treatment of systolic HR; however, they should be started after the patient's symptoms have resolved and be initiated at low doses.

The Agency for Health Care Policy and Research (AHCPR) provides guidelines for the approach to treatment of systolic heart failure (U.S. DHHS, 1994). In general, all patients should be given a trial of ACE inhibitor therapy unless contraindications exist. Those with contraindications should be given hydralazine and isosorbide. Diuretics are started in the patient with overt symptoms, and digoxin is added in those who continue to have symptoms despite ACE inhibitor and diuretic therapy (Konstam et al., 1994). The approach to the patient with diastolic failure is less clear. As mentioned previously, beta-blockers and calcium channel blockers may be useful in reducing HR, with subsequent improvement in diastolic filling.

Nonpharmacological Therapy

Other therapeutic interventions include the use of supplemental oxygen and mechanical ventilation. Oxygen should be given to maintain an oxygen saturation of > 90% and a PaO_2 > 60–70. Intubation and the use of mechanical ventilation may be necessary to ease the work of breathing, especially if the patient is restless and agitated. Positioning the patient upright with the feet dangling promotes diuresis and helps relieve some of the breathing difficulty associated with HF. Another intervention in the critically ill patient is the use of mechanical support with an IABP. The use of IABP counterpulsation restores perfusion to the systemic circulation by reducing afterload, decreasing myocardial oxygen demand, and increasing coronary artery perfusion. This may be most beneficial in those who experienced an acute MI prior to the onset of HF.

Lastly, counseling the patient about the disease process; medications, including issues of compliance; activity; and dietary restrictions should be initiated in the CCU. As mentioned previously, the shortened length of hospital stay necessitates that education begin as early as feasible.

ARRHYTHMIAS

Sinus node dysfunction, common in the elderly, may lead to sinus bradycardia, sinus pauses, and bradycardia-tachycardia syndrome. It is often associated with diffuse conduction disease and atrial arrhythmias. Atrial pacing or dual chamber pacemakers may be warranted. Sinus node automaticity, HR variability, and maximal HR achieved with exercise decline with age. In combination with CHD, which may affect the conduction system; cardiac medications that may slow conduction; fibrosis of the conduction system; and calcific degeneration of the aortic or mitral valves, sinoatrial block, AV block, and BBB may result (Rials, Marinchak, & Kowey, 1992). All forms of symptomatic block are treated with pacing. Right bundle branch block (RBBB) plus left anterior hemiblock implies structural disease and worse prognosis, and LBBB is strongly associated with CHD.

Supraventricular arrhythmias are common in the elderly. Although supraventricular tachyarrhythmias, except for AF, are of little importance in the absence of structural heart disease, ischemic changes and LVH are associated with an increased mortality risk, with the underlying disease determining prognosis. Sinus tachycardia is a common physiological response to a number of pathological states: fever, pain, anemia, dehydration (Rials et al., 1992). It is best treated by correcting the underlying condition. Digoxin toxicity, to which the elderly are susceptible because of poor renal function, should be considered in the presence of paroxysmal atrial or junctional tachycardia. Multifocal atrial tachycardia is frequently seen in the setting of COPD. Digoxin may increase automaticity and further aggravate the arrhythmia (Rials et al., 1992). Treatment often includes beta-blockers, verapamil or magnesium.

Atrial flutter (AF) is usually seen with organic heart disease (Rials et al., 1992). Treatment includes controlling ventricular rate followed by attempts to convert to normal sinus rhythm (NSR), class 1 antiarrhythmics, electric cardioversion, or rapid atrial pacing. At rates less than 300 beats per minute or a ratio > 2:1, in absence of drug therapy, conduction system defects should be suspected and the risk of bradycardia or heart block at time of conversion should be anticipated (Rials et al., 1992).

AF is common in the elderly and is an important cause of stroke. It is frequently associated with CHD, HTN, and valvular and thyroid diseases; however, it can occur in the absence of structural heart disease (Rials et al., 1992). Mortality usually results from the underlying disease and thromboembolism. Patients frequently present with palpitations, fatigue, dyspnea, and dizziness. Management of ventricular rate is the first priority. Digoxin, beta-blockers (esmolol, propranolol, or metoprolol), and calcium channel blockers (diltiazem or verapamil), along with treatment of any underlying conditions, such as ischemia, HF, and thyroid disease, should be promptly instituted (AHA, 1996). In patients with chest pain or HF resulting from the rapid rate, these drugs may be administered intravenously. However, hypotension and HF may result from IV administration; therefore, in asymptomatic patients, they are administered orally, with preference for calcium and beta-blockers over digoxin (AHA, 1996). If hypotension, severe HF, or anginal chest pain are present, direct current cardioversion is usually necessitated (Ferrick & Fisher, 1999).

Once the ventricular rate has been controlled, conversion to sinus rhythm with class 1 antiarrhythmic agents may be attempted in hemodynamically stable patients, although they rarely terminate AF (AHA, 1996). Long-term antiarrhythmic medication should be titrated slowly upward. Proarrhythmia (sinus bradycardia, bradyarrhythmias, and torsades de pointes) is a common problem and should be carefully assessed for in the elderly, who frequently have multiple risk factors: structural heart disease, HF, LV dysfunction, hypokalemia, LVH, and prolonged QT interval. Proarrhythmia can be seen initially or during the 24–48 hours following initiation of therapy. Use of short-acting barbiturates or benzodiazipines during cardioversion will require careful monitoring in the elderly individual. As with atrial flutter, if AF is associated with a slow ventricular response in the absence of drug therapy, conduction system disease should be suspected. The need for temporary pacing should be anticipated as a prolonged period of asystole, or high-grade AV block may result from cardioversion. At present, the agent that can provide the best long-term maintenance of sinus rhythm has not been established.

Prevention of thromboembolism is the third goal of management. The patient should be anticoagulated for 3 weeks prior to cardioversion, and this should be continued for 4 weeks following if AF has been present more than 48 hours or if time of onset is unknown. Drug interactions between digioxin and warfarin should be closely assessed. In low-risk patients or those at high risk, who cannot safely receive anticoagulation, aspirin at a dose of 325 mg/d should be administered. In patients at high risk for thromboembolism, warfarin is recommended. Although the recommended International Normalized Ratio (INR) ranges from 2–3, close observation should be made in the elderly, who may require lower INR levels because of an increased risk of bleeding.

As many as 70–80% of elderly individuals have ventricular arrhythmias (Tresch & Thakur, 1999). As with AF, in the absence of underlying heart disease, ventricular arrhythmias are not associated with an increased mortality risk (Fleg & Kennedy, 1982). Several recent trials have demonstrated an increase in mortality and sudden cardiac death in post-MI patients treated with encainide, flecainide, moricizine, and D-sotalol (Cardiac Arrhythmia Suppression Trial [CAST] Investigators Preliminary Report, 1989; CAST II Trial Investigators, 1992; Waldo et al., 1996). Routine long-term use of antiarrhythmic medication for asymptomatic ventricular ectopy, therefore, is not recommended, and treatment of symptomatic ventricular ectopy may be treated with beta-blockers without intrinsic sympathomimetic activity or with amiodarone (Cairns et al., 1997; Julilan et al., 1997; Kennedy et al., 1994). Amiodarone, however, is associated with significant adverse effects—hypothyroidism, hyperthyroidism, pulmonary fibrosis—that require special precautions in the elderly.

Patients with sustained VT, which is commonly seen with structural and ischemic heart disease, receive antiarrhythmic medications, the administration of which is guided by electrophysiology testing. Antiarrhythmic therapy may be associated with adverse reactions in the elderly, especially in the setting of other systemic illnesses. Therefore, careful assessment of side effects should be ongoing and should be included as part of patient and caregiver teaching. The overall approach to management of ventricular arrhythmias includes correction of reversible underlying conditions (ischemia, electrolyte abnormalities, medications), evaluation for and treatment of underlying heart disease, and assessment of prognostic factors (Tresch & Thakkur, 1999). Patients at moderate risk may then be followed closely, whereas those at high risk, based on signal-averaged ECG, results of LVEF, and type of ventricular ectopy, will usually receive more aggressive treatment, including amiodarone and an implantable cardioverter-defibrillator (ICD) if medication is unsuccessful in controlling the arrhythmia.

REFERENCES

The Acute Infarction Ramipril Efficacy Study Investigators. (1993). Effect of rampril on mortality and morbidity of survivors of acute myocardial infarction with clinical evidence of heart failure. The AIRE Study. *Lancet, 342,* 821–828.

Ades, P. A., & Grunvald, M. H. (1990). Cardiopulmonary exercise testing before and after conditioning in older coronary patients. *American Heart Journal, 120,* 585–589.

Ades, P. A., Waldmann, M. L., McCann, W. J., & Weaver, S. O. (1992). Predictors of CR participation in older coronary patients. *Archives of Internal Medicine, 152,* 1033–1035.

Ades, P. A., Waldmann, M. L., Polk, D. M., & Coflesky, J. T. (1992). Referral patterns and exercise response in the rehabilitation of female coronary patients aged > 62 years. *American Journal of Cardiology, 69,* 1422–1425.

American Heart Association. (1995). Preventing heart attack and death in patients with coronary disease. *Circulation, 2,* 2–4.

American Heart Association. (1996). *Management of patients with atrial fibrillation.* Dallas, TX: American Heart Association.

American Heart Association. (1997). Guide to primary prevention of cardiovascular diseases. *Circulation, 95,* 2329–2331.

American Heart Association. (1998). *Heart and stroke facts and statistics.* Dallas, TX: American Heart Association.

American Heart Association. (1999). *1999 Update: ACC/AHA guidelines for the management of patients with acute myocardial infarction.* Dallas, TX: American Heart Association.

Antiplatelet Trialists' Collaboration. (1988). Secondary prevention of vascular disease by prolonged antiplatelet treatment. *British Medical Journal, 296,* 320–331.

Applegate, W. B., Graves, S., Collins, S., Zwaag, R. V., & Akins, D. (1984). Acute myocardial infarction in elderly patients. *Southern Medical Journal, 77* (9), 1127–1129.

Aronow, W. S. (1987). Prevalence of presenting symptoms of recognized acute myocardial infarction and of unrecognized healed myocardial infarction in elderly patients. *American Journal of Cardiology, 60* (14), 1182.

Aronow, W. S. (1999). Management of the older person with atrial fibrillation. *Journal of the American Geriatrics Society, 47,* 740–748.

Backes, R. J., & Gersh, B. J. (1992). Cardiomyopathies in the elderly. In D. T. Lowenthal (Ed.), *Geriatric cardiology.* Philadelphia: F. A. Davis.

Barzilay, J. I., & Kronmal, R. A. (1998). Coronary heart disease in diabetic and nondiabetic patients with lower extremity arterial disease. *American Heart Journal, 135,* 1055–1062.

Bayer, A. J., Chadha, J. S., Farag, R. R., & Pathy, M. S. (1986). Changing presentations of myocardial infarction with increasing old age. *Journal of the American Geriatrics Society, 34* (4), 263–266.

Berkman, L. F., Leo-Summers, L., & Horowitz, R. (1992). Emotional support and survival after myocardial infarction: A prospective population based study of the elderly. *Annals of Internal Medicine, 117,* 1003–1009.

Berkman, L. F., & Syme, S. L. (1979). Social networks, host resistance, and mortality: A nine-year follow-up study of Alameda County residents. *American Journal of Epidemiology, 109,* 186–204.

Burrows, B., Alpert, J. S., & Ross, J. C. (1987). Pulmonary heart disease. *Journal of the American College of Cardiology, 10,* 63A–65A.

Cairns, J. A., Connolly, S. J., Roberts, R., & Gent, M., for the Canadian Amiodarone Myocardial Infarction Arrhythmia Trial Investigators. (1997). Randomized trial of outcome after myocardial infarction in patients with frequent or repetitive ventricular premature depolarizations: CAMIAT. *Lancet, 349,* 675–682.

Cardiac Arrhythmia Suppression Trial (CAST) Investigators. (1992). Preliminary report. Effect of encainide and flecainide on mortality in a randomized trial of arrhythmia suppression after myocardial infarction. *New England Journal of Medicine, 321,* 406–412.

CAST II Trial investigators. (1989). Effect of the anti-arrhythmic agent moricizine on survival after myocardial infarction. *New England Journal of Medicine, 327,* 227–233.

Chakko, S., & Kessler, K. M. (1992). Changes with aging as reflected in noninvasive cardiac studies. In D. T. Lowenthal (Ed.), *Geriatric cardiology.* Philadelphia: F.A. Davis.

Chen, Y. T., Vaccarino, V., Williams, C. S., Butler, J., Berkman, L. F., & Krumholz, H. M. (1999). Risk factors for heart failure in the elderly: A prospective community-based study. *American Journal of Medicine, 106,* 605–612.

Chung, M. K., Bosner, M. S., McKenzie, J. P., Shen, J., & Rich, M. W. (1995). Prognosis of patients > 70 years of age with non-Q-wave acute MI compared with younger patients with similar infarcts and with patients > 70 years of age with Q-wave acute MI. *American Journal of Cardiology, 75,* 18–22.

Chyun, D. (1998). The prognostic importance of diabetes mellitus in elderly patients with myocardial infarction. *Dissertation Abstracts International.*

Chyun, D., Vaccarino, V., Young, L. H., & Krumholz, H. M. (1999). Abstract: Heart failure and recurrent MI in the elderly with diabetes. *Circulation, 100* (Suppl. 1).

Constans, T., Bacq, Y., & Brechot, J. F. (1992). Protein-energy malnutrition in elderly medical patients. *Journal of the American Geriatrics Society, 40,* 263–268.

Dracup, K., & Moser, D. K. (1991). Treatment-seeking behavior among those with signs and symptoms of acute myocardial infarction. *Heart and Lung, 20,* 570–575.

Ferrick, K. J., & Fisher, J. D. (1999). Management of supraventricular tachycardia in the elderly. In D. D. Tresch & W. S. Aronow (Eds.), *Cardiovascular disease in the elderly patient.* New York: Marcel Dekker.

Fleg, J. L. (1999). Electrocardiographic findings in older persons without clinical heart disease. In D. D. Tresch & W. S. Aronow (Eds.), *Cardiovascular disease in the elderly patient.* New York: Marcel Dekker.

Fleg, J. L., & Kennedy, H. L. (1982). Cardiac arrhythmia in a healthy elderly population. Detection by 24-hour ambulatory electrocardiography. *Chest, 81,* 302–307.

Frasure-Smith, N., Lesperance, F., & Talajic, M. (1993). Depression following myocardial infarction: Impact on 6 month survival. *JAMA, 270,* 1819–1825.

Gill, T. M., Williams, C. S., Mendes de Leon, C. F., & Tinettit, M. E. (1997). The role of change in physical performance in determining risk of dependence in ADLs among nondisabled community-living elderly persons. *Journal of Clinical Epidemiology, 60,* 765–772.

Gillum, R. F. (1993). Trends in acute myocardial infarction and coronary heart disease death in the United States. *Journal of American College of Cardiology, 23,* 1273–1277.

Goldberg, R. J., Gore, J. M., Gurwitz, J. H., Alpert, J. S., Brady, P., Strohsnitter, W., Chen, Z., & Dalen, J. E. (1989). The impact of age on the incidence and prognosis of initial acute MI: The Worcester Heart Attack Study. *American Heart Journal, 117,* 543–549.

Graves, E. J. (1992). *National Hospital Discharge Survey: Annual Summary, 1990.* Hyattsville, MD: National Center for Health Statistics, Public Health Service, Vital and Health Statistics. Series 13, no. 112.

Grines, C. L., Browne, K. F., & Marco, J. (1993). A comparison of immediate angioplasty with thrombolytic therapy for acute myocardial infarction. *New England Journal of Medicine, 328,* 673–679.

Gurwitz, J. H., Osganian, V., Goldberg, R. J., Chen, Z. Y., Gore, J. M., & Alpert, J. S. (1991). Diagnostic testing in acute myocardial infarction. *American Journal of Epidemiology, 134,* 948–957.

The GUSTO Angiographic Investigators. (1993). The effects of tissue plasminogen activator, streptokinase, or both on coronary artery patency, ventricular function, and survival after acute myocardial infarction. *New England Journal of Medicine, 329,* 673–682.

Ho, K. L., Pinsky, J. L., Kannel, W. B., & Levy, D. (1993). The epidemiology of heart failure: The Framingham study. *Journal of the American College of Cardiology, 22* (suppl. A), 6A–13A.

Inouye, S., Viscoli, C. M., Horowitz, R. I., Hurst, L., & Tinetti, M. E. (1993). A predictive model for delirium in hospitalized elderly medical patients based in admission characteristics. *Annals of Internal Medicine, 119,* 474–481.

Julian, D. G., Camm, A. J., Frangin, G., Janse, M. J., Munoz, A., Schwartz, P. J., & Simon, P., for the European Myocardial Infarct Amiodarone Trial Investigators. (1997). Randomized trial of effect of amiodarone on mortality in patients with left-ventricular dysfunction after recent myocardial infarction: EMIAT. *Lancet, 349,* 667–674.

ISIS-2 (Second International Study of Infarct Survival) Collaborative Group. (1988). Randomized trial of intravenous streptokinase, oral aspirin, both, or neither among 17,187 cases of suspected acute myocardial infarction: ISIS-2. *Lancet, 2* (8607), 349–360.

Kannel, W. B., & Abbott, R. D. (1984). Incidence and prognosis of unrecognized myocardial infarction. *The New England Journal of Medicine, 311,* 1144–1147.

Kennedy, H. L., Brooks, M. M., Barker, A. H., Bergstrand, R., Hother, M. L., Beanlands, D. S., Bigger, J. T., & Goldstein, S. (1994). Beta-blocker therapy in the Cardiac Arrhythmia Suppression Trial. *American Journal of Cardiology, 74,* 674–680.

Kolibash, A. J., Kilman, J. W., & Bush, C. A. (1986). Evidence for progression from mild to severe mitral regurgitation in mitral valve prolapse. *American Journal of Cardiology, 58,* 762–765.

Konstam, M., Dracup, K., Bottoroff, M. B., Brooks, N. H., Dacey, R. A., Dunbar, S. B., Jackson, A. B., & Jessup, M. (1994). *Heart failure: Management of patients with left-ventricular systolic dysfunction. Quick reference guide for clinicians No. 11* (AHCPR Publication No. 94-0613). Rockville, MD: U.S. Department of Health and Human Services.

Konu, V. (1977). Myocardial infarction in the elderly: A clinical and epidemiologic study with 1 year follow-up. *Acta Medica Scandinavia, 604* (suppl.), 3–68.

Kotler, M. N., Jacobs, L. E., & Ioli, A. (1992). Evaluation of valvular heart disease in patients older than 65. In D. T. Lowenthal (Ed.), *Geriatric cardiology.* Philadelphia: F.A. Davis.

Kovar, M. G., Fitti, J. E., & Chyba, M. M. (1992). *The longitudinal study of aging 1984–1990.* Hyattsville, MD: National Center for Health Statistics.

Lavie, C., & Milani, R. V. (1995). Effects of cardiac rehabilitation programs on exercise capacity, coronary risk factors, behavioral characteristics, and quality of life in a large elderly cohort. *American Journal of Cardiology, 76,* 177–179.

Lavie, C. J., Milani, R. V., & Littman, A. B. (1993). Benefits of cardiac rehabilitation and exercise training in secondary coronary prevention in the elderly. *Journal of the American College of Cardiology, 22,* 678–683.

Lernfelt, B., Wikstrand, J., & Svanborg, A. (1991). Aging and left ventricular function in elderly healthy people. *American Journal of Cardiology, 68*, 547–549.

Levy, D., Anderson, K. M., Savage, D. D., Kannel, W. B., Christiansen, J. C., & Castelli, W. P. (1988). Echocardiographically detected left ventricular hypertrophy: Prevalence and risk factors. The Framingham Heart Study. *Annals of Internal Medicine, 108*, 7–13.

Levy, D., Garrison, R. J., Savage, D. D., Kannel, W. B., & Castelli, W. P. (1989). Left ventricular mass and incidence of coronary heart disease in an elderly cohort. *Annals of Internal Medicine, 110*, 101–107.

Lewis, J. F., & Maron, B. J. (1992). Cardiovascular consequences of the aging process. In D. T. Lowenthal (Ed.), *Geriatric cardiology.* Philadelphia: F. A. Davis.

Lombard, J. T., & Selzer, A. (1987). Valvular aortic stenosis. A clinical and hemodynamic profile of patients. *Annals of Internal Medicine, 106*, 292–295.

Luchi R. J. (1997). Cardiomyopathies in the elderly. In F. E. Kaiser, J. E. Morley, & R. M. Coe (Eds.), *Cardiovascular diseases in older people.* New York: Springer Publishing.

Lusiani, L., Perrone, A., Pesevanto, R., & Conte, G. (1994). Prevalence, clinical features, and acute course of atypical myocardial infarction. *Angiology, 41* (1), 49–55.

MacDonald, J. B. (1984). Presentation of acute myocardial infarction in the elderly. *Age and Aging, 13*, 196–200.

Marcus, F. I., Friday, K., McCans, J., Moon, T., Hahn, E., Cobb, L., Edwards, J., & Kuller, L. (1990). Age related prognosis after acute myocardial infarction. The Multicenter Diltiazem Postinfarction Trial. *American Journal of Cardiology, 65*, 559–566.

Mayer-Oakes, S. A., Oye, R. K., & Leake, B. (1991). Predictors of mortality in older patients with acute pulmonary edema and normal ejection fraction after acute myocardial infarction. *Journal of the American Geriatrics Society, 39*, 862–868.

Meischke, H., Eisenberg, M. S., & Larsens, M. P. (1993). Prehospital delay interval for patients who use emergency medical services: The effect of heart-related medical conditions and demographic variables. *Annals of Emergency Medicine, 22*, 1597–1601.

Mittlemark, M. B., Psaty, B. M., Rautaharju, P. M., Fried, L. P., Borhani, N. O., Tracy, R. P., Gardin, J. M., & O'Leary, D. H. (1993). *The American Journal of Epidemiology, 137*, 311–317.

Muller, R. T., Gould, L. A., Betzu, R., Vacek, T., & Pradeep, V. (1990). Painless myocardial infarction in the elderly. *American Heart Journal, 199*, 202–203.

Nadelman, J., Frishman, W. H., Ooi, W. L., Tepper, D., Greenberg, S., Guzik, H., Lazar, E. J., Heiman, M., & Aronson, M. (1990). Prevalence, incidence, and prognosis of recognized and unrecognized myocardial infarction in persons aged 75 years and older: The Bronx Aging Study. *American Journal of Cardiology, 66*, 533–537.

Narain, P., Rubenstein, L. Z., Wieland, A. D., Rushbrook, R., Strome, L. S., Pietrusaka, F., & Mosley, J. E. (1988). Predictors of immediate and 6 month outcomes in hospitalized elderly patients. The importance of functional status. *Journal of the American Geriatric Society, 36*, 775–873.

Naylor, M., Brooten, D., Jones, R., Lavizzo-Mourey, R., Mezey, M., & Pauly, M. (1994). Comprehensive discharge planning for hospitalized elderly. *Annals of Internal Medicine, 120*, 999–1006.

Nestico, P. F., Depace, N. L., Morganroth, J., Kotler, M. N., & Ross, J. (1984). Mitral annular calcification: Clinical, pathophysiology, and echocardiographic review. *American Heart Journal, 107*, 989–992.

Normand, S. T., Glickman, M. E., Sharma, R. G. V. R. K., & McNeil, B. J. (1996). Using admission characteristics to predict short-term mortality from myocardial infarction in elderly patients. *JAMA, 275,* 1322–1328.

Pathy, M. S. (1967). Clinical presentation of myocardial infarction in the elderly. *British Heart Journal, 29,* 190–199.

Pepine, C. J. (1986). Silent myocardial ischemia; definition, magnitude and scope of the problem. *Cardiology Clinics, 4,* 577–581.

Pernenkil, R., Vinson, J. M., Shah, A. S., Beckham, V., Wittenberg, C., & Rich, M. W. (1997). Course and prognosis in patients > 70 years of age with congestive heart failure and normal versus abnormal left ventricular ejection fraction. *American Journal of Cardiology, 79,* 216–219.

Pfeffer, M. A., Braunwald, E., Moye, L. A., Basta, L., Brown, E. J., Cuddy, T. E., Davis, B. R., Geltman, E. M., Goldman, S., Flaker, B. L., and the SAVE Investigators. (1992). Effect of captopril on mortality and morbidity in patients with left ventricular dysfunction after myocardial infarction. Results of the Survival and Ventricular Enlargement trial. *New England Journal of Medicine, 327,* 669–677.

Reilly, A., Dracup, K., & Dattolo, J. (1994). Factors influencing prehospital delay in patients experiencing chest pain. *American Journal of Critical Care, 3,* 300–306.

Rials, S. J., Marinchak, R. A., & Kowey, P. R. (1992). Arrhythmias in the elderly. In D. T. Lowenthal (Ed.), *Geriatric cardiology.* Philadelphia: F. A. Davis.

Rich, M. W. (1997). Epidemiology, pathophysiology, and etiology of congestive heart failure in older adults. *Journal of the American Geriatrics Society, 45,* 968–974.

Rich, M. W., Bosner, M. S., Chung, M. K., Shen, J., & McKenzie, J. P. (1992). Is age an independent predictor of early and late mortality in patients with acute myocardial infarction? *American Journal of Medicine, 92,* 7–13.

Rich, M. W., Beckham, V., Wittenburg, C., Leven, C., Freddland, K., & Carney, R. (1995). A multidisciplinary intervention to prevent readmission of elderly patients with congestive heart failure. *The New England Journal of Medicine, 333,* 1190–1195.

Savage, D. D., Garrison, R. J., & Castelli, W. P. (1983). Prevalence of submitral (annular) calcium and its correlates in a general population-based sample (The Framingham Study). *American Journal of Cardiology, 51,* 1375–1378.

Schulman, S. P. (1999). Normal aging changes of the cardiovascular system. In D. D. Tresch & W. S. Aronow (Eds.), *Cardiovascular disease in the elderly patient.* New York: Marcel Dekker.

Seeman, T. E., Kaplan, G. A., Knudsen, L., Cohen, R., & Guralnik, J. (1987). Social network ties and mortality among the elderly in the Alameda County Study. *American Journal of Epidemiology, 126,* 714–723.

Singh, M., Thompson, R. C., & Holmes, D. R. (1999). In D. D. Tresch & W. S. Aronow (Eds.), *Cardiovascular disease in the elderly patient.* New York: Marcel Dekker.

Solomon, C. G., Lee, T. H., Cook, E. F., Weisberg, M. C., Brand, D. A., Rouan, G. W., & Goldman, L. (1989). Comparison of clinical presentation of acute myocardial infarction in patients older than 65 years of age to younger patients: The Multicenter Chest Pain Study Experience. *The American Journal of Cardiology, 63,* 772–776.

Soufer, R., Wohlgelernter D., Vita, N. A., Amuchestegui, M., Sostman, H. D., Berger, H. J., & Zaret, B. L. (1985). Intact systolic left ventricular function in clinical congestive heart failure. *American Journal of Cardiology, 55,* 1032–1036.

Steel, K., Gertman, P. M., & Crescenzi, A. J. (1981). Iatrogenic illness on a general medical service at a university hospital. *New England Journal of Medicine, 304,* 638–642.

Sullivan, D., & Lipschitz, D. (1997). Evaluating and treating nutritional problems in older patients. *Clinics in Geriatric Medicine, 13,* 753–768.

Tinker, G. M. (1981). Clinical presentation of myocardial infarction in the elderly. *Age and Aging, 10,* 237–240.

Tresch, D. C. (1987). Atypical presentation of cardiovascular disorders in the elderly. *Geriatrics, 42* (10), 31.

Tresch, D. D. (1998). Management of the older patient with acute myocardial infarction: Difference in clinical presentation between older and younger patients. *Journal of the American Geriatrics Society, 46,* 1157–1162.

Tresh, D. D., & Thakur, R. K. (1999). Ventricular arrhythmias in the elderly. In D. D. Tresch & W. S. Aronow (Eds.), *Cardiovascular disease in the elderly patient.* New York: Marcel Dekker.

Turi, Z. G., Stone, P. H., Muller, J. E., Parker, C., Rude, R. E., Raabe, D. E., Jaffe, A. S., Hartwell, T. D., Robertson, T. L., & Braumwald, E. (1986). Implications for acute intervention related to time of hospital arrival in acute myocardial infarction. *The American Journal of Cardiology, 58,* 203–208.

Uretsky, B. F., Farquhar, D. S., Berezin, A. F., & Hood, W. B. (1977). Symptomatic myocardial infarction without chest pain: Prevalence and clinical course. *The American Journal of Cardiology, 40,* 498–503.

U.S. Department of Health and Human Services. (1994). *Clinical practice guidelines #11: Congestive heart failure: Evaluation and care of patients with left ventricular systolic dysfunction* (AHCPR publication No. 94-0612). Rockville, MD: U.S. DHHS.

U.S. Department of Health and Human Services. (1995). *Clinical practice guidelines #17: Cardiac rehabilitation* (AHCPR publication No. 96-0672). Rockville, MD: U.S. DHHS.

Venner, G., & Solitro-Seelbinder, J. (1996). Team management of congestive heart failure across the continuum. *Journal of Cardiovascular Nursing, 10* (2), 71–84.

Waldo, A. L. Camm, A. J., deRuyter, H., Friedman, P. L., MacNeil, D. J., Pauls, J. F., Pitt, B., Pratt, C. M., Schwartz, P. J., Vettri, E. P., for the SWORD investigators. (1996). Effect of d-sotalol on mortality in patients with left ventricular dysfunction after recent and remote myocardial infarction. *Lancet, 348,* 7–12.

Wei, J. Y. (1994). Heart failure. In W. R. Hazzard, J. P. Blass, W. H. Ettinger, J. B. Holter, & J. G. Ouslander (Eds.), *Principles of geriatric medicine and gerontology* (3rd ed., p. 679). New York: McGraw-Hill.

Wei, J. Y. (1999). Advanced aging and the cardiovascular system. In N. K. Wenger (Ed.), *Cardiovascular disease in the octogenarian and beyond.* Cambridge: Cambridge University Press.

Weinberger, J., Silvers, T., & Adam, R. (1999). Cerebrovascular disease in the elderly (pp. 83–108). In D. D. Tresch & W. S. Aronow (Eds.), *Cardiovascular disease in the elderly patient.* New York: Marcel Dekker.

Yusuf, S., Collins, R., MacMahon, S., & Peto, R. (1988). Effect of intravenous nitrates on mortality in acute myocardial infarction: An overview of randomized trials. *Lancet, 1* (8594), 1088–1092.

PART IV

Social and Policy Issues

18

Ethical Decision Making

Ethel Mitty

Nurses caring for critically ill elderly are in the unique, but not necessarily enviable, position of managing the interaction of social policy, bioethics, patient health care goals, and cultural diversity. The context of acute care for the elderly is suffused with differing opinions about age indicators for aggressive interventions, the goals of medicine, cure versus care, definitions of quality of life, decisional capacity to make health care choices, and the necessity of advance directives. In the midst of these cross-currents, the nurse is a moral agent of and in society; practice is guided by the combination of principle-based ethics and an ethics of care. The nurse—the "one caring"—helps the patient (or a surrogate) determine what is best in accordance with the patient's beliefs, goals, and preferences in a morally ambiguous situation. The ability to reach a principled solution requires identification of the "oughts" and "shoulds" of moral reasoning; draws on nursing's professional code of ethics; seeks knowledge of the legal, historical, and evidence-based ways of decision making; and uses the process of ethical decision making. This chapter discusses the bioethical principles in the context of care of the critically ill elderly, the bedside dilemmas that confound them, and the moral, principled approaches to resolve them.

MORAL PRINCIPLES AND AN ETHICS OF AGING

There are basically four moral principles that underlie rational ethical decision making. However, it must be kept in mind that each can be interpreted somewhat differently and enacted by different cultures and societies.

1. *Autonomy* contains the concept of self-determination and, by extension, the *right* to make an informed choice. It has been suggested that

autonomy, the right to say "no" is a post-Nuremberg phenomenon. Autonomy is also the right to say "yes" to choices that an individual is offered. In the United States, autonomy and self-determination are codified in the federal Patient Self-Determination Act (1991), which declares the right of patients to receive information about mechanisms to ensure that their end-of-life care wishes will be respected and honored. As such, institutions receiving Medicare and Medicaid reimbursement are required to educate patients as well as staff about advance planning in general and advance directives in particular.

2.   *Respect for Persons* is held by some ethicists to be a component of or superordinate to the autonomy principle; it includes *veracity* or truth telling, *confidentiality,* and *fidelity* or keeping promises. Veracity and confidentiality have implications for the locus of decision making: patient centered or family centered. World views on truth telling vary from that of individual responsibility and the right to know everything to the view that giving bad news directly to patients causes pain, increases their burden, and might even hasten death (Braun, Pietsch, & Blanchette, 2000; Crow, Matheson, & Steed, 2000).

3.   *Beneficence and Nonmaleficence* mean doing good and preventing harm and crystallize as the alleviation of suffering and preservation of life, but not necessarily at all costs. Cost can be construed as the benefits and burdens to the particular patient in the particular circumstance. The notion of *beneficent paternalism* seeks to justify a paternalistic intervention that respects autonomy and does not override it (Beauchamp & Childress, 1994). This approach does not incorporate an individual's consent but rather proceeds from the assumption that a person at significant risk of damage or loss can be helped by an action that has a high probability of preventing such damage or loss *and* would not incur significant risks, costs, or burdens to the person. The justification for not fully disclosing information to the patient (but fully disclosing to a family member) is couched in beneficent paternalism. Congruent with nonmaleficence (the duty to do no harm), as the likelihood of risk or irreversible harm increases, the justification for a paternalistic intervention also increases. For many health care professionals, the least autonomy-restricting option that will achieve the predicted benefits and reduce or avoid the identified risks is the approach taken and, in their view, is morally justified as a beneficent action.

4.   *Justice* is a complex principle that traditionally has been concerned with the fair distribution of benefits and burdens in the allocation of resources. Recent conceptions of justice include concerns about access to health care services and rationing. Cost containment and its almost inevitable corollary, rationing, viewed in the context of an aging society, includes the allocation of funding for chronic care of fragile elderly as well as the more sensational issue of use of (access to) advanced medical technology to support and sustain life. Callahan (1999) argues that the elderly are not served by positing that it is lack of resources or political power that stands

between them and living longer. The question is not whether we have succeeded in giving longer life to the aged but, rather, whether medicine has helped make old age a decent and honorable time of life. Callahan (1999) suggests that government (and medical science) should help people live out a "natural life span," beyond which society's obligation is to relieve suffering, not to provide life-extending technology. Needless to say, there is considerable debate about what constitutes a natural life span. Outcomes research of costly interventions should occur in all age groups; distributive justice demands at least that.

Access to and receipt of quality health care is a right of and a duty owed to the elderly as well as younger individuals and groups in society. In terms of quality of care, the same standard of care, although not necessarily the same type of care, applies. Election of a less aggressive course of care or refusal of care (directly or via an advance directive instruction) swings the pendulum from cure to care and heightens the need for quality, wrap-around palliative or comfort care. Overall function, prognosis, and those elusive, idiosyncratic, and highly personal notions of quality of life should direct our caregiving. Age alone and many diagnostic labels (e.g., Alzheimer's disease and Parkinson's disease) are poor descriptors and predictors of functional status and well-being.

AN ETHICS OF AGING

An *ethics of aging* is grounded on the respect for and autonomy of older people to exercise control over their own lives even in the face of confusion and forgetfulness. A corollary right is that an older person can voluntarily grant decision-making authority to another, presumably one who knows the person's values and wishes and is trusted by the person. In thinking about an ethics of aging in the context of critical care nursing, perhaps the most difficult situations are those in which medicine and nursing have different perspectives about the goals of care for the particular patient, his or her previously stated wishes and present capacity to make decisions, the benefits and burdens associated with treatment options, and the manner and time of death. "Old people are old only incidentally . . . people whose rights, protections and responsibilities do not wither at age sixty-five. First among those rights is the prerogative to chart the course of their own lives . . . they have the right to make their own mistakes" (Dubler & Nimmons, 1993, p. 193). Tethered to intravenous (IV) lines, tubes, and wires and tied down with restraints, we trample upon those rights for their "self-preservation" under the guise of beneficence and nonmaleficence. The "ethical tightrope" in caring for acutely ill elderly strands us between empowering and abandoning them. We justify removing the IV and paraphernalia of treatment and life support not only because the patient is railing and tearing at them but also because these acts are consistent with past known decisions; we are empowering the patient. Are we not also abandoning them because we know that the patient's decision failed to adequately consider the potential risks of nontreatment?

It can be very difficult to discriminate between mental impairments and personality, compounded by hearing loss and vision impairment. Without a family member at the bedside to differentiate a new disability or dysfunction from lifetime behavior and personality characteristics, an acutely ill older adult might be treated more (or less) aggressively. The hectic pace and constantly changing faces of acute care are precisely the obstacles that conspire against taking the time to learn about the elderly patient's preferences and personality, peculiarities and values. Our collective duty to prevent harm demands strenuous efforts, perhaps even more so than with a younger patient, to learn as much as we can about the patient prior to the acute event. Dubler and Nimmons (1993) urge practitioners to talk to the patient first before deferring to the spouse or offspring for information and decision; the patient can "make known in a myriad of ways who they are and what they want" (p. 215). Old people have the right to take risks; they have a lifetime of learning from experience.

Nursing's *Professional Code of Ethics*, first issued in 1976, revised in 1985, and currently undergoing review and revision, reflects the ethical principles in its articulation about "respect for human dignity and the uniqueness of the client," safeguarding the patient's right to privacy, health care, and safe practice; maintaining competence; and improving standards in practice (American Nurses Association [ANA], 1985). Drawing on explicit and implicit formulations in the *Code,* nursing care of the older person should be that of support, protection, and nurturance while meeting basic human needs, provision of useful and understandable information, reduction of fear of isolation and abandonment, communication that is effective and culturally sensitive, and advocacy for reflective and compassionate patient-centered decision making. Our responsibility to older patients lies in assisting people with identifying their values and beliefs relevant to the situation or choices to be made; acknowledging the validity of their beliefs and values; providing them with sufficient information to choose among alternatives; helping them express their beliefs and choices; *and* advocating for them when they lack the ability, power, or resources to have those values and choices honored. The fact that an older patient chooses to refuse care or rejects an option proffered by the health care team is not, in and of itself, evidence that the person lacks decision-making capacity.

ETHICAL CONUNDRUMS IN CRITICAL CARE
FOR THE ELDERLY

Despite the oft-heard public sentiment that people want to die at home, most people die in hospitals and nursing homes. It was not until midway into the 20th century, with the advent of major technological advances in medical science and pharmacotherapeutics, that people moved from dying at home to dying in institutional settings. The knowledge that modern medicine cannot cure everything does not stop the attempt to try. Consequently, "the dying and the recovering share the technology, and often even physicians cannot tell them apart" (Hall et al., 1999, p. 301). Life processes are sustained; death is prolonged. In the past, families had no control over the course of an illness but had control over the environment in which illness ran its course and death occurred. Bioethics emerged out of a setting in which medicine sought control over the illness and the family controlled nothing. Whether to use the medical armamentarium often comes down to a philosophical as well as a medical decision. The presence of managed care as a player in the decision suggests that it may be an economic decision, as well (Hall et al., 1999).

An ethical dilemma in the practice of medicine becomes, almost always, an ethical issue for nurses. Distinctions between withholding and withdrawing treatment, active and passive euthanasia, ordinary and extraordinary treatment, notions of medical futility, the doctrine of double effect, and the implementation of DNR orders engages nursing time, concern, code of ethics, conscience, and a burgeoning literature by nurse researchers and ethicists. The limitations of this chapter do not allow full discussion of these enormously significant subjects; once again, the reader is urged to learn more not only for at-the-bedside understanding but also to contribute to the discourse in ethics committees and public policy decisions.

Independent of medical ethics, culpability for *acting and failing to act* is based on common law doctrine, which holds that there is no general *duty to rescue.* However, the act/nonact distinction does not fit as comfortably with regard to medical decisions to *withdraw or withhold* treatment. (Note: the issue is not withdrawal or withholding of "care.") The courts sometimes permit withholding and characterize it as an "omission" but hold withdrawing impermissible and characterize it as an "act." Avoiding liability on the basis of acting or failing to act confuses the legal and ethical analysis (Hall et al., 1999). The notion that withholding treatment is an act of omission and hence more defensible than withdrawal belies medicine's (and nursing's) obligation to provide beneficial therapy to patients. Most legal cases of treatment termination authorize withdrawal rather than withholding of treatment on the grounds that the LST has already begun and any action on it involves withdrawal. The President's Commission (1982) held that distinctions between withdrawal and withholding are a slippery slope and should not be used. Continuing a treatment long after its beneficial use has disappeared out of fear that discontinuing will require special justification is as "pernicious" as not starting a treatment with some potential for therapeutic gain out of fear that the treatment cannot be stopped even if its effect was less than hoped (Hall et al., 1999). As such, legal scholars and bioethicists consider treatment withdrawal and withholding the same.

Euthanasia, commonly known as "mercy killing," recognizes that the intent that caused the death of another was motivated by compassion. It is important to recognize that legal authorization to terminate treatment is not euthanasia, even though treatment termination leads to death. Classic understanding and legal acceptance of the basic premise of euthanasia is based on the motivation of the agent; that is, compassion and mercy versus some egregious reason. Active euthanasia is illegal; passive euthanasia is not illegal and can encompass any intentional nontreatment, from withholding or withdrawing to, in some cases, the "doctrine of double effect." The impact of Oregon's legalization of assisted suicide in 1998 (which allows a "health care provider" to prescribe and administer a lethal medication) on nursing practice, its Code of Ethics, and nursing services policies is, as yet, unknown but has to be addressed as more states consider legislation and codification of what many feel is a basic human right.

The *doctrine of double effect* holds that the "intent" behind administration of morphine is to relieve pain and suffering and increase comfort; the death of the patient pursuant to morphine administration is not intended, and, therefore, the act is not wrong. It would be more accurate to say that the "motive" for morphine administration was compassion—to relieve pain, not to kill—and reflects a beneficent ethic. Hall and colleagues (1999) comment that if death ("killing," p. 317) as a result of a compassionate act is acceptable, then euthanasia becomes more justifiable.

The distinction between *ordinary* and *extraordinary treatment* was explicated by the Catholic church and has support in Judaism and other major religions. Its usefulness in cases of treatment termination or administration proved elusive, as noted by the Quinlan court. What is ordinary in one case might be extraordinary in another; the usefulness of the distinction has to be in the context in which the treatment would be provided. Ordinary is defined as all medicines, treatments, and surgeries that offer a reasonable hope of benefit obtained without excessive pain, expense, or other hardship. Extraordinary means are those medicines, treatments, and surgeries that cannot be obtained without excessive pain or cost (etc.) *or,* if used, that do not have a reasonable potential for benefit (Hall et al., 1999). Elaboration on this distinction holds that assessment of the burden of treatment on the patient or family, consideration of the patient's own interest in treatment termination, and "disproportionate" investment in equipment or personnel must be considered, also. The President's Commission (1982) opined that the distinction was applicable, perhaps, at the summation of an ethical discussion, not at the outset or as a contributor to it.

A claim that a treatment option is *medically futile* removes it from the range of options available to the patient or family, agent, or surrogate. Typically, the statement made is not that the treatment or intervention will harm the patient but, rather, that it will not produce the sought-after benefit. The ethical obligation to provide a medical benefit is thus canceled by a claim of medical futility. Definitions of medical futility include the assertion that the procedure cannot be performed because of the patient's condition, that it will not produce the intended physiological effect and benefits, and that the anticipated benefits will be outweighed by the burdens, harms, and costs of the treatment. Recourse to scientific data is used differentially; some physicians claim that an intervention is futile if it has zero chance of effectiveness; others hold futility at 1 to 13% chance of success. A variety of voices are heard: the benefit that the physician feels is unlikely to be achieved may not, in fact, be the benefit that the patient wants (Beauchamp & Childress, 1994); patients and families should not be offered futile treatment and "false choices" (Tomlinson & Brody, 1990); futility claims are dishonest and deny options to patients who might be willing to live with a compromised quality of life (Truog, Brett, & Frader, 1992).

The issues surrounding DNR and CPR include assessment of futile care, beneficence and nonmaleficence, self-determination, and disclosure. Consent to resuscitation is presumed; a DNR order requires consent to withhold treatment. Yet, it can be argued that if resuscitation would not provide a medical benefit and might even harm the patient, then physicians should not be required to discuss this option with the patient or family. Critical care nurses have probably been exposed to situations in which the patient or family, or both, was informed about CPR and then subjected to information and influence that it would produce no benefit. Rather than enhancing autonomy by implying that a meaningful choice is possible, it destroys it. It is axiomatic that a physician is under no moral obligation to provide a medical benefit (i.e., intervention) if no medical benefit exists, despite patient or family demand for it. As suggested by Hall and colleagues (1999), other than the small number of cases of absolute medical futility from a physiological perspective only, the much larger number of remaining cases are not an issue of medical futility but involve value judgments about individuals and the allocation of health care resources.

In caring for the critically ill elderly, especially those whose quality of life by every value-free objective measure seems minimal or absent, nurses have to be aware of the possibility that an advance directive (or clear and convincing evidence) for LSTs is not being honored. Similarly, nurses have to be alert to coercive influence on an elderly patient or their family to forego aggressive treatment. The pervasive concern among acute and long-term care nurses that a DNR order is, ipso facto, consent to "do not treat" is not dissuaded by the paucity of studies looking at aggressiveness of (comfort/palliative) care for patients with DNR orders.

ORGANIZATIONAL ETHICS AND WHISTLE-BLOWING

Health care organizations are not immune from an "ethics gap"—the difference between what is ethical and the actions necessary for business success—

particularly in the presence and aftermath of downsizing and restructuring. Organizational ethics has a different focus than clinical ethics has. It seeks to identify, educate, and facilitate internalization of institutional values and beliefs. Leaders and followers must subscribe to commonly shared values that are then realized in the policies, programs, and systems of the organization. Tainted values or "dirty hands" occur when one acts morally incorrectly because of another's immorality (Mohr & Mahon, 1996). The informal culture of an organization, its norms of (rewarded) behavior, and the failure of the formal organization to monitor practice are the source of the dirty hands phenomenon. Dirty hands include falsifying services or charges, not reporting a medication or surgical error, failure to report or document a patient fall, providing services or conducting tests that are not necessary, inadequate personal care for patients, incomplete treatments, and documenting a team meeting that never occurred.

Whistle-blowing indicates the failure or absence of an ethical infrastructure for the organization. It represents a breakdown in accountability, the highest tenet of nursing's social contract with the public. Staff concerns about patient welfare must be addressed by the organization. In the absence of internal procedures to address concerns, whistle-blowing becomes a moral action, albeit one of last resort. It is important to differentiate whistle-blowing from reporting, wherein the latter is an internal process and the former is an external act in response to an unresponsive organization (Sellin, 1995). Whistle-blowing is a morally courageous act after all avenues to resolution of an issue, properly followed, have been ignored or refuted. The moral justification for whistle-blowing includes the continuing presence of serious wrongdoing despite repeated attempts to draw organizational attention to the issue, justification of the act by recourse to ethical principles and the facts of the situation, and the considered assumption that patients will not be harmed by the act and could benefit by it. Perhaps the most painful aspect of whistle-blowing is the need to decide that loyalty to one's patients overrides loyalty to the organization and one's colleagues.

Nurses faced with ethical conundrums and dilemmas in patient care, professionalism, and organizational behavior can create, if they do not already exist, mechanisms and forums for ethically informed discussion and decisions. The Joint Commission for Accreditation of Healthcare Organizations (JCAHO), the professional codes for nurses and other health care providers, and even institutional ethics committees are beginning to address organizational ethics: "the intentional use of values to guide the decisions of a system" (Potter, 1996, p. 4). It is essential to be knowledgeable about and gain the skills of ethical decision making, which, in many ways, is not dissimilar from the scientific process.

ETHICAL DECISION-MAKING PROCESS

The law-and-ethics consultant team headed by Nancy Dubler at The Montifiore Hospital Medical Center developed a pathway to follow every time they are called into a case: *facts*—obtain and clarify the medical facts of the situation and ensure that all parties understand them; *options*—identify the consequences of each alternative, including doing nothing; *values*—identify the values inherent in each option and the meaning of those values for each participant in the decision; and finally move to the *four concentric circles of decision*—start with the patient, then move to advance directives, other decision makers (i.e., substitute judgment, best interest), and as a last resort, the courts (Dubler & Nimmons, 1993). Being with the patient means determining their decisional capacity to make a health care decision, that is, their understanding is sufficient to appreciate the situation, processing it within a personal framework, and communicating it.

There is no one dominant model of ethical decision making; each model tries to bring some order to the chaos surrounding medical decision making. Most suggest the following order of steps presented sequentially, but that in no way implies rigid adherence; there is always movement in and between steps, sometimes occurring concurrently. The first step, however should always be to

1. gather the medical facts and other relevant information; determine if the patient is decisionally capable

    ascertain patient preferences, including advance directives, known wishes

    collect the views of family members and significant others; identify who is the spokesperson or key person in decision-making participation

    identify applicable law, hospital policies, and potential liabilities
2. name the ethical dilemma (it may be a legal issue or one involving poor communication and have no ethical aspects)

    What are the values in conflict?
3. identify the options and the risks, benefits and consequences of each and present these to the patient first (if capacitated), then to the proxy (if one is appointed), family, surrogate, *and* the health care team
4. reach consensus about the best or most agreeable (least disagreeable) solution (Ross, 1986).

An *ethics consultant* seeks to facilitate resolution of an ethical dilemma by (1) supporting, protecting, and empowering the patient to make health care decisions that reflect the patients values and preferences and (2) acknowledging the rights and legitimate interests of the family and the health-team professionals. When a patient is incapacitated and without an advance directive or family, another individual or committee (i.e., a surrogate) is authorized to make decisions using the best interest standard. The consultant follows essentially the same steps outlined earlier and generally begins by meeting with the person requesting the consultation to discuss the broad contours of the case. In addition to meeting with the patient, proxy, family, and members of the team, the consultant could seek input from social work, psychiatry, risk management, and pastoral care, as appropriate. Some consultants will present a "principled solution" to the involved parties, whereas other consultants attempt to elicit this from the concerned parties themselves. A consultant's responsibilities include clarification of the agreed-upon solution, the principles that support it, and any consequences that might flow from it. In addition, the consultant can suggest how the solution should be implemented, including a timetable and follow-up steps. The consultant should document the consultation in the patient's medical record and return to the patient to determine that the solution was, in fact, implemented. Most hospitals require risk management notification when a consultation involves an incapacitated patient without advance directives, family, or other surrogate and withholding or withdrawing life-sustaining treatments.

All hospitals are required to have an ethics committee; an ethics consultant or team is adjunct and advisory. Most committees include nurses whose contribution is enhanced if they have some formal ethics training, several years of clinical experience, master's level of education, and tenure on the committee of at least one year (Oddi & Cassidy, 1990). The functions of ethics committees are education, policy development or review, and case consultation or review. Policy development is an important function because it helps define the organization's mission and the structures and processes that will support it. It is the interface between government regulation, cost-containment, and individual patients and decision makers. Three modes of institutional compliance are available to health care organizations. The first makes it optional whether or not to consult the ethics committee; compliance with committee recommendations is left to professional's discretion. A second model requires the committee's mandatory review of certain decisions, such as DNR for incapacitated patients, but the clinician retains authority for the final decision. The third and least recommended model requires mandatory review and compliance with ethics committee recommendations. Whereas the first model risks that committee decisions will be ignored, the third model has legal ramifications in the dispersion of clinical decision-making responsibility from the clinicians at the bedside to the more remote members of the ethics committee (some of whom might be clinicians).

CONCLUSION

The best resolutions to ethical dilemmas are those that begin with patient values, preferences, and wishes and emerge from dialogue with the patient, proxy, family, and the professionals who care for them. The courts should not become the center and source of ethical decision making. The fact that the courts often assume this responsibility reflects the failure of health care professionals to anticipate, appreciate, and analyze potential ethical dilemmas and decisions. Nurses from all settings of care for the elderly should join together to describe the multiple faces of autonomy within dependency, shared decision making, enlightened benevolence and thoughtful distributive justice. "We are, after all . . . old people in training" (Dubler & Nimmons, 1993, p. 193). Empowered and educated to articulate what ethical principles look like in practice, nurses can inform and significantly influence social and health care policy for the elderly.

REFERENCES

American Nurses Association. (1985). *Code for nurses with interpretive statements.* Washington, DC: American Nurses Association.

Beauchamp, T. L., & Childress, J. F. (1994). *Principles of bioethics* (4th ed.). New York: Oxford Press.

Braun, K. L., Pietsch, J. H., & Blanchette, P. L. (2000). *Cultural issues in end-of-life decision making.* Thousand Oaks, CA: Sage.

Callahan, D. (1999). A miscellany of hard choices. Rationing health care according to age. In J. D. Arras & B. Steinbock (Eds.), *Ethical issues in modern medicine* (5th ed., pp. 652–658). Mountain View, CA: Mayfield.

Crow, K., Matheson, L., & Steed, A. (2000). Informed consent and truth-telling. Cultural directions for healthcare providers. *Journal of Nursing Administration, 30,* 148–152.

Dresser, R., & Whitehouse, P. J. (1994). The incompetent patient on the slippery slope. *Hastings Center Report, 24* (4), 6–12.

Dubler, N., & Nimmons, D. (1993). *Ethics on call. Taking charge of life-and-death choices in today's health care system.* New York: Vintage Books.

Eleazer, G. P., Hornung, C. A., Egbert, C. B., Egbert, J. R., Eng, C., Hedgepeth, J., McCann, R., Strothers, H., Sapir, M., Wei, M., & Wilson M. (1996). The relationship between ethnicity and advance directives in a frail older population. Journal of the American Geriatrics Society, 44, 38–43.

Hall, M. A., Ellman, I. M., & Strouse, D. S. (1999). *Health care law and ethics.* St. Paul, MN: West Group.

Mohr, W. K., & Mahon, M. M. (1996). Dirty hands: The underside of marketplace health care. *Advances in Nursing Science, 19* (1), 28–37.

Oddi, L. F., & Cassidy, V. R. (1990). Participation and perceptions of nurse members in the hospital ethics committee. *Western Journal of Nursing Research, 12,* 307–317.

Omnibus Budget Reconciliation Act of 1990, Pub L. No. 101-508.

Potter, R. L. (1996). From clinical ethic to organizational ethics: The second stage of the evolution of bioethics. *Bioethics Forum, 12* (2), 3–12.

President's Commission for the Study of Ethical Problems in Medicine and Biomedical and Behavioral Research. (1982). *Making health care decisions.* Washington, DC: U.S. Government Printing Office.

Ross, J. (1986). *Handbook for hospital ethics committees.* Chicago: American Hospital Publishing.

Sellin, S. C. (1995). Out on a limb: A qualitative study of patient advocacy in institutional nursing. *Nursing Ethics: An International Journal for Health Care Professionals, 2* (1), 19–29.

Tomlinson, J. B., & Brody, H. (1990). Futility and the ethics of resuscitation. *Journal of the American Medical Association, 264,* 1276–1280.

Truog, R. D., Brett, A. S., & Frader, J. (1992). Sounding board: The problem with futility. *New England Journal of Medicine, 362,* 1560–1564.

19

End-of-Life Care

Linda E. Moody

The dying need but little, dear—
A glass of water's all,
A flower's unobtrusive face
To punctuate the wall,
A fan, perhaps, a friend's regret . . .

—Dickinson

HISTORY OF PALLIATIVE CARE AND NURSING

Poet Emily Dickinson expresses simply and elegantly what the dying person needs. Nursing's role in palliative care can be traced as far back as Florence Nightingale's work during the Crimean War. Nightingale's philosophy was based on caring for the physical, emotional, spiritual, and environmental needs of the dying patient and expressed the notion that nursing's role was to "put the patient in the best possible position for nature to act upon him" (Light, 1997, p. 33). Another major influence on nursing's "caring" focus was Virginia Henderson, one of the first nursing theorists to include care of the dying in her philosophy of nursing. She described it as "assisting the individual, sick or well, in the performance of those activities contributing to health or its recovery, or to a peaceful death, that he would perform unaided if he had the necessary strength, will, or knowledge" (Halloran, 1996, p. 19).

A major force in shaping nursing's caring role in the early 1970s was psychologist Abraham Maslow, whose theory purports that basic physical and security needs must be met before one can turn one's attention to the higher cognitive and spiritual needs. This principle is particularly applicable to the care of the dying. Other more contemporary scholars of the "caring" aspects of nursing are Patricia Benner and colleagues. Benner's focus on the phenomenologic view has helped provide a fuller understanding of the meaning of events, the person, the concept of caring, and the context of care delivery in critical care nursing (Benner & Wrubel, 1989).

Hospice versus Palliative Care: *Ars Moriendi* and the Good Death

The term hospice dates back to medieval times and originally meant a refuge or place of comfort for weary travelers. It was later adopted by the health system in Great Britain to denote places that provided respite to those who were near death. It was Dame Cicely Saunders, founder of the modern hospice movement who expanded the concept to include pain control and spiritual, emotional, and psychological care (Gurfolino & Dumas, 1994). The popularity of hospice care spread to the United States in the early 1980s and the U.S. health system established regulations for reimbursement for hospice care in 1982. Palliative care is a term that has been used to denote a philosophy of "alleviation of suffering" but has no tie to reimbursement with the formal health care system in the United States (Johnson, 1998). Both philosophies share a focus on improving quality of life, honoring choices of the patient and family, and alleviating pain and suffering through an interdisciplinary team approach. Palliative care is replacing the term hospice care in many areas because it is not tied to prognosis (6 months of projected remaining life) or to reimbursement (Gurfolino & Dumas, 1994). Both terms, hospice care and palliative care, are used synonymously, and both aim to help the individual achieve "*ars moriendi*" (the art of dying) and the good death. The good death is defined by each individual, shaped by sociocultural background, and holds a unique meaning for each person (Bertman, 1998).

The Terminally Ill Elderly in Critical Care: Paradoxical Goals?

Although it may seem paradoxical at first that an elderly patient who is near the end of life might be admitted to a critical care unit, there are a number of reasons why it occurs. Elders in critical care who were transferred from a nursing home are often admitted for one or more of these problems: urinary tract infection (UTI), sepsis (most often secondary to UTIs or pressure sores), pneumonia or respiratory failure, and delirium or acute confusional state. The issues surrounding end-of-life care for the terminally ill elderly in intensive care units are complex and not easily resolved, requiring a team of specialists who above all, keep the patient's wishes and best interests in the forefront of all decision making. In some cases, the elderly resident is admitted because the nursing home team has depleted its repertoire of interventions, and this admission represents a last effort to save the patient's life, to provide comfort, or to reassure the family that something is being done, or a combination of these.

Shifting Paradigms: From Curing to Caring

Although the use of hospice care by residents in nursing homes and other settings has increased in the last few years, it is speculated that more effective use of hospice care, or a "palliative approach," would result in more appropriate and dignified care toward the end of life. In the United States, patients must have a prognosis of 6 months or less to receive hospice care under the Medicare Hospice Benefit. Ethical dilemmas include the difficulty in predicting accurately a patient's prognosis of 6 months or less and the obligation to provide patients and families with full information about their illness, treatment, and prognosis (Kinzbrunner, 1995). Hence, it is not unusual to find that critical care units encounter elderly patients who are admitted under hospice care. This often requires the critical care team to shift from the "curing" paradigm to the "caring" paradigm reflected in the palliative care approach.

ISSUES SURROUNDING END-OF-LIFE CARE: BARRIERS TO TIMELY ACCESS

Some of the issues regarding end-of-life care revolve around formal hospice care and psychological support, such as barriers to timely access, reimbursement issues, how to apply benefits of hospice care, and how to sustain the hope and quality of life of the patient and family. The "technological imperative ethic," defined as the need to do everything regardless of potential adverse effects, costs, or benefits, still drives many care providers toward overaggressive treatment of dying patients (Moody, Lunney, & Grady, 1999). Concerns about litigation may promote the use of "defensive" medicine. Many providers are reluctant to admit patients to hospice care until they are convinced that treatment will no longer benefit the patient. There is also concern that early referral to hospice may diminish the level of hope for the patient and family. Clearly, the critical care nurse can assist the patient and family in understanding the purpose and philosophy of hospice care and in making appropriate and timely referrals.

Hospice Referral and the Medicare Reimbursement System

The Health Care Financing and Administration reimbursement structure, Medicare, requires a prognosis of 6 months or less and a terminal illness for admission to hospice care. For those with end-stage chronic diseases involving the heart, lung, kidneys, liver, and some types of cancer, prognosis is often difficult to predict to within 6 months. Practitioners readily admit the difficulty in predicting survival time in end-stage chronic diseases such as congestive heart failure or end-stage lung disease. These types of conditions pose problems for patients and families who often require hospice care longer than 6 months. However, providers, regardless of health-care setting, must be made aware of the many factors affecting palliative care, including predicting death and anticipating the need to change the goals of care as therapeutic trials and interventions fail, anticipating and treating troubling symptoms of dying patients, and recognizing that family support and frequent close contact between the dying patient and family can facilitate better decision making and acceptance of death (Moody et al., 1999).

END-OF-LIFE CARE NEEDS: NURSING CAN MAKE A DIFFERENCE

What are the special needs of dying, elderly patients in critical care units? What are the needs of their family members? Research studies in nursing have identified two areas where nursing can have a major impact on end-of-life care: (1) communication and support in decision making and (2) relief of suffering through pain and symptom management (Moody et al., 1999). The remainder of this chapter focuses on these essential areas of end of life care and identifies some of the special nursing needs that the elderly and their families may face.

Advance Directives

In most instances, advance directives documents include the following essential elements that direct the preferences of the patient:

- Living will
- Do not resuscitate
- Feeding and fluids
- Artificial ventilation

Often, the patient and family may not be able to specify preferences beyond "do not resuscitate" and will need to be guided by the physician and nurse through informed consent about feeding and fluids, medications, and other preferences. Even though health care durable power of attorneys may have been designated and advance directives completed, previous research indicates that implementation is often not congruent with the patient's or surrogate's directives. Research indicates that often providers make decisions regarding treatment based on their own personal values

(Teno et al., 1994). For more information on the legal and ethical aspects of honoring the preferences of advance directives, see chapters 18 and 22. In addition, the reference notebook for consumers, developed from a grant by the American Association of Critical Care Nurses and the University of Southern California School of Nursing (1998), assists patients and families in developing and completing Living wills and Advance Directives. This complete notebook kit was developed especially for use in critical care units.

Assessment and Management of Suffering

An essential aspect of palliative and hospice care is relief of suffering. Alleviation of suffering can only be accomplished by adequate assessment and management of the patient, the psychological and spiritual aspects as well as the symptoms associated with the terminal illness or condition (Weitzner, Moody, & McMillan, 1997). As Byock (1996) points out, suffering is not confined to just the symptoms associated with the terminal condition, and despite our vocalizations of "holistic care," the Cartesian separation of mind and body still pervades clinical practice. Developing a rapport with the patient and family and "knowing" the particular needs of the patient are essential to providing alleviation of pain and suffering.

Assessment and Management of Common Symptoms and Conditions

Some of the most common symptoms and conditions experienced by patients with terminal illness are dyspnea, fatigue, nausea, opioid-induced constipation, and insomnia (Weitzner et al., 1997). Farncombe (1997) found that patients experiencing dyspnea were 39% more likely to complain of other symptoms than were patients with no shortness of breath and were 55% more likely to report other symptoms as being severe. Assessment and management of these symptoms can be approached in a manner similar to that of pain assessment and management. A graphic rating scale can be used to assess the severity of the symptom (dyspnea, nausea, insomnia, etc.) followed by qualitative assessment of the degree of distress the symptom is causing the patient.

- *Dyspnea* Dyspnea, or breathlessness, is a common symptom for patients who are terminally ill with cancer or end-stage lung, heart, liver, or kidney disease. Assessment of dyspnea is often poorly conducted, but it should be done on a regular basis, like pain assessment (Farncombe, 1997). Dyspnea can interfere significantly with the quality of life, sleep, and fatigue level of the patient. Pharmacological measures are aimed at reducing the root cause of the dyspnea if possible or at treating the underlying problem most proximal to the condition. For example, in congestive heart failure or ascites, use of diuretics may help; in end-stage lung disease, use of systemic steroids may alleviate the dyspnea. Common pharmacological measures include inhaled or systemic steroids, opioids, benzodiazepines, oxygen, and, in some cases, inhaled morphine (Zeppetella, 1998). Nursing measures to relieve dyspnea include use of high Fowler's position, sitting in a chair or on the side of the bed with elbows resting on the overbed table, increased ventilation with cool air by a small fan directed toward the face, a cold washcloth to the face, and other measures identified by the patient and family that seem to work. Pacing the activities of the patient is important, and providing meals that are small, frequent, and easy to chew can help conserve energy.

- *Agitation, Anxiety, and Depression* These symptoms may be related to hypoxemia, pain, or fear. The patient may have an agitated depression and exhibit anxiety and agitation. Many of the newer antidepressants such as paroxetine are also anxiolytic and may be effective. Some analgesics and antiemetic medications may also have an anxiolytic effect. Choice of drugs for the elderly includes paroxetine or citalopram. As always, one should check for potential drug interactions with the patient's current therapy (Taylor, 1997).

- *Nausea* Determining the most proximal cause of the nausea is the first step toward selecting the intervention. In the case of chemotherapy or a medication that the patient needs to continue to receive, and adjusting the dosage or switching to another type is not an option, the antiemetic drugs may have to be administered parenterally, intravenously, or by dermal patch (Thompson, 1999). Control of nausea and vomiting is important because uncontrolled it can lead to serious complications, such as aspiration, dehydration, electrolyte disturbances, and disruption of the underlying therapy. A recent study found that the use of intravenous dexamethasone significantly decreased the incidence of nausea and vomiting after epidural morphine (Wang et al., 1999). Choices for antinausea medications include prochlorperazine, metoclopramide, and cisapride. Droperidol intravenously or intramuscularly may be used for refractory vomiting. Dosage of these drugs is individualized according to the age, weight, and overall condition of the patient (Taylor, 1997). Keeping the environment as free as possible from noxious odors may also help reduce nausea. Reminding staff and visitors not to wear perfumes or colognes that might be offensive may also help.

- *Constipation* The patient may be constipated naturally or it may be related to inadequate fluid intake, opioid use, inactivity, or bowel obstruction. Severe constipation may lead to fecal impaction and result in urinary frequency or incontinence, loss of appetite, and nausea. It is important to know the patient's history regarding bowel habits. If it is impossible to increase fluids and fiber, choices of drugs include milk of magnesia, stool softeners (docusate sodium), motility agents (metoclopramide or bisacodyl), and enemas. Patients on opioids should be checked often for stool production and for impaction.

- *Bladder Problems* Urinary retention may be treated with intermittent catheterizations and avoidance of chronic catheterization, if possible, to reduce chances of infection. Assessment of urinary spasm should begin with evaluating the possibility of overdistention. Symptoms may be treated with cholinergic agents, such as oxybutynin.

- *Insomnia* Treating some of the underlying symptoms such as pain, nausea, dyspnea, anxiety, and depression may result in improved sleep patterns for the patient. If not, other causes of the insomnia must be examined and treated when possible. If the patient has extreme fears and anxiety or depression, a psychiatric consult or spiritual counseling, depending on the patient's preferences, may help in alleviating the patient's concern and lead to better sleep. If all of these measures fail, pharmacological measures include the use of antihistamines such as diphenhydramine at bedtime. The use of phenobarbital sedatives is not recommended because they tend to accumulate faster in the body because of physiological changes in the elderly. Appropriate sedatives include the group of benzodiazapenes in the lowest dose possible to prevent confusion and dizziness (Taylor, 1997). Nonpharmacological measures include sitting at the bedside and allowing the patient to talk, use of choice of music via headphones at bedtime, or a relaxing back massage.

- *Confusion and Delirium* The initial treatment of delirium or acute confusional state is aimed at first treating the most proximal identifiable cause. Potential causes include drug interactions, fever, electrolyte imbalance, and protracted insomnia. It is estimated that in more than 50% of terminal cases, no identifiable cause can be found (Fainsinger & Bruera, 1992). Adams (1988) advocates quick and aggressive intervention (a combination of a neuroleptic such as haloperidol, a benzodiazepine, and a narcotic via the intravenous route) in the early phase of delirium followed by decreasing drug doses to maintenance levels when the behavioral manifestations are resolved. Typically, therapy is begun with haloperidol 3 mg, lorazepam 0.5 mg, and hydromorphone 0.5 mg; the hydromorphone is given every 3 hours and haloperidol and lozaepam are given every 20 minutes until an adequate response is achieved. When the patient is sedated, the lorazepam is discontinued and the haloperidol is decreased to 50% of the dose over the previous 24 hours. The patient should be observed for extrapyramidal side effects, hypotension, and excessive sedation. The patient should be assigned increased nursing supervision, and the staff should avoid using physical restraints, which often increase agitation and lead to injury. Delirium and agitation are often frightening for the patient and the family, and adequate control of the delirium provides a great relief for both.

- *Nutritional Support*   Because food and fluids are perceived as signs of hope and life and have many psychosocial and cultural meanings, this area can be one of the most distressing and can provoke many emotions from patients, families, and providers. Too often, withholding food and fluids is viewed as an act of despair or abandonment. The patient with terminal illness or the health care surrogate should guide the amount and type of nutrition received. It should be explained to patients and families that studies have shown that forced feeding may cause distention and discomfort and may prolong suffering by speeding the rate of cancer growth. Alert patients, who are anorexic, should be evaluated for pain control, oral candidiasis, depression, and constipation. Symptoms of dry mouth may be treated with glycerine swabs, mouthwash or viscous lidocaine. Thirst may be relieved with ice chips or sips of water. The basis of nutritional support is guided by whatever the patient can tolerate and likes in terms of food and fluid preferences (Taylor, 1997). Allowing the family to bring in a special, favorite food can have great meaning to the patient and family.

READINESS FOR DEATH ISSUES

A recent study examining patients' preferences at the end of life found that there are wide fluctuations in the patients' will to live (Chochinov, 1999). The will to live, readiness for death, and depression are three concepts that are not easily understood in those who are near death (Moody, Beckie, Long, & Edmonds, 1999). Signs that the patient has accepted that death is near may be similar to some of the signs of depression and loss of will to live: giving away cherished items, disengagement, loss of appetite, and increased sleep. It is important to try to distinguish between the two. Assessment with one of the standard depression tools can be helpful in detecting clinical depression and if present appropriate treatment with antidepressants may be warranted.

A study in a hospice in England by Oxenham and Cornbleet (1998) revealed that the auxiliary nursing staff, not the physicians or professional nurses, were most accurate in predicting imminent death and theorized that the reason was the amount of time spent at the bedside of the patient that allowed them to know the patients more intimately. No similar studies have been done in the critical care units in the United States, but one might also speculate that the professional critical care nurses at the bedside would be more able to predict imminent death for the same reason. In the study by Benner and Wrubel (1989), many critical care nurses reported that they learned to develop a "sixth sense" about patients' impending death. Although formal study of this area is needed, if critical care nurses are able to sense impending death, it would be important to try to bring patients and families closer together during this time to resolve any issues and to say their goodbyes.

DNR and Resuscitation of Elderly Hospice Patients

Studies suggest that when CPR is attempted, about 14% survive to discharge and 86% die acutely. Certain groups have a much lower survival rate. For example, the elderly have a survival rate ranging from 0 to 6.5%. Those with metastatic cancer have a survival rate of 0% (Taylor, 1997). Patients and families who choose not to be resuscitated should be reassured that other treatments will not be affected by this decision.

Withholding versus Withdrawing Treatment

Ethically, there is no difference between withholding and withdrawing care that cannot or has not achieved its desired effect. However, withdrawing care has a different effect on providers, patient, and family because it is more difficult to take something away, and it may be perceived as giving up. It is critical that there be clear expectations among all parties about treatment withholding and withdrawal. Patients and families must be assisted in identifying the positives and negatives of an intervention through the informed consent process, known as the "benefits versus burdens" approach. Generally, the notion of "benefits versus burdens" is the guiding principle in selecting a diagnostic or therapeutic intervention (Finucane & Harper, 1996) and explaining the benefits and risks of each intervention applied or each intervention that is withdrawn. This is a very complex process and may be very difficult to apply in discussions with cognitively impaired elderly patients and elderly spouses. The critical care nurse can help facilitate communication and understanding in this ongoing process.

Assisting the Patient and Family Near Death

Providing relief or alleviation of suffering and comfort are two foremost goals that, if accomplished, will help ensure a compassionate ending for the patient and family (Moore, 1997). The assessment and management of symptoms is considered effective if the patient is comfortable and the mentation is not adversely affected by opiates, sedatives, or other drugs. Making special arrangements to accommodate the preferences of the patient and family regarding pastoral or spiritual comfort is very important in relieving suffering and helping the patient and family come to terms with the meaning of the impending death (Frankl, 1984). It is an understatement to say that sometimes the most important thing the nurse can do is listen.

Bereavement counseling is often offered to families by hospice services. Many families may benefit by referral to bereavement services or support groups to assist them in coping with their grief.

Future Research on End-of-Life Care

In the last 5 years, several private and government funding agencies have focused their research priorities in the area of end-of-life care issues. Most studies have focused on the areas of advance directives and pain management. Other areas for future research, especially in the critical care area, lie in the areas of communication and decision making, symptom management, and needs of near-death patients and their families (Moody et al., 1999). There is great potential in the critical care units to study these issues and add to our repertoire of knowledge in this important area at the end of life.

REFERENCES

Adams, F. (1988). Neuropsychiatric evaluation and treatment of delirium in cancer patients. *Advances in Psychosomatic Medicine, 18,* 26–36.

American Association of Critical Care Nurses/University Southern California School of Nursing. (1998). *Critical care choices guide.* Aliso Viego, CA: Author.

Benner, P., & Wrubel, J. (1989). *The primacy of caring: Stress and coping in health and illness.* Menlo Park: Addison-Wesley.

Bertman, S. (1998). *Ars moriendi:* Illuminations on "The Good Death" from the arts and humanities. *Hospice Journal, 13,* 5–28.

Byock, I. (1996). The nature of suffering and the nature of opportunity at the end of life. *Clinics in Geriatric Medicine, 12,* 237–252.

Chochinov, H. (1999). Will to live fluctuates among dying patients. *Lancet, 354,* 816–819.

Dickinson, E. (1960). The dying need but little dear. In T. Johnson (Ed.), *The complete poems of Emily Dickinson.* Boston: Little Brown.

Fainsinger, R., & Bruera, E. (1992). Treatment of delirium in a terminally ill patient. *Journal of Pain and Symptom Management, 7,* 54–56.

Farncombe, M. (1997). Dyspnea: Assessment and treatment. *Comment in: Support Care Cancer, 5,* 94–99.

Finucane, T. E., & Harper, M. (1996). Ethical decision-making near the end of life. *Clinical Geriatric Medicine, 12,* 369–377.

Frankl, V. (1984). *Man's search for meaning.* New York: Washington Square Press.

Gurfolino, V., & Dumas, L. (1994). Hospice nursing: The concept of palliative care. *Nursing Clinics of North America, 29,* 533–546.

Halloran, E. J. (Ed.). (1996). Virginia Henderson and her timeless writings. *Journal of Advanced Nursing, 23* (1), 17–19.

Johnson, C. (1998). Hospice: What gets in the way of appropriate and timely access. *Holistic Nursing Practice, 13* (1), 8–21.

Kinzbrunner, B. M. (1995). Ethical dilemmas in hospice and palliative care. *Supportive Care in Cancer, 37* (1), 28–36.

Light, K. (1997). Florence Nightingale and holistic philosophy. *Journal of Holistic Nursing, 15* (1), 25–40.

Moody, L., Lunney, J., & Grady, P. (1999). Nursing perspective on end-of-life care research and policy issues. *Journal of Health Care Law and Policy, 2,* 243–257.

Moody, L., Beckie, T., Long, C., & Edmonds, A., & Andrews, S. (1999). Psychometric properties of the revised readiness for death instrument. *Hospice Journal, 15*, 49–65.

Moore, J. (1997). Complementary therapies in hospice care: Compassionate endings. *American Journal of Hospice & Palliative Care, Mar/Apr*, 75–80.

Oxenham, D., & Cornbleet, M. A. (1998). Accuracy of prediction of survival by different professional groups in a hospice. *Palliative Medicine, 12*, 117–118.

Taylor, R. B. (1997). *Manual of family practice.* Boston: Little, Brown.

Teno, J. M., Lynn, J., Phillips, R. S., Murphy, D., Younger, S. J., Bellamy, P., Connors, A. F., Desbiens, N. A., Fulkerson, W., & Knaus, W. A. (1994). Do formal advance directives affect resuscitation decisions and the use of resources for seriously ill patients? SUPPORT Investigators. Study to Understand Prognoses and Preferences for Outcomes and Risks of Treatments. *Journal of Clinical Ethics, 5* (1), 23–30.

Thompson, H. J. (1999). The management of post-operative nausea and vomiting. *Journal of Advanced Nursing, 29*, 1130–1136.

Wang, J. J., Ho, S. T., Liu, Y. H., Ho, C. M., Liu, K., & Chia, Y. Y. (1999). Dexamethasone decreases epidural morphine-related nausea and vomiting. *Anesthesia & Analgesia, 89*, 117–120.

Weitzner, M., Moody, L., & McMillan, S. (1997). Issues in hospice care research. *American Journal of Hospice & Palliative Care, 14*, 190–195.

Zeppetella, G. (1998). The palliation of dyspnea in terminal disease. *American Journal of Hospice & Palliative Care, 15*, 322–330.

20

Spiritual and Religious Care

Martha E. F. Highfield

Nursing's focus on caring for the whole person uniquely positions us to help older adults address their spiritual and attendant religious concerns. Spiritual longings often come sharply into focus for persons confronting either a life-threatening illness or the losses associated with aging (Burnard, 1987; Moberg, 1990; Reed 1992; Walton, 1999). Thus, the older adult in critical care, who is faced with both situations, may be among those most in need of spiritual assistance. Additionally, as nurses care for persons in crisis and work to facilitate spiritual need fulfillment of patients, they come face to face with their own spiritual needs and issues (Highfield, Taylor, & Amenta, 2000).

Although research and literature on spiritual needs and caregiving is growing, little research is available about the spiritual needs of critical care patients either in general or in older cohorts. Therefore, in this chapter concepts related to spirituality and religion are defined, spirituality and religion among older adults are discussed, and applications to the critical care setting are recommended with the hope that others will test these recommendations in practice. Special challenges to patients' spiritual well-being that are posed by aging and the critical care setting are discussed, as well as recommendations for nurse self-examination, nursing diagnosis, and specific ways in which nurses can promote the spiritual well-being of the critically ill older adult.

SPIRITUALITY OF OLDER ADULTS

Spiritual Well-Being

Growing old physically can be a time of growing up spiritually. As adults age and face increasing physical limitations and losses, the spiritual task of finding meaning in one's life becomes increasingly important (Burnard, 1987). Self-transcendence is a process that promotes finding meaning and includes the human capacity to step outside of physical and temporal boundaries and to understand oneself as more than present events and activities or a physical body. For the elderly this means developing a healthy introspection, altruism, and an integration of "perceptions of one's past and future to enhance the present" (Reed, 1991a, p. 5). Through self-transcendence, the realities of aging are not denied but imbued with a sense of meaning that is spiritual at its core.

This developmental understanding of spirituality of the older adult is at the heart of Reed's articulation of nursing's "emerging paradigm" (1992, p. 349) of spirituality. Spirituality, she concluded, is understood by nursing as

the propensity to make meaning through a sense of relatedness to dimensions that transcend the self. . . . This [empowering] relatedness may be experienced intrapersonally (as a connectedness within oneself), interpersonally (in the context of others and the natural environment), and transpersonally (referring to a sense of relatedness to the unseen, God, or power greater than the self and ordinary resources). (p. 350)

Spirituality, according to Reed, is the effort to find meaning in life within the context of relationships. Healthy spirituality, we may conclude, requires sustaining relationships and results in interpreting the whole of life as meaningful.

These ideas build on the work of other disciplines. Two decades ago the National Interfaith Coalition on Aging (NICA) formulated a definition of spiritual well-being among the elderly as

the affirmation of life in a relationship with God, self, community and environment that nurtures and celebrates wholeness. . . . [Further], the *spiritual* is not one dimension among many in life; rather, it permeates and gives meaning to all life. The term spiritual well-being therefore, indicates wholeness in contrast to fragmentation and isolation. (as cited in Cook, 1980, p. xiii)

As Tournier reflected, "[God is] leading me along the new paths of old age. It is He who has made the unity of my life" (1972, p. 214).

Within the NICA definition of spiritual well-being are overlapping religious and existential aspects. The religious or vertical dimension of spiritual well-being focuses on developing a sustaining and meaningful relationship with God or the supernatural and the existential or horizontal dimension focuses on purpose in and satisfaction with life. Both are important to positive spiritual well-being, and each occurs along a continuum of greater to lesser well-being. Together they may be collectively exhaustive of the concept of spiritual well-being but are not mutually exclusive (Ellison, 1983).

Religion and Spiritual Well-Being

Religion differs from spirituality but is complementary to it. Spirituality is the search to find meaning and connectedness; religion is an answer. When formal religion is not a part of a person's life, a secular system of values, beliefs, and symbols serves as an answer (O'Brien, 1999). Although the concept of religion has often been reduced to specific, external doctrines and ritualized behaviors, NICA and others more properly recognize its broader role in supporting and expressing spiritual well-being and in answering the ultimate questions of meaning and one's place in the universe (Byrne & Price, 1979; Cook, 1980; Ellison, 1983; O'Brien, 1999).

Religion can be understood as those values, beliefs, practices, and symbols that are adopted as a response to spiritual needs (Byrne & Price, 1979; Ellison, 1983; Highfield, 1992). Often the term religion refers to an organized local or global community of faith that provides psychosocial and spiritual support; opportunity for worship; sacraments to connect with the divine or activities to connect with the transcendent; rituals and rites of passage; and proscriptions and prohibitions concerning how one should live and relate intrapersonally, interpersonally, and transpersonally. Some authors have noted that spirituality can be expressed in many ways other than formal religion (Burkhardt & Nagai-Jacobson, 1997) and that a secular life philosophy can also be effective in satisfying spiritual needs (Amenta, 1986). In this latter sense, life philosophy, with its attendant values, beliefs, practices, and symbols, functions as religion (O'Brien, 1999).

Having a religion or secular life philosophy, however, does not always create a high level of spiritual well-being. The healthiness or unhealthiness of a value and belief system is seen in the outcomes it produces. Salugenic or healthy values and beliefs promote higher spiritual well-being by helping the person to find meaning and to strengthen relationships (Allport, 1959; Clinebell, 1979). In contrast, pathogenic values and beliefs interfere with meeting spiritual needs by disrupting relationships with self, others, and God or higher power (Clinebell, 1979). Waldfogel (1997) observed that religious and spiritual practices may lead to increased stress, marginalization of the ill person, or a sense that suffering is God's punishment.

Persons with pathogenic religion may live inconsistently with their values or may behave religiously without inner conviction. Such individuals use their religion or philosophy for personal gain; self-justification; self-gratification; or magical thinking that borders on, or can become, psychopathological (Allport, 1959; Clinebell, 1979; Fallon et al., as cited in Matthews, Larson, & Barry, 1993; Field & Wilkerson, 1973). Salugenic religion creates spiritual well-being through life-affirming relationships; pathogenic religion creates "fragmentation and isolation" (NICA, as cited in Cook, 1980, p. xiii).

Religion and Older Adults

Salugenic religion and spiritual values can provide considerable support to older persons. Multiple studies document the importance of religious faith and practices among the elderly (Matthews et al., 1983). Approximately 50 years of Gallup survey data in the United States reveal that many older adults and more older than younger adults consider religion important in their lives, "seek God's will through prayer" (Moberg, 1990, p. 180), frequently attend religious services, and often express their spirituality through traditionally western beliefs and practices. Additionally, older adults value and practice prayer more often than younger adults do (Levin & Taylor, 1997). Despite the claim of some that secular values and beliefs will increase within the population as our scientific knowledge increases, data suggest otherwise. In the United States, religious faith and practice continue to grow with each new generation of elders (Moberg, 1990), and whereas the baby boomers who are soon to be elders may not feel strong ties to any one religious group, they are returning to churches in a search for spiritual connectedness and meaning (Roof, 1994).

Although ideas abound about what creates the high level of religiousness observed among older adults, none has been empirically substantiated. Reasons are probably multiple, integrated, and complex. Perhaps release from career and family responsibilities allows more time to focus on faith and prayer, or the elderly are closer to death and receive comfort from religion, or the poor compensate for their poverty and the unemployed for a sense of uselessness through religion (Moberg, 1990).

One hypothesis is that the more religious simply outlive their less religious counterparts because of the psychosocial and physical benefits of faith-based values and beliefs (Moberg, 1990). A corollary to this is that women outlive men and are more religious than men are (Levin & Taylor, 1997). In further support of this hypothesis, studies repeatedly demonstrate the benefits of religious commitment, including lower mortality and morbidity, improved mood, lower death anxiety, fewer hospital admissions, shorter inpatient stays, lower blood pressure, and other positive physical and psychosocial health outcomes for older adults (Fehring, Miller, & Shaw, 1997; Koenig & Larson, 1998; Matthews et al., 1993). Additionally, although controversial, other studies suggest, and many patients and providers believe, that prayer by the patient or by others on the patient's behalf improves physical and psychosocial outcomes (Benson, 1996; Dossey, 1993, 1996; Jaret, 1998; Matthews et al., 1993; Shelly & Miller, 1999; Targ, 1997; Walton, 1999).

Regardless of why they are more religious, older adults do find comfort in a salugenic life philosophy or religion that provides "strength in the face of the unknown or in times of crisis" (Byrne & Price, 1979, p. 6). For example, in one study of adult caregivers, the more difficult the caregiving situation became, the more adult caregivers relied on religious values, beliefs, and practices as a coping strategy (Picot, Debanne, Namazi, & Wykle, 1997). Data from other studies suggest that both families and patients use spiritual values, beliefs, and practices to cope with serious illness (Emblen & Halstead, 1993; Fehring et al., 1997; O'Brien, 1999; Reed, 1991b; Rukholm, Bailey, Coutu-Wakulczyk, & Bailey, 1991; Sodestrom & Martinson, 1987; Walton, 1999).

One example of this was uncovered during an unrelated study on the effects of income on aging. The unsolicited and consistent reports of sustaining faith from 50 elderly, poor, Black women resulted in unanticipated research conclusions about the effectiveness of religious beliefs in coping with suffering.

> Their hardship had meaning because they interpreted it as a measure of their strength, imbued it with divine purpose and foresaw a just end. . . . Their life [sic], no matter how difficult, was part of a divine plan that will bring rewards both in this life and the next. . . . Faith in God was more than a coping mechanism for a difficult life. It was an active, very living, viable partnership. (Black as cited in Briggs, 1999, p. D10)

Among these women and other individuals, religious faith has demonstrated a role in creating and supporting a robust sense of spiritual wellbeing under the most adverse circumstances, including a personal or family member's terminal, acute, critical, and chronic illnesses (Conco, 1995; Fryback, 1993; Highfield, 1997; O'Brien, 1999; Picot et al., 1997; Shelly & Miller, 1999; Walton, 1999).

It is not fully clear whether hardship and aging themselves create a higher sense of religiousness or simply enhance focus on the more fundamental issues arising from the spirit. Based on case studies, Derrickson (1996) concluded that persons might not become more religious during terminal illness but that they do become more spiritually focused on healing of broken relationships and on reframing their lives as meaningful. Those who are devout may become more focused on their preexisting religious beliefs and practices, and those who are not religious find meaning and connect with the transcendent in other ways (Burnard, 1987; Derrickson, 1996). Earlier Weisman (1979) and Amenta (1986) also affirmed from their clinical observations that people approach death as they have approached life.

NURSING DIAGNOSES

Because spirituality and religiousness positively influence the health and coping of older adults, critical care nurses need to find ways to mobilize these resources. In addition to the nurse's spiritual self-examination, which will be discussed later, the first step is to assess accurately the person's spiritual health status. To facilitate assessment, the North American Nursing Diagnosis Association (NANDA) (1999) has listed clusters of patient verbal and nonverbal behaviors that help professionals to differentiate the spiritually healthy from the spiritually distressed.

Diagnostic Cues

Using NANDA criteria, the nurse can determine whether a person has a higher level of spiritual well-being that would lead to a diagnosis of the *"Potential for Enhanced Spiritual Well-Being,"* or whether the person has a lower level of spiritual well-being suggestive of *"Spiritual Distress"* (Carpenito, 1997; NANDA, 1999). NANDA's conceptual definition of a healthy sense of spiritual well-being is "the process of an individual's . . . unfolding of mystery [surrounding the struggles, uncertainty, and meaning of life] through harmonious interconnectedness [with others, God, self, and environment] that springs from inner strengths" (1999, p. 68). The resulting indicators for the diagnosis of *Potential for Enhanced Spiritual Well-Being* include patient expressions of

- an inner strength that nurtures trust, self-awareness, peace, integration, and "sacred source" (Carpenito, 1997, p. 870)
- an "intangible motivation and commitment directed toward values of love, meaning, hope, beauty, and truth . . .
- [a trusting relationship] with or in the transcendent that provides a basis for meaning and hope . . . and love" (p. 870)
- meaning and purpose in life

Spiritually, healthy elders may draw on their spiritual strengths during serious physical illness in two ways. First, a high level of spiritual well-being may serve a health-promoting, stress-preventing function by facilitating interpretation of potentially stressful events as manageable (Picot et al., 1997). Second, when the person does experience life events as stressful, spirituality as expressed through values, beliefs, and practices may serve as an effective coping resource (O'Brien, 1999; Picot et al., 1997; Sodestrom & Martinson, 1987; Walton, 1999).

Other elders will react less positively to confrontation with critical illness and its attendant negative pathophysiological, situational, developmental, or treatment-related events (Carpenito, 1997). As a result of one or a combination of these triggering events they may experience *Spiritual Distress,* a "disruption in the life principle that pervades a person's entire being and that integrates and transcends one's biological and psychosocial nature" (NANDA, 1999, p. 67). Individuals in spiritual distress will exhibit the behavioral clusters listed in Table 20.1, including conflicts between faith and treatment, disturbing religious doubts, or frank rejection of previously held values, beliefs, and practices. Past value and belief systems are at least temporarily inadequate to maintain inner strength or hope and to find meaning in the circumstance of life-threatening illness and care (Carpenito, 1997).

Difficulties in Diagnosis

The diagnostic process is not easy, particularly when the individual does not express spiritual issues in religious terms. The first difficulty is in differentiating those who are at risk for spiritual distress from those with actual distress. The intense search for meaning and a sense of connectedness that is triggered by negative events is not pathological but instead is a risk factor and indicator of potential distress. The hopelessness that comes when a person's search results in a sense of meaninglessness and alienation is spiritually pathological and constitutes actual distress (Burnard, 1987; Carpenito, 1997; NANDA, 1999).

The second diagnostic difficulty is that some indicators of spiritual distress, such as anxiety, grief, and sleep disturbances, may also occur as a

TABLE 20.1 Defining Characteristics of Spiritual Distress

Must be present:
"Expresses concern with meaning of life/death and/or belief systems" (NANDA, 1999, p. 67)
"Experiences a disturbance in belief system [that provides hope, meaning, & strength]" (Carpenito, 1997, p. 852)

May be present:
"Questions moral/ethical implications of therapeutic regimen
Description of nightmares/sleep disturbances
Verbalizes inner conflict about beliefs
Verbalizes concern about relationships with deity
Unable to participate in usual religious practices
Seeks spiritual assistance
Questions meaning of suffering . . . [and] own existence
Displacement of anger toward religious representatives
Anger toward God
Alteration in behavior/mood evidenced by anger, crying, withdrawal, preoccupation, anxiety, hostility, apathy, etc.
Gallows humor" (NANDA, 1999, p. 67)
"Chooses not to practice usual religious rituals . . .
Expresses that he has no reason for living . . .
Feels a sense of spiritual emptiness" (Carpenito, 1997, p. 852)

result of psychosocial or physical issues. The noisy, busy, and sometimes depersonalizing environment of a unit assaults the senses, emotions, and intellect through sleep deprivation, loss of privacy, and a host of other negative factors. These factors can create a complex matrix of unhealthy patient outcomes that make it difficult to sort out spiritual issues from others. Similarly, indicators of a high level of spiritual well-being are also expressed through behaviors that are closely related to psychosocial and physical status.

These diagnostic difficulties arise because humans are not neatly compartmentalized into physical, psychosocial, and spiritual dimensions of being. All dimensions are intertwined, and health or distress in one dimension results in a corresponding health or distress in other dimensions. For example, pain can result in depression and a sense that God is absent; loss of meaning and hope can result in suicide or physical illness. As a further complicating issue, the only way that we know about either the psychosocial or the spiritual status of persons is as those dimensions are revealed to us by the patient through physical actions and spoken words.

Twibell, Wieseke, Marine, and Schoger's (1996) research highlighted the difficulty of differentiating spiritual and psychosocial nursing diagnoses among critical care patients. They investigated how critical care nurses used the indicators for the NANDA diagnoses of both spiritual distress and psychosocial ineffective individual coping. Their convenience sample of 59 nurses validated the importance of seven major indicators of spiritual distress (i.e., spiritual emptiness, disturbance in beliefs, no reason for living, request for spiritual assistance, concern over life's meaning, questioning, or doubting beliefs) and two minor ones (i.e., unable to practice rituals and detachment from self). At the same time, respondents used two NANDA indicators of spiritual distress (i.e., shows emotional detachment from self and others and expresses no reason for living) to diagnose ineffective individual coping. The authors suggested that indicators probably do overlap and that their respondents probably did not reject NANDA indicators, but had incomplete knowledge of them. The outcome of redundancy among indicators, they concluded, may be that nurses omit these diagnoses from a plan of care, rather than taking the time to sort out whether a problem is primarily spiritual or psychosocial.

SPIRITUAL DISTRESS AND HEALTH IN CRITICAL CARE

Barriers to Healthy Spirituality

In assessing patient spirituality, nurses must recognize not only the behavioral outcomes that reflect spiritual status, but also the positive and negative factors that put the patient at risk for distress or that support well-being. The elderly in critical care are subject to many factors that can disrupt spiritual well-being. Some of these potential barriers are physical, patho-physiological and treatment-related issues that are shared by other age groups (Table 20.2), and some are developmental and psychosocial issues more likely to occur with increased age (Table 20.3).

These potential barriers can create adverse and uncertain circumstances within which the person must meet the spiritual needs of finding meaning and maintaining connectedness. Establishing or maintaining "the affirmation of life in a relationship with God, self, community and environment that nurtures and celebrates wholeness" (NICA, as cited in Cook, 1980, p. xiii) in critical care becomes no small task, requiring all of the patient's

TABLE 20.2 Critical Care–Related Barriers to Spiritual Well-Being

- Separation from loved ones and the familiar
- Imminent fear of pain, death, and suffering
- Disruption of meaningful religious routines and practices
- Disruption of connections with religious community
- Conflict between treatment and values/belief system
- Sense of helplessness resulting from dependence upon strangers, technology, and medical interventions
- Lack of privacy and repeated invasion of personal space by strangers
- Noise and sleep disruption
- Pain and other negative symptoms
- Requests to participate in clinical trials; feeling like a "guinea pig"
- Toxicities from drugs, electrolyte imbalances
- Activation of physiological stress response
- Requests to decide on code status and advance directive planning
- Observing emergency procedures performed on a nearby person
- Transfer anxiety
- Fear that a nurse will "pull the plug" during a time of deteriorating physical health
- Inability to communicate needs verbally

Adapted from Carpenito (1997) and O'Brien (1999).

TABLE 20.3 Aging-Related Barriers to Spiritual Well-Being

- Loss of autonomy
- Limited financial resources
- Sensory deficits
- Social isolation
- Loss of significant others
- Loss of body part(s) or function(s)
- Terminal illness
- Chronic comorbid pathology or psychopathology

Adapted from Carpenito (1997) and O'Brien (1999).

internal and external spiritual resources, including nursing support. For the older person, who has less energy and stamina than a younger person has, these demands can be significant. The need to face multiple negative circumstances simultaneously may place all older, critically ill patients at risk for spiritual distress.

In addition to the potential barriers related to critical care and age, other characteristics of particular elders may also promote spiritual distress. Spiritual well-being may previously have been diminished by pathogenic religion or philosophy or by cumulative grief from multiple losses of friends, spouse, sensory acuity, financial security, or employment. Earlier developmental tasks of establishing a sense of self-identity and intimate relationships that would have prepared the older person for the tasks associated with aging may never have been met. Additionally, preexisting cognitive or emotional impairment may limit the benefits of a past sustaining faith. Any combination of these factors may overwhelm some elders during the crisis of critical illness, with its accompanying inevitable sense of powerlessness, anger, or anxiety and its unavoidable ultimate spiritual questions of meaning and connectedness, such as, "Am I still valuable?" "What is the meaning of this illness and my life?" and "Why must I suffer or die?"

Patient Responses

Critical illness and treatment themselves, of course, are not spiritual problems, just as aging is not a spiritual problem. The problem, or lack of it, is in how the individual responds. Over the course of their lifetimes, many older adults have developed healthy characteristics that are assets to spiritual well-being (Table 20.4). Perhaps as a result, some patients immediately respond to a heart attack with more peace and confidence and others with more anxiety and fear (Walton, 1999).

TABLE 20.4 Age-Related Factors Supporting Spiritual Well-Being

- Introspection focusing on inner spirituality
- Generativity and altruism
- Finding meaning through integration of past, present, and future
- Self-transcendence, including seeing self as more than a body and physical ailments
- Time to pray
- Decreased stresses from job and career-building
- Wisdom
- Experience in coping with past crises
- Endurance of past hardships
- Strong religious commitment

Adapted from Moberg (1990), O'Brien (1999), and Reed (1991a).

Crisis theory may help to explain radically differing patient responses. Aguilera (1994) has proposed that ordinarily persons establish a healthy, dynamic balance in dealing with their life situations. However, when confronted with threatening developmental (e.g., losses associated with aging) or situational (e.g., critical illness and hospitalization) stressors, equilibrium is disturbed and a new balance must be achieved. Three factors can help an individual to maintain or regain equilibrium: a realistic perception of events, available support systems, and effective coping strategies, particularly those used to overcome past difficulties. In contrast, if the person has an unrealistic perception, lacks support, or possesses inadequate coping strategies, then the individual will be overwhelmed and immobilized by negative life events.

If Aguilera's (1994) ideas are applied to the spiritual responses of persons to critical illness and care, then it is reasonable to assume that the spiritually healthy elder would

- use previously effective values, beliefs, practices, and symbols to cope
- draw on effective support from nurses, family, friends, faith community, or other sources
- accurately comprehend information and make effective decisions within the context of life's meaning and purpose

Anecdotal reports (Bardanouve, 1994) and research (Walton, 1999) suggest that the religious do deal effectively with life-threatening illness in the preceding three ways. Walton (1999) found that religious faith facilitated the ability of patients recovering from myocardial infarction to process information and make decisions, to draw on inner coping strategies effectively, and to receive support from a community of family, friends, and other believers. It would be consistent with Aguilera (1994) to suggest that those with salugenic secular values, support systems, and coping strategies would also be able to have a realistic perception of events and avoid crisis.

By eliminating or minimizing critical care and age-related barriers to spiritual health and by facilitating effective coping strategies, support systems, and information processing, nurses can assist older adults toward improved spiritual well-being. Although these activities are often understood as psychosocial, they are spiritual to the extent that they help to affirm meaning and relationships with self, others, environment, and the transcendent.

THE CONTEXT OF SPIRITUAL CARE

Nurse Characteristics

Nurses should become aware of their own characteristics, which may influence their spiritual assessment, diagnosis, and care. Although research has yet to elucidate fully the effect of nurse characteristics on spiritual care-giving, current findings and anecdotal reports suggest the following may be important: the nurse's cultural background and beliefs (Martsolf, 1997), nurse ethnicity (Highfield, 1992), the capacity of the nurse to be present with patients (Osterman & Schwartz-Barcott, 1996), nurse spirituality, nurse religiousness, education in spiritual care, basic nursing preparation, area of specialty practice, frequency of attendance at religious services, perceived ability to provide care, and whether spiritual caregiving is valued (Boutell & Bozett, 1990; Carson, Wilkelstein, Soeken, & Brunins, 1986; Piles, 1990; Taylor, Highfield, & Amenta, 1999).

Unknown is whether these characteristics of nurses may be effects, causes, or both in relation to patient interaction. In one national study of hospice and oncology nurses, nurse spirituality was often influenced positively by caring for seriously or terminally ill patients, and nurse spirituality in turn was positively related to the frequency of, ability in, and comfort with spiritual caregiving (Highfield et al., 2000). This type of complicated relationship may also be present in other nurse characteristics.

Self-examination of values, beliefs, and practices and how these have been shaped by personal and educational experiences is a prerequisite to effective care. The most effective nurse spiritual caregivers will be those who positively value spirituality and who understand spiritual well-being as a healthy and integrative force in helping older patients achieve wholeness when their physical bodies are failing. These nurses understand that meaning; integration of the past, present, and future; connectedness with self, others, and environment; and the transcendent occur within the context of a specific culture and a religious or secular heritage. They will be aware of the influence of their own culture and heritage on their own spirituality and will be able to differentiate these personal values and beliefs from those of the patient (Carpenito, 1997; Dorff, 1993; Martsolf, 1997; O'Brien, 1999; Tripp-Reimer, Johnson, & Sorofman, 1999).

In contrast to those nurses who fully accept their own and their patients' spirituality, others may believe that spirituality is limited to a psychosocial or cultural phenomenon and will address spiritual concerns from the perspectives of those disciplines and theories. This approach may reduce spiritual needs to empirically observable, psychological, or sociological behaviors, rather than appreciating them as unique and transpersonal. It interprets psychosocially expressed evidence of the human spirit as evidence of the psyche. This view of the spiritual as psychology conflicts with the personal experiences of patients and the consensus of a growing body of health professionals (Barnum, 1996; Burkhardt & Nagai-Jacobson, 1997; Carson, 1989; Larson & Larson, 1994; O'Brien, 1999; Waldfogel, 1997).

Other nurses believe that spirituality is outside the realm of professional nursing and so avoid discussing any religious, spiritual, or values questions raised by patients. From a historical perspective, this position ignores the religious origins of health care, and from a practical standpoint, professional silence on religious and spiritual issues "dehumanizes both [nurse and patient]" (Dorff, 1993, p. 57). If nurses fail to recognize spiritual needs or retreat into a personally disconnected pseudoprofessionalism (Evans, 1993) or into the "glamour and power of high-technology" (Donley, 1991, p. 178), the results can be spiritually devastating for the patient, whose efforts to connect meaningfully with the nurse as another human being have failed.

Some of these nurses and others who do value patient spirituality may believe that the only appropriate spiritual intervention is referral to clergy or spiritual advisors. Carpenito (1997) warns against this, noting that it is well within the professional role of nurses to listen nonjudgmentally, to provide resources and time for the practice of religious activities, and to assist persons to meet spiritual needs. Patients and nurses agree (Barnum, 1996; Broten, 1997; Boutell & Bozett, 1990; Carson, 1989; Conco, 1995; Donley, 1991; Emblen & Halstead, 1993; Highfield et al., 1999; O'Brien, 1999; Reed, 1992; Shelly & Miller, 1999; Sodestrom & Martinson, 1987; Taylor, Amenta, & Highfield, 1995).

In other instances, nurses may be so unaware of spiritual issues that they do not recognize patient expressions of spiritual well-being and distress. When patients say that they are suffering, these nurses might provide only physical comfort measures or reassurances that the person's physical progress is going as planned. In these instances, the milieu of the nurse-patient relationship is task oriented rather than spiritually attentive. The rush to complete demanding nursing tasks within the critical care environment may also create a similar short-circuiting response in which spiritual issues may be recognized but are neglected.

Many sources are available to assist the nurse in developing self-awareness. Authors with traditional and nontraditional religious values have provided overlapping definitions and explanations of the spiritual dimension that is present in both nurse and patient (Amenta, 1986; Barnum, 1996; Burkhardt & Nagai-Jacobson, 1997; O'Brien, 1999; Reed, 1992; Stoll, 1989). Some of these authors and others give the nurse information with which to compare personal convictions by outlining differing world views, beliefs, and practices of various religions (Barrett, 1994; Carpenito, 1997; Gerardi, 1989; Martin, 1989; Tripp-Reimer et al., 1999). Further, Martsolf (1997) offers specific questions for nurse self-assessment about the impact of culture on personal spirituality, including with what cultural group one most identifies, how and where did one learn life's meaning and what is most important, what interpersonal and transpersonal relationships and experiences one has had, how and to whom would one explain these, and whether one's life story is parallel to the story of a particular group of people.

Diversity

Nurses and patients and their significant others reflect the diversity of the surrounding population. This means that these individuals vary widely in terms of religious or secular values, beliefs, and practices, as well as in age, education, ethnicity, gender, country of origin, and cultural heritage. Nurses struggling to provide care that is sensitive to older patients and to those whose spiritual values beliefs and practices differ from their own will find it a Herculean task to understand and accommodate the intricacies of these differences without some general guidelines.

Berlin and Fowkes (as cited in Tripp-Reimer et al., 1999) have proposed the LEARN model as a way to guide culturally sensitive care in a family practice setting (Table 20.5). The scope of this model makes it potentially applicable to patient and family care that is sensitive to age-related values and religious or secular values, beliefs, meaningful symbols, and important practices.

Although it would require evaluation for usefulness in the critical care setting, LEARN has potential to guide dialogue and planning with significant others and with the patient who is able to communicate. The strengths of this model, listening and negotiation, also constitute its weaknesses in potential application to the critically ill older adult for whom its use is restricted by intubation, altered consciousness, anxiety, exhaustion, sleep deprivation, and limited patient physical energy. In such instances, family, friends, and spiritual advisors may work with nurses on behalf of the patient.

PROMOTING SPIRITUAL WELL-BEING

The intertwined biophysical-psychosocial-spiritual nature of persons means that every nursing action can promote or undermine spiritual well-being. This assumption can account for the otherwise surprising range of activities that patients and nurses have identified as spiritual interventions. In various studies, patients have provided the following list of spiritual care interventions: explain procedures, remain hopeful, be alert to patient needs (Martin, Burrows, & Pomilio, 1976/1988), facilitate time with family or significant others, facilitate religious practices, facilitate religious service

TABLE 20.5   LEARN Model

L:	Listen with understanding to the patient's perception of the problem and to his or her notions of the best way to treat it
E:	Explain your perception of the problem.
A:	Acknowledge and discuss the differences and similarities between your viewpoints
R:	Recommend a treatment plan within the constraints of your ideas and those of the patient.
N:	Negotiate an agreement (that may not be the first choice of either party)

Adapted from Berlin and Fowkes as cited in "Cultural Dimensions in Gerontological Nursing," by T. Tripp-Reimer, R. Johnson, & B. Sorofman in *Gerontological Nursing: A Health Promotion/Protection Approach*, 2nd ed., by M. Stanley & P. G. Beare (Eds.), 1999, Philadelphia: F. A. Davis.

attendance, provide inspirational reading material (Reed, 1991b), share personal beliefs (Belcher, Dettmore, & Holzemer, 1989; Conco, 1995; Reed, 1991b), ask about feelings (Highfield, 1997), respect patient beliefs, listen (Belcher et al., 1989; Clark & Heidenreich, 1995; Martin et al., 1976/1988; Sodestrom & Martinson, 1987), provide competent technical care, display a caring attitude (Conco, 1995; Clark & Heidenreich, 1995; Emblen & Halstead, 1993; Martin et al., 1976/1988; Sodestrom & Martinson, 1987), arrange visits with clergy, allow time for personal prayer, pray with patient (Emblen & Halstead, 1993; Martin et al., 1976/1988; Reed, 1991b; Sodestrom & Martinson, 1987), talk, touch, smile, assess needs, be compassionate, and be present (Conco, 1995; Emblen & Halstead, 1993; Clark & Heidenreich, 1995). Nurses (Boutell & Bozett, 1990; Emblen & Halstead, 1993; Sodestrom & Martinson, 1987) and chaplains (Emblen & Halstead, 1993) agree.

Although a discussion of these and other activities within the context of the spiritual dimension is warranted, the following section will focus selectively on a few. The choice and description of the particular approaches is not comprehensive nor does it necessarily capture those actions of highest spiritual priority. It is intended to stimulate questions, dialogue, and research related to spiritual care of the critically ill older adult.

Collaborating with Clergy

Nurse spiritual caregiving should complement the role of chaplains and spiritual advisors, just as nurse physical caregiving complements the role of medical colleagues. Because nurses are the main source of interpersonal contact 24 hours a day, are present during acute health crises, and establish intimate physical and psychosocial relationships with patients, they are uniquely positioned to address spiritual issues. Nurses are often the first to assess spiritual concerns, particularly in situations in which the person may be unwilling to reveal doubts or worries to significant others or when time with significant others is severely limited. Nurses can communicate patients' spiritual and religious needs to chaplains, schedule pain medications and treatments to accommodate clerical visits, provide privacy for religious activities, and explain special physical care considerations, such as isolation procedures or level of acuity, to clergy (Shelly & Fish, 1988).

Several issues are unique to working with clergy from the community. When a patient asks the nurse to call a spiritual advisor who is not a hospital employee, professional courtesy dictates that the nurse involve hospital chaplains in making such contacts (Vandecreek, 1997). Also, because community clergy may not be comfortable in a high technology environment, the nurse may need to provide careful direction and information regarding anything that may facilitate or constrain the visit or religious activities. For example, nurses may wish to explain alarms and noises or that the clergyperson should assume that the nonresponsive patient will hear his or her conversation, readings, or prayers. Additionally, in the unlikely event that a nurse observes that clergy are upsetting to the patient, the nurse should involve hospital chaplains in any assessment and resolution of the problem (Shelly & Fish, 1988).

Visits from clergy can provide a sense of transpersonal connectedness with God or a higher power. The clergy symbolize the divine or forces greater than the self, and as such they are empowered to administer sacraments, such as Baptism and Holy Communion, and to provide the patient with official religious information on exemptions from religious practices for the sick (Shelly & Fish, 1988). These activities can ameliorate spiritual distress by preempting or resolving conflicts between religious practices and beliefs and treatment.

In contrast, some individuals do not want visits from religious representatives. The nurse must assess patient wishes before recommending any religious referral and should not assume that the patient's stated religious affiliation or culture represents closeness to a particular faith community. Some individuals have stated that they prefer spiritual support from family, friends, physicians, nurses, social workers, a pet, bartender, or patient advocate (Highfield, 1992). In other settings where chaplains routinely visit all patients, patients who have previously rejected clerical visits may find a particular clergyperson to be a preferred source of comfort (Hunter; 1991; O'Brien, 1999).

Facilitating Life Review

Temporal integration, a weaving together of past, present, and future into a meaningful pattern, is important to the health of older adults (Reed, 1991a). Reminiscence or life review by the older adult can strengthen a sense of intrapersonal connectedness through a deeper understanding of the self and the life lived (O'Brien, 1999). Past intrapersonal, interpersonal, or transpersonal conflicts may be recognized and resolved, wisdom shared, and meaning uncovered. For some religious persons, God's continual faithfulness may become evident and provide a basis for peace, hope, and meaning (Lashley, 1992; Walton, 1999), and the person may reconcile relationships by giving and by receiving forgiveness (Derrickson, 1996; O'Brien, 1999). Critically ill persons may recall how they have coped successfully with past crises and may gain both confidence and direction for dealing with the present (O'Brien, 1999). Just as there was a future to those events, the older adult may be able to gain hope by seeing a future beyond the present difficulties.

Critical care nurses can facilitate reminiscence by providing an empathetic interpersonal environment—if not a quiet physical one—in which the older adult can reflect aloud about significant family, friends, pets, events, faith, symbols, and values. This requires eye contact, a nonjudgmental attitude, a genuine interest in the person in the bed (not simply on the body to be healed), and a "focusing of both mind and body on the other person" (Lashley, 1992, p. 7) from the nurse. It does not require that the nurse say anything in particular or answer a patient's rhetorical or reflective questions. Being physically, spiritually, and psychosocially available to the patient is most important (Conco, 1995; Corcoran, 1993; O'Brien, 1999).

The spiritual need to reminisce can be blocked by demands on both nurse and patient. Providing a listening environment can be difficult for the critical care nurse, who is managing complex technology, communicating with various disciplines, coordinating care, and burdened by his or her own tiredness and stresses. Additionally, the older patient may not have the energy to speak or may be intubated or sedated. In these situations, nurses can support the patient's sense of connectedness that might otherwise be met through reminiscence by keeping meaningful pictures and symbols, such as photos of pets or religious items, nearby or taped to the bed. Friends and family can be encouraged to read favorite secular or religious literature or to tell family stories. Bardanouve (1994) recounts her experience of remembering precise details of every Biblical passage read to her and prayers said for her by family during a critical illness, although she remembered nothing else.

Integrating one's life into a whole that has meaning reassures the patient that this illness is one event within the context of the person's entire life and does not define who they are. The "MI in bed 8" can maintain identity as a father, brother, tennis player, executive. The result is integration, rather than fragmentation and alienation.

Praying

Prayer meets spiritual needs by creating a transpersonal connection between older adults and the divine (Levin & Taylor, 1997; Moberg, 1990) and an interpersonal connection with others (Walton, 1999). Communicating with God can provide a source of comfort among elders (O'Brien, 1999) and among those experiencing life-threatening illnesses. Those who are aware that others are praying for them feel hope and a part of a larger community (Bardanouve, 1994; Walton, 1999). By providing opportunities for prayer and sometimes participating in prayer, the nurse can facilitate spiritual well-being.

"Prayer is as unique as the individual who prays" (O'Brien, 1999, p. 105). Prayers may be said alone or with others, aloud or in silence, on behalf of self or others, and benevolently or, sadly, malevolently (Dossey, 1993). They may have a conversational, rational, affective, meditative, worshipful, ritual, or focusing dimension (Wright as cited in O'Brien, 1999). The content and form of prayer will be strongly influenced by the patient's usual religious symbols, beliefs, and practices (Barrett, 1994), and more elaborate prayers may evolve during the course of illness into simple repeated two- to three-word phrases near death (Taylor, 1998). One terminally ill Christian de-scribed the evolution of his prayers from early petitions for healing to those for finding meaning and purpose in suffering and finally to a prayer for endurance and faithfulness (Highfield, 1997).

One commonly used classification of prayers groups them into meditative prayer that focuses on the presence of the divine, intercessory prayer that makes requests on behalf of others, ritual prayer of religiously prescribed words and accompanying activities, petitional prayer that requests the meet-ing of one's own needs, and colloquial prayer that asks for guidance in decisions (Waldfogel, 1997). Patients who practice these types of prayer perceive a relationship in which God or a higher personal power will respond to their verbally or nonverbally articulated needs. Meditation can be a form of prayer but also may be more secular and more focused on the self (Waldfogel, 1997).

Not all types of prayer have demonstrated equivalent health benefits. For example, exclusive use of petitionary and ritualistic prayer is associated with less positive psychosocial outcomes than is colloquial prayer (Poloma & Pendleton as cited in Waldfogel, 1997).

Patients may ask the nurse to pray aloud for them, may speak or silently articulate a prayer themselves in a way that is personally meaningful, may call on clergy or significant others to pray aloud with them (Barrett, 1994), or may ask for ongoing intercessory prayer by others. Selection will depend on patient preferences, compatibility of nurse and patient values (Barrett, 1994), and physical ability of the patient to decide and pray.

Anecdotal and research reports consistently suggest that most providers and patients agree that prayer or assistance with prayer is an acceptable spiritual intervention on the part of nurses and other health care providers (Benson, 1996; Castellaw et al., 1999; Dossey, 1993, 1996; Emblen & Hal-stead, 1993; Highfield, 1997; Martin et al., 1976/1988; O'Brien, 1999; Reed, 1991b; Shelly & Miller, 1999; Sodestrom & Martinson, 1987). Rare is the patient who objects to intercessory prayer, even when the individual does not ordinarily practice prayer (Dossey, 1993, 1996). Nonetheless, nurses report that they rarely pray aloud with their patients.

Nurses do report praying frequently *for* their patients (O'Brien, 1999). In a survey of oncology nurses, well over half report that they often pray privately for patients and that they often encourage patients to pray. Most, however, rarely prayed or offered to pray *with* patients (Taylor et al., 1995). These oncology nurse responses parallel findings among psychiatric nurses (Roberts, Sato, & Southwick, 1999).

From a physical and psychosocial perspective both psychic healing and benevolent prayers for and with patients have been associated with a multi-plicity of improved outcomes (Dossey, 1993; Sicher, Targ, Moore, & Smith, 1998; Targ, 1997), and malevolent prayers have been associated with nega-tive ones (Dossey, 1993). Although these cause-and-effect observations have suggested that prayer "works," they have not explained how.

Scientists assume that prayer can be studied empirically as part of cause-and-effect phenomena; believers submit their requests and meditations to a powerful and personal force at work in the universe. Scientifically, prayer's effectiveness has been understood as a possible intangible placebo effect (Benson, 1996) or ill-defined nonlocal event in which healer and patient are connected without being together physically or temporally (Dossey, 1993, 1996). Theologically, prayer's effectiveness is understood as divine intervention (Barrett, 1994; Blazer as cited in Jaret, 1998; Lewis, 1958/ 1980; Shelly & Miller, 1999). Current empirical, scientific studies of prayer and other types of distant healing are plagued with methodological and theoretical difficulties (Targ, 1997), whereas older adults and the critically ill continue to report a sense of connectedness, peace, and comfort from practicing prayer (Levin & Taylor, 1997; O'Brien, 1999; Walton, 1999).

Being Present

Presence, the process of being physically, psychosocially, and spiritually open and available to patients, facilitates meeting the spiritual need for interpersonal connectedness. Critically ill patients rely on nurses for life-saving physiological, emotionally sustaining psychosocial, and meaningful spiritual support. Except for a few minutes of daily visiting hours with significant others, the patients are surrounded by frightening, unfamiliar technology and strangers. The critical care nurse-stranger, who assumes physiological care of an older adult, becomes that person's most available connection with another human being and a key source of spiritual support. Being present with the suffering person and helping the person to find meaning in the experience is a primary nursing intervention (Donley, 1991; Travelbee, 1971).

Although critical care nurses are almost continually physically present with their patients, they may not be psychologically and spiritually present. Based on observations of nurse interactions with seriously ill, disabled patients, Osterman and Schwartz-Barcott (1996) have suggested that nurses can be present in four increasingly involved ways:

- physically present but self-absorbed in activities unrelated to the patient
- task-oriented without self-introduction, information sharing, or interaction
- interpersonally focused within a reciprocal relationship of sharing, empathy, and compassion
- transcendent-focused, which "moves beyond the interactional to the transpersonal" (p. 28) and gives to the nurse a subjective sense of a connectedness within self and with a force greater than self, as well as a subjective sense of oneness with the patient. Both nurse and patient experience increased peace, comfort, openness, enhanced energy, relaxation, and sense of spiritual connectedness.

This fourth level of presence is best suited to helping older adults to achieve the spiritual well-being described by NICA (as cited in Cook, 1980).

Pettigrew (1990) describes two critical components of effective presence for intensive care nurses. First, presence requires nurse vulnerability and a willingness to resist the temptation to answer the patient's unanswerable questions. Nurses must recognize that sometimes a person's suffering cannot be fixed with words or actions. By spiritually accompanying the person through suffering, sometimes silently and always compassionately, nurses can communicate their solidarity and common humanity with the patient in gesture of spiritual connectedness (Donley, 1991; Pettigrew, 1990). Nurses must learn simply "to be there in the midst of a helpless situation" (Pettigrew, 1990, p. 505) no matter how awkward it feels. Being present requires focus on the patient as person, not focus on conversation. Second, "presence takes place only at the invitation of the one suffering [and] . . . is a privilege" (Pettigrew, 1990, p. 505). Patients become vulnerable during presence, and nurses must be attentively available until patients trust them.

Again, responsiveness and energy level of the patient are not necessary for the nurse to be present with the patient. Some nurses may talk with the patient while watching for nonverbal cues (Osterman & Schwartz-Barcott, 1996), others are quietly attentive to patient needs, and still others believe that prayer on a patient's behalf allows them to be present with their patients during physical separation, such as when the patient is in the operating room (O'Brien, 1999).

Historically, presence has been a religious concept implying the imminent presence of God, but it has evolved into a psychosocial concept that focuses on nurse-patient relationships. Yet, despite the secularization of "being present," Osterman and Schwartz-Barcott (1996) observed that nurses, who were most present, transformed nurse–patient relationships by spiritualizing them. This recognition and the reclaiming of nurse–patient interactions as spiritual desecularizes and sanctifies presence (Donley, 1991; O'Brien, 1999; Shelly & Miller, 1999).

Supporting Religious Practices

Nurses must assess patient religious practices for two reasons. First, they can assist in avoiding conflicts between beliefs and health care, and second they can facilitate important religious practices, an activity valued by critical care patients and families (O'Brien, 1999; Rukholm et al., 1991). Seeking clergy to interpret religious exceptions for the sick, such as exemption from fasting in order to take medications, can eliminate conflict. Keeping religious symbols, objects, or written prayers or scriptures nearby can provide a sense of connection with God and faith.

A trilevel religiospiritual assessment is suggested, including religious affiliation, personal religious beliefs and values, and spiritual health status. Assessing the patient's religious preference may give the nurse a sense of the patient's history and worldview. Second, identifying particular religious beliefs and practices that are important in maintaining health and treating disease allows early identification of potential sources of healing or conflict. Third, observing for NANDA behavioral indicators and the etiology of any distress provides information about underlying spiritual health status.

Nurses cannot assume that a written religious preference on the chart captures the patient's entire value and belief system. Sometimes individuals use differing religious and cultural beliefs to complement one another as in the case of a Roman Catholic Hispanic, who may trust both priest and *curandero* folk healer (O'Brien, 1999), or the Native American healer, who believes that there is a place for traditional and western medicine (Dossey, 1993). At other times illness may create religious conflict within individuals and families, such as when a Christian Scientist seeks traditional, western medical care rather than religious healing practices.

Nurses should not expect to become experts in all world religions, nor should they be expected to violate their own values in attempting to deliver religiously and culturally sensitive care. Patients and families may be eager to share their religious or cultural beliefs and practices. In one study relatives of critical care patients indicated that it was important to their own spiritual health to tell about the patient's spiritual beliefs (Rukholm et al., 1991). Other resources for understanding and delivering appropriate care include chaplains, nurses who profess the same religious faith or have the same ethnic background as patients, and the patients themselves. Nurses are asked to participate in few religious rituals beyond prayer, and patients report that they are helped spiritually when nurses simply facilitate their religious practices (Sodestrom & Martinson, 1987).

Integrating Music

Music is a potential source of spiritual healing for the elderly in critical care. One experienced surgeon used the art and rhythm of words to express how valuable the introduction of the arts could be to caregiver and hospitalized patient alike. Guzzetta notes that spiritual distress is a nursing diagnosis "compatible with music therapy interventions" (1997, p. 200) and agrees that music may inspire peace, joy, comfort, and relaxing images. Yet, many units have not taken advantage of the benefits of this medium that demonstrates a capacity to connect a person's physiology, psychology, and spirit.

Most research focuses on psychophysiological rather than holistic models to interpret music. Aldridge's (1994) summary of such studies suggests that music is beneficial for the elderly and for the critical care patient. For persons with Alzheimer's, music improves quality of life and communication, and among other elders it may reduce use of hypnotics and tranquilizers. Based on findings of the positive effect of music on mental health and the aged, Aldridge recommends that music be used to enhance interaction, improve mood, stimulate speech, and improve cognitive function among older adults.

Aldridge (1994) also summarized the effects of music therapy on the critically ill. Listening to music may positively influence heart rate and rhythm, particularly when the tempo of the music is matched to the heart rate of the patient. When listening to music was coupled with relaxation, the stress-reducing effects were greater within the experimental group than among controls or among those using relaxation alone, and respiratory rates have been synchronized with music when patients tapped out its rhythm. Patients have also reported that music is calming, invokes "inner peace" (Aldridge, 1994, p. 208) and is soothing when played in the operating room environment. Listening to music reduces pain among some cancer patients and improves outcomes of aphasia therapy after neurological trauma. In one study, the therapist's singing with the breathing patterns of comatose patients induced improved clinical consciousness as measured by a coma scale (Aldridge, 1994).

More recently in their summary of research, Chlan and Tracy (1999) added the following to the list of music's benefits: lowered blood pressure, buffering of unpleasant environmental noises, alleviation of boredom, and enhanced mood and expression of feelings. They emphasized, however, that nurses should carefully assess what type of music, if any, would be helpful to the patient. Music is a highly personal experience.

Involving Significant Others

Seriously ill patients name family and friends among their most preferred sources of spiritual support (Highfield, 1992). These significant others have often provided interpersonal continuity through the ups and downs of life circumstances, and the critically ill patient is likely to rely on them for continued caring. Family and friends are already trusted and may quickly be invited by the patients to be present with them through suffering.

The patient's relationships with family and friends can meet the spiritual needs for interpersonal connectedness with others, as well as intrapersonal and transpersonal connectedness. Interpersonally, family members and patient may share a common history, traditions, culture, faith, and family rituals. They are part of the patient's life story and, thus, meaning. Intrapersonally, individuals understand themselves within the context of their roles and relationships with others. The older patient will have experienced many meaningful roles and relationships and continues to develop new ones over a lifetime (Murray & Zentner, 1997; Reed, 1991a). Finally, the patient's transpersonal relationship with God or a higher power may be fostered as a family articulates prayers and reads scriptures for the patient when the patient is physically unable to do so (Bardanouve, 1994).

Involving significant others in spiritually supporting the patient requires that the nurse attend to their spiritual needs in addition to those of the patient. Family and friends experience the same spiritual needs for connectedness and meaning, as do patients, and the critical care environment and patient's illness may be equally anxiety provoking for them. In one Canadian study, spiritual needs and situational anxiety explained much of the variation in whether families of critical care patients felt a variety of their needs were met (Rukholm et al., 1991). Spiritual interventions with families may include facilitation of familiar religious practices, providing information, compassion, presence, prayer, religious readings, visits from clergy, listening (O'Brien, 1999), recognizing the family, providing an opportunity for the family to communicate the patient's spiritual values, and communicating to families that the patient is valued (Rukholm et al., 1991). Besides constituting direct care to families, these actions provide indirect care to patients by strengthening the capacity of significant others to support the ill person (Kupferschmid, Briones, Dawson, & Drongowski, 1991).

From a spiritual care perspective, it is more important to identify and support those who are significant to the patient than it is to determine whether they fit a particular definition of family or friend. Understandings of family vary within and between cultures and generations. Some who are not biologically or legally connected to an ill person may assume roles and responsibilities associated with families. Examples include gay or unmarried heterosexual partners; godparents; or, in Latino culture, a *compadrazgo*, a role of coparenthood with the biological parents (Murray & Zentner, 1997). Additionally, a religious (O'Brien, 1999) or secular community may serve as extended family.

Observations of who visits when and of the patient's reactions to these visits will help the nurse to identify those best able to provide spiritual support and those most in need of support themselves. Although generally viewed as psychosocial interventions, support and involvement of significant others promotes spiritual well-being in the elderly as articulated by NICA (as cited in Cook, 1980, p. xiii).

The influence of families and significant others, however, is not universally positive. Old hurts and conflicts may be remembered in the context of serious illness and imminent death, and forgiveness may be given or withheld by families and by patients. Critical illness may remind family members of their own mortality, and they may retreat emotionally and spiritually from the patient even when physically present. Preexisting problems in family relationships may be heightened, and religious conflicts or pressure to adopt a particular value or belief system may surface as family members express their concern for the life and destiny of the ill person.

Nurses should not expect to resolve such problems alone. These issues require interdisciplinary work with chaplains, mental health specialists, other appropriate disciplines, patients, and the families themselves. Nurses should avoid the temptation to ignore families or to view them as obstacles. Promoting a positive sense of connectedness among family members is one way to support patients spiritually.

SUMMARY

The spiritual well-being of the elderly requires maintaining a sense of meaning and of life-affirming intrapersonal, interpersonal, and transpersonal connectedness. Most older adults find religious beliefs and practices helpful in sustaining spiritual well-being, but some prefer a secular value or belief system. It is appropriate for nurses to support their patients' spiritual well-being by reducing barriers to spiritual well-being that occur within the critical care setting and by facilitating meaningful religious and spiritual activities.

REFERENCES

Aguilera, D. C. (1994). *Crisis intervention: Theory & methodology* (7th ed.). St. Louis, MO: Mosby.

Aldridge, D. (1994). An overview of music therapy in research. *Complementary Therapies in Medicine, 2,* 204–216.

Allport, G. (1959). *The individual and his religion.* New York: Macmillan.

Amenta, M. O. (1986). Spiritual concerns. In M. O. Amenta & N. L. Bohner (Eds.), *Nursing care of the terminally ill* (pp. 115–172). Boston: Little, Brown.

Bardanouve, V. E. (1994). Spiritual ministry in the ICU. *Journal of Christian Nursing, 11* (4), 28–29.

Barnum, B. S. (1996). *Spirituality in nursing: From traditional to new age.* New York: Springer.

Barrett, S. L. (1994). Effect of Christian and Jewish beliefs on nursing practice. *CAET Journal, 13* (4), 21–24.

Belcher, A. E., Dettmore, D., & Holzemer, S. P. (1989). Spirituality and sense of well-being in persons with AIDS. *Holistic Nursing Practice, 3* (4), 16–25.

Benson, H. (with Stark, M.). (1996). *Timeless healing: The power and biology of belief.* New York: Simon & Schuster.

Boutell, K. A., & Bozett, F. W. (1990). Nurses' assessment of patients' spirituality: Continuing education implications. *Journal of Continuing Education in Nursing, 21,* 172–176.

Broten, P. J. (1997). Spiritual care documentation: Where is it? *Journal of Christian Nursing, 14* (2), 29–31.

Burkhardt, M. A., & Nagai-Jacobson, M. G. (1997). In B. M. Dossey (Ed.), *Core curriculum for holistic nursing* (pp. 42–51). Gaithersburg, MD: Aspen.

Burnard, P. (1987). Spiritual distress and the nursing response: Theoretical considerations and counseling skills. *Journal of Advanced Nursing Practice, 12,* 377–382.

Byrne, J. T., & Price, J. H. (1979). In sickness and in health: The effects of religion. *Health Education, 10* (1), 6–10.

Carpenito, L. J. (1997). *Nursing diagnosis: Application to clinical practice* (7th ed.). Philadelphia: Lippincott.

Carson, V. B. (Ed.). (1989). *Spiritual dimensions of nursing practice.* Philadelphia: Lippincott.

Carson, V. B., Wilkelstein, M., Soeken, K., & Brunins, M. (1986). The effect of didactic teaching on spiritual attitudes. *Image, 18,* 161–164.

Castellaw, L. S., Wicks, M. N., & Martin, J. C. (1999). Spirituality in white older women with arthritis. *Graduate Research in Nursing, 1* (2), [On-line], Available: http://www.graduateresearch.com/wicks.htm

Chlan, L., & Tracy, M. F. (1999). Music therapy in critical care: Indications and guidelines for intervention. *Critical Care Nurse, 19*, 35–41.

Clark, C., & Heidenreich, T. (1995). Spiritual care for the critically ill. *American Journal of Critical Care, 4* (1), 77–81

Clinebell, H. (1979). *Growth counseling: Hope-centered methods of actualizing human wholeness.* Nashville: Abingdon.

Conco, D. (1995). Christian patients' views of spiritual care. *Western Journal of Nursing Research, 17*, 266–276.

Cook, T. C. (1980). Preface. In J. A. Thorson & T. C. Cook (Eds.), *Spiritual well-being of the elderly* (pp. xiii–xviii). Springfield, IL: C. C Thomas Publisher.

Corcoran, E. (1993). Spirituality: An important aspect of emergency nursing. *Journal of Emergency Nursing, 19*, 183–184.

Derrickson, B. S. (1996). The spiritual work of the dying: A framework and case studies. *Hospice Journal, 11* (2), 11–30.

Donley, Sr. R. (1991). Spiritual dimensions of health care: Nursing's mission. *Nursing & Health Care, 12*, 178–183.

Dorff, E. N. (1993). Religion at a time of crisis. In M. Z. Cohen & M. B. Whedon (Eds.), Spiritual well-being. *Quality of life: A nursing challenge monograph, 2* (3), 56–59.

Dossey, L. (1993). *Healing words: The power of prayer and the practice of medicine.* New York: HarperCollins.

Dossey, L. (1996). *Prayer is good medicine.* New York: HarperCollins.

Ellison, C. W. (1983). Spiritual well-being: Conceptualization and measurement. *Journal of Psychology and Theology, 11*, 330–339.

Emblen, J. D., & Halstead, L. (1993). Spiritual needs and interventions: Comparing the views of patients, nurses, and chaplains. *Clinical Nurse Specialist, 7*, 175–182.

Evans, K. (1993). Patientview: A mother asks, "Where is your compassion." *Journal of Christian Nursing, 10* (2), 20–22.

Fehring, R. J., Miller, J. F., & Shaw, C. (1997). Spiritual well-being, religiosity, hope, depression, and other mood states in elderly people coping with cancer. *Oncology Nursing Forum, 24*, 663–671.

Field, W. E., & Wilkerson, S. (1973). Religiosity as a psychiatric symptom. *Perspectives in Psychiatric Care, 11*, 99–105.

Fryback, P. B. (1993). Health for people with a terminal diagnosis. *Nursing Science Quarterly, 6*, 147–159.

Gerardi, R. (1989). Western spirituality and health care. In V. B. Carson (Ed.), *Spiritual dimensions of nursing practice* (pp. 76–112). Philadelphia: W. B. Saunders.

Guzzetta, C. E. (1997). Music therapy. In B. M. Dossey (Ed.), *Core curriculum for holistic nursing* (pp. 196–204). Gaithersburg, MD: Aspen Publishers.

Highfield, M. F. (1992). Spiritual health of oncology patients: Nurse and patient perspectives. *Cancer Nursing, 15*, 1–8.

Highfield, M. F. (1997). Spiritual assessment across the cancer trajectory: Methods and reflections. *Seminars in Oncology Nursing, 13*, 237–241.

Highfield, M. E. F., Taylor, E. J., & Amete, M. O. (2000). Preparation to care: The spiritual care education of oncology and hospice nurses. *Journal of Hospice & Palliative Nursing, 2* (2), 53–63.

Hunter, L. L. (1991). *Nursing: A channel for spiritual care* [Videotape]. Tampa, FL: H. Lee Moffitt Cancer Center & Research Institute.

Jaret, P. (1998). Alternatives: Can prayer heal? *Health, 12* (2), 48–49, 54.

Koenig, H. G., & Larson, D. B. (1998). Use of hospital services, religious attendance, and religious affiliation. *Southern Medical Journal, 91,* 925–932.

Kupferschmid, B. J., Briones, T. L., Dawson, C., & Drongowski, C. (1991). Families: A link or a liability? *AACN Clinical Issues in Critical Care Nursing, 2,* 252–257.

Larson, D. B., & Larson, S. S. (1994). *The forgotten factor in physical and mental health: What does the research show? An independent study seminar.* Rockville, MD: National Institute for Healthcare Research.

Lashley, M. E. (1992). Reminiscence: A Biblical basis for telling our stories. *Journal of Christian Nursing, 9* (3), 4–8.

Levin, J. S., & Taylor, R. J. (1997). Age differences in patterns and correlates of the frequency of prayer. *The Gerontologist, 37,* 75–88.

Lewis, C. S. (1980, April). The efficacy of prayer. *HIS Magazine, 40* (7), 16–18. (Reprinted from *The World's Last Night and Other Essays* by C. S. Lewis, 1958, Harcourt Brace Jovanovich, Inc.).

Martin, J. P. (1989). Eastern spirituality and health care. In V. B. Carson (Ed.), *Spiritual dimensions of nursing practice* (pp. 113–131). Philadelphia: W. B. Saunders.

Martin, C., Burrows, C., & Pomilio, J. (1976/1988). Spiritual needs of patients' study. In J. A. Shelly & S. Fish (Eds.), *Spiritual care: The nurse's role* (3rd ed., pp. 160–176). Downers Grove, IL: InterVarsity Press.

Martsolf, D. S. (1997). Cultural aspects of spirituality in cancer care. *Seminars in Oncology Nursing, 13,* 231–236.

Matthews, D. A., Larson, D. B., & Barry, C. P. (Eds.). (1993). *The faith factor: An annotated bibliography of clinical research on spiritual subjects* (Vol. 1). Rockville, MD: National Institute for Healthcare Research.

Moberg, D. O. (1990). Religion and aging. In K. F. Ferraro (Ed.), *Gerontology: Perspectives and issues* (pp. 179–204). New York: Springer Publishing Co.

Murray, R. B., & Zentner, J. P. (1997). *Health assessment & promotion strategies through the life span* (6th ed.). Stamford, CT: Appleton-Lange.

North American Nursing Diagnosis Association. (1999). *Nursing diagnoses: Definitions & classification 1999–2000.* Philadelphia: Author.

Osterman, P., & Schwartz-Barcott, D. (1996). Presence: Four ways of being there. *Nursing Forum, 31,* 23–30.

Pettigrew, J. (1990). Intensive nursing care: The ministry of presence. *Critical Care Nursing Clinics of North America, 2,* 503–508.

Picot, S. J., Debanne, S. M., Namazi, K. H., & Wykle, M. L. (1997). Religiosity and perceived rewards of black and white caregivers. *The Gerontologist, 37,* 89–101.

Piles, C. L. (1990). Providing spiritual care. *Nurse Educator, 15* (1), 36–41.

Reed, P. G. (1991a). Self-transcendence and mental health in oldest-old adults. *Nursing Research, 40,* 5–11.

Reed, P. G. (1991b). Preferences for spiritually related nursing interventions among terminally ill and nonterminally ill hospitalized adults and well adults. *Applied Nursing Research, 4,* 122–128.

Reed, P. G. (1992). An emerging paradigm for the investigation of spirituality in nursing. *Research in Nursing & Health, 15,* 349–357.

Roberts, J. M., Sato, A., & Southwick, W. E. (1999). Spiritual care: A study on the views and practices of psychiatric nurses. *Research for Nursing Practice* [On-line]. Available: http://www.graduateresearch.com/mcroberts.htm

Roof, W. C. (with Greer, B., Johnson, M., Leibson, A., Loeb, K., & Souza, E.). (1994). *A generation of seekers: The spiritual journeys of the baby boom generation.* New York: HarperCollins Publishers.

Rukholm, E., Bailey, P., Coutu-Wakulczyk, G., & Bailey, W. B. (1991). Needs and anxiety levels in relatives of intensive care unit patients. *Journal of Advanced Nursing, 16,* 920–928.

Shelly, J. A., & Fish, S. (1988). *Spiritual care: The nurse's role* (3rd ed.). Downers Grove, IL: Intervarsity Press.

Shelly, J. A., & Miller, A. B. (1999). *Called to care: A Christian theology of nursing.* Downers Grove, IL: Intervarsity Press.

Sicher, F., Targ, E., Moore, D. 2nd, & Smith, H. S. (1998). A randomized double-blind study of the effect of distant healing in a population with advanced AIDS. Report of a small scale study. [On-line abstract]. *Western Journal of Medicine, 169,* 356–363. Available: http://firstsearch.oclc.org/

Sodestrom, K. E., & Martinson I. M. (1987). Patients' spiritual coping strategies: A study of nurse and patient perspectives. *Oncology Nursing Forum, 14,* 41–46.

Stoll, R. I. (1989) The essence of spirituality. In V. B. Carson (Ed.), *Spiritual dimensions of nursing practice* (pp. 4–23). Philadelphia: W. B. Saunders.

Targ, E. (1997). Evaluating distant healing: A research review. *Alternative Therapies in Health and Medicine, 3* (6), 74–78.

Taylor, E. J. (1998). Spiritual and ethical end-of-life concerns [CD-ROM]. In S. L. Groenwald, M. H. Frogge, M. Goodman, & C. H. Yarbro (Eds.), *Cancer nursing: Principles and practice* (4th ed.). Sudbury, MA: Jones and Bartlett Publishers.

Taylor, E. J., Amenta, M., & Highfield, M. (1995). Spiritual care practices of oncology nurses. *Oncology Nursing Forum, 22,* 31–39.

Taylor, E. J., Highfield, M. F., & Amenta, M. (1999). Predictors of oncology and hospice nurses' spiritual care perspectives and practices. *Applied Nursing Research, 12,* 30–37.

Tournier, P. (1972). *Learn to grow old.* New York: Harper & Row.

Travelbee, J. (1971). *Interpersonal aspects of nursing* (2nd ed.). Philadelphia: F. A. Davis.

Tripp-Reimer, T., Johnson, R., & Sorofman, B. (1999). Cultural dimensions in gerontological nursing. In M. Stanley & P. G. Beare (Eds.), *Gerontological nursing: A health promotion/protection approach* (2nd ed., pp. 21–36). Philadelphia: F. A. Davis.

Twibell, R. S., Wieseke, A. W., Marine, M., & Schoger, J. (1996). Spiritual and coping needs of critically ill patients: Validation of nursing diagnoses. *Dimensions of Critical Care Nursing, 15,* 245–253.

Vandecreek, L. (1997). Collaboration between nurses and chaplains for spiritual caregiving. *Seminars in Oncology Nursing, 13,* 279–280.

Waldfogel, S. (1997). Spirituality in medicine. *Primary Care, 24,* 963–976.

Walton, J. (1999). Spirituality of patients recovering from an acute myocardial infarction: A grounded theory study. *Journal of Holistic Nursing, 17,* 34–53.

Weisman, A. D. (1979). *Coping with cancer.* New York: McGraw-Hill.

21

Ethnogeriatric Issues in Critical Care

Lisa Skemp Kelley, Toni Tripp-Reimer, Eunice Choi, and Janet Enslein

Over the past 15 years, critical care nurses have increasingly recognized the importance of patient- and family-centered approaches to the delivery of effective and satisfactory care. Despite this advancement, little formal consideration has been given to the cultural dimension of patient- and family-centered care. For example, the overwhelming majority of recent texts on critical care nursing have ignored the topic of culture. As a result of three interrelated factors, this omission is particularly unfortunate when addressing the needs of critically ill ethnic elders: (a) patient and family cognitions and behaviors are rooted in culture, (b) beliefs related to illness and death are foundationally related to cultural systems, and (c) values concerning life itself, such as autonomy versus dependence, individualism versus family collectivity, and spiritual directions derive from a cultural context. These patterns are seen in the surface structure of behaviors such as communication patterns, pain response, family visitation preferences, patient and family coping styles, and family evaluation of professional care. Critical care nurses generally have little formal preparation in the skills needed to competently address the needs of ethnic/minority patients. Specifically, skills related to modifying interpersonal communication styles, partnering with interpreters, conducting targeted cultural assessments, and negotiating culturally congruent interventions and outcomes are essential for competent critical care practice with ethnic/minority patients.

The proportion of elders in the general population is increasing rapidly, and the proportion of ethnic elders is demonstrating an even faster rate of increase. In 1990 minority elders represented only 13% of all elders in the United States; however, this is projected to increase to 22% by 2020, and 33% by 2050 (United States Department of Health and Human Services, 1993).

Nurses who understand and incorporate cultural aspects into their practice are in a better position to meet the critical care needs of ethnic elders and their families. Ethnogeriatrics is the branch of gerontology that intersects the concepts of aging, health, and ethnicity (Klein, 1995). To enhance the practice of critical care nursing, this chapter first provides an overview of culture and ethnicity. Cultural issues central to the critical care context will then be highlighted. Finally, an overview of assessment and intervention skills essential for the provision of competent care to ethnic elders and their families is presented.

OVERVIEW

Before discussing ethnogeriatric issues in critical care it is important to clarify terms. When discussing ethnic elders a variety of terms are employed including "culture," "race," and "ethnicity." Culture refers to a set of shared beliefs, values, and patterns of behavior of a group of people. The term "ethnicity" is preferred for this chapter because it is a broader concept that encompasses commonalities based on any of the following: national origin (e.g., Greece), race (e.g., Black), religion (e.g., Jewish), or language (e.g., Spanish). Additionally, it is important to recognize intraethnic diversity. Knowing that there is as much variation within groups as between them will mitigate the tendency to stereotype members.

ETHNOGERIATRIC ISSUES IN CRITICAL CARE

Ethnicity is a critical variable in how the care experience is perceived and treated by the patient and family. Cultural factors mediate preferred patterns of interaction. For instance, the meaning of critical illness; whether a particular critical condition is stigmatized or accepted; ways in which symptoms are identified and interpreted, patterns of decision making and preferences for end-of-life care, appropriate modes of expression of pain and discomfort; the use of rituals, traditional healers, and healing practices; and whether the dependency that accompanies an illness is disvalued or considered part of the normal cycle of life. Clearly, ethnicity merits careful consideration in critical care to ensure optimal outcomes.

MEANING OF CRITICAL ILLNESS AND CRITICAL CARE

Ethnicity strongly influences one's definition, recognition, and evaluation of health situations. Determining whether symptoms are sufficiently serious to warrant urgent attention is affected by both ethnicity and age. Ethnic elders often attribute their symptoms to the effects of age, rather than to an illness (Goodwin, Black, & Satish, 1999; Keller, Leventhal, Prohaska, & Leventhal, 1989). For example, elderly Native Americans tend to accept ill health as a part of their old age (Saravanabhavan & Marshall, 1994), and many elderly African Americans do not define a condition as an illness unless it interferes with their functioning (Brangman, 1995). This in part explains the delay in seeking care for urgent health problems. For example, there is considerable variation in the ways different ethnic groups think about and respond to the symptom of chest pain (Goodwin et al., 1999; Kosko & Flaskerud, 1986; Neill. 1993; Strogatz, 1990).

Ethnic groups also differ in the impact of co-morbid conditions on perceived appropriateness of intensive care (ICU) admissions. Considering ICU admissions for persons with dementia, fewer than 50% of Anglos but more than 80% of Mexican Americans endorsed such admissions (Caralis, Davis, Wright, & Marcial, 1993).

Cultural norms affect patients' perception of self in a health crisis. In a study of Taiwanese and Chinese American perceptions of self in an ICU, the majority of patients described a sense of abnormality and loss of face (Shih, 1997). This sense of shame was associated with ICU experiences such as the elders' attempts to remove equipment (e.g., E-T tube) when they were not fully conscious. Other potentially stigmatizing conditions for patients and/or families include diagnoses of elder abuse, suicide attempts, cirrhosis, or cancer (Cheung & Snowden, 1990; Moon & Williams, 1993). Further, although the ICU is viewed as a life-saving environment, it also may be stressful. In a recent study, 90% of Taiwanese ICU patients reported stress resulting from uncertainty and an unfriendly environment. The unfriendly environment included noise, light, lack of privacy, as well as treatment procedures. Beyond the urgent aspects of care, the meaning of the illness, hospitalization, and environment are key considerations in care.

BELIEF SYSTEMS AND ILLNESS BEHAVIORS OF ETHNIC ELDERS AND THEIR FAMILIES

Beliefs

There are multiple complex systems of illness beliefs in each culture that affect the family and ethnic elder's illness behaviors, such as expression of pain and desired/expected treatments (Haley, Han, & Henderson, 1998). All ethnic groups have indigenous health care systems that include methods of prevention, diagnosis, and treatment of health problems as they are diagnosed by and for members of that group. Lay systems of treatment include care by self, family, lay healers (such as herbalists) or indigenous specialists (such as Native American shamen or Mexican American curanderos). Traditional illness beliefs can generally be clustered into those caused by a natural imbalance or supernatural forces. Common examples of imbalance include the hot/cold taxonomy of the circum-Mediterranean area, Mexico, and Central and South American, and the yin/yang taxonomy of Chinese and other Asian groups. Examples of supernatural causes include soul loss or susto among Mexican Americans, evil eye (matiasma) among Greeks, and "castigo" or illness being caused as punishment for sins among Spanish, castigo. Other sources of imbalance include an intrusion of cold into the body through drafts or winds: "mal aire" in Spanish or "wind" (*pung*) in Chinese. When imbalance is the basis for illness, common treatments include herbs, foods, teas, and tonics. When illness results from supernatural causes, therapies are most often of a religious nature, needing the expertise of special healers such as a medicine man or curandero. Beliefs regarding death show wide variation across cultures. For some groups death is a termination or end, for others a transition from one state to another, and for still others a cycle of rebirth and regeneration. For many Christian and Moslem adherents, death is a time of transition into a final stage of eternal life; whereas for many Hindus, death is part of an ongoing cycle of reincarnation.

Beliefs regarding treatments and procedures in the ICU may also vary by ethnic group. For example, beliefs regarding autopsy have been reported to vary dramatically between Anglos and Mexican Americans. In a recent study, Anglos reported that autopsies advance science and improve patient care, whereas Mexican Americans contended that they offered no useful information unless they could help families understand a mysterious death. Further, Mexican Americans reported that discussion of such decisions could be harmful, possibly hastening death. Finally, Anglos reported no harm coming to the deceased person from an autopsy, whereas Mexican Americans believed that the soul remains near the body and can feel the pain associated with the autopsy (Perkins, Supik, & Hazuda, 1993).

The extent to which ethnic elders ascribe to these traditional belief systems and corresponding illness behaviors depends on multiple interacting factors including the elder's generation of immigration, English-language proficiency, access to traditional and scientific practitioners, level of education, and gender. An understanding of the range of illness beliefs and cultural norms provides the basis for understanding patient and family responses to illness and treatment options.

Illness Behaviors

Pain

An understanding of how ethnicity may influence an elder's response to pain is crucial to competent critical care practice. Although all people tend to have about the same threshold for pain (Greenwald, 1991), the expression and interpretation of pain varies dramatically among ethnic groups (Ross, 2000; Zborowski, 1952). Villarruel (1995) found that central aspects of Mexican American's pain experiences included an obligation to bear pain stoically. This contrasts with elder Russian èmigrès who, because of having to demand care assertively in Russia in order to receive scarce health services, often have exaggerated reports of pain (Brod & Heurtin-Roberts, 1992). Ethnic elders' behaviors depend in part on whether stoicism or expressivity is the culturally sanctioned response to pain. Reizian and Meleis (1986) point out that Arab Americans tend to be expressive and vocal in response to pain, but are more expressive with family than with clinicians. They further note that it is the role of family members (more than patients) to request pain medications. If patients do not report discomfort during generally painful situations, it may reflect a cultural norm of stoicism, a reluctance to talk about pain, a difficulty in describing the pain state (e.g., language fluency), an expectation that practitioners should anticipate pain needs and that family members will request pain relief, or that no pain exists. An exaggerated report of pain may reflect a culturally learned behavior of acquiring assistance and health resources, heightened fear that pain relief will not be forthcoming, or that severe pain exists.

Research has advanced our understanding of ethnic pain responses to promote informed care assessment and treatment strategies. In his classic studies, Zborowski (1952, 1969) investigated the relationship among pain, meaning, and behavior in four ethnic groups. Through this work he drew two generalizations: (a) similar reactions to pain manifested by members of different ethnic groups do not necessarily reflect similar attitudes to pain, and (b) reactive behaviors to pain may have different functions and serve different purposes within various cultural groups. Zola (1966) reported on how people from different ethnic groups represent pain symptoms differently. He speculated that ways of communicating illness may reflect major values and preferred ways of handling problems within the culture itself. Subsequent investigations concerned ethnic variation in the meaning of acute versus chronic pain, the implications of the dependency that may accompany severe pain, and variation in pain response (Koopman, Eisenthal, & Stoeckle, 1984; Lipton & Marbach, 1984). In assessing pain, then, it is important to be aware of common patterns of pain expression for various cultural groups. Otherwise, individuals who freely express pain may receive excessive medication and those who are stoic may be undermedicated for pain. Knowledge of the different cultural meanings of and responses to pain can serve as the basis for effective pain control and therapy. The information regarding cultural trends toward stoicism or expressivity provide a foundation for assessment of pain behaviors of the critically ill ethnic elder.

FAMILY SYSTEMS

Patient and family stress occurs with the hospitalization of a critically ill elder, and their coping styles and strategies will be affected by their ethnic affiliation (Rukholm, Bailey, & Coutu-Wakulczyk, 1991). Although particular structural features vary among different ethnic groups, the concept of family is universal. For every ethnic group, the family usually constitutes the most important support system for the elder and provides the social context within which illness occurs. Several diverse features in family structure have direct relevance in critical care units (CCUs). The structure and organization of the family varies widely among American ethnic groups. The identification of the specific individuals who constitute the family is a crucial area of assessment. Family composition and structure will likely influence the support available, how health decisions are made, the availability of persons to stay with and care for a family member, and even who should have visitation rights. A good example of differing familial compositions emerges when examining kinship systems. Among some Native American tribes, first cousins are treated as siblings and some children may have more than two sets of grandparents. Similarly, fictive kin such as godparents or co-parents are highly important in many families of Southern Mediterranean origin (e.g., Greek and Italian). Informal fictive kin are also common in many African American families. These fictive kin may be active family members. Thus, it is important to understand that family members may be broadly defined and do not necessarily conform to the nuclear family or legal boundaries. Two examples of ethnic families will be described to illustrate diversity in structure, organization, and social support. The traditional Mexican American family is very heterogeneous with respect to class, urbanization, and degree of acculturation. Although the multigenerational household has never been the norm for Mexican Americans, the Mexican American elder is substantially more likely than the Anglo elder to live with relatives, and less likely to reside alone or in long-term-care facilities. In traditional rural Mexican American families, three core values have been identified as having particular salience. The first core value is *familism*, an ethic in which the family collective supersedes the needs of any individual family member. Embedded in this concept are the ideals that mutual support (financial, material, caregiving, and social) is available first from the extended kin network. The second core value is *machismo*, which stresses the importance of a man in ensuring the security of the family. Although this value has primarily received a negative portrayal, it more accurately depicts an ethic of courage, honor, and protection of and respect for the family. The third core value is *jerarquismo* (hierarchy) in which the younger family members are subordinate to the older family members, to whom they owe *respecto* (respect). Not only are the elderly supposed to be more highly respected than younger family members, but older siblings have higher authority than younger ones (Burlingame, 1999; Sotomayor, 1990).

On the other hand, Asian societies are typically characterized by a Confucian-influenced ethic of filial piety termed *Hyo* in Korean, *Hsiao* in Chinese, and *Ko* in Japanese (Sung, 1990). For example, in Korea the ethic of filial piety serves as a keystone of social support for the elderly. This norm dictates that elders should be respected and cared for because of their past contributions and sacrifices for the family. Components of filial piety include respect for one's parents, filial responsibility and sacrifice, and maintenance of harmony within the family.

Family definition and structure will influence preferred visitation patterns in the ICU. Many ethnic groups (e.g., Mexican Americans, Hmong, and Old Order Amish) expect family and significant others (some times up to 20 visitors) to accompany an elder to the hospital and for a family member to remain with them during their stay (Mardiros, 1984). Lopez and Hendrickson (1990) reported that physiological improvements in patients occurred during family visits. They attributed this finding to a stress-buffering effect from family social support. Although more research needs to be conducted on visitation effects, nursing assessments can evaluate the effect of visitation on the patient and tailor visitation patterns accordingly. A stabilization of vital signs with visitation likely indicates a salutary effect, whereas increased anxiety and vital-sign destabilization may indicate a need to reduce visitation.

Finally, for a wide variety of ethnic elderly, religion and a sense of spirituality serve as major supports in daily living as well as in times of adversity. Further, local churches and synagogues have increasingly provided more nonreligious social services (Putnam, 2000). These sources of social support—the family, friends, and religious institutions—are significant, particularly for ethnic elderly. As such, they merit inclusion in decision-making aspects of care in areas regarding advanced directives, consent, and visitation.

DECISION MAKING

The principles of autonomy, beneficence, justice, veracity, and fidelity ground Western biomedical ethical standards, promoting patients' rights to be informed and to participate in health decisions. In contrast to Western notions of autonomy, for many ethnic elders the family constitutes the most important social context in which decision making regarding illness, care, consent, and advanced directives occurs and is resolved (Blackhall, Murphy, Frank, Michel, & Azen, 1995). For example, in Japan, harmony and interdependence generally have greater importance than individual autonomy. Individualism is suppressed so that the feelings of togetherness and relatedness have primacy. This emphasis on harmony and interdependence conflicts with the Western bioethics of autonomy, and instead stresses the need for people to be dependent on others such as their family.

All of the structural and organizational features of the family influence patterns of decision making regarding health matters at every stage of an elder's illness, from defining whether the elder is ill, selecting lay consultants or professional practitioners, accepting recommended therapy, and determining whether life-sustaining efforts are warranted. For example, among Hmong, the decision to enter a hospital is often reached only after a family conference (Boult & Boult, 1995). There are important reasons for group decisions in cases dealing with medical treatment. Illness is more than a biological disorder; it is a potential social and economic problem for the entire social group. Because illness affects the entire family it is only logical that the family should be expected to participate in the decision making. This contrasts dramatically with Norwegian Americans who place a high value on individualism and autonomy, and who tend to be much less interdependent in health matters (Tripp-Reimer, 1999).

Health care providers' decisions about who to inform regarding medical diagnoses, terminal illness, treatment risks, and advanced directives requires knowledge of cultural beliefs and norms. Informed consent is grounded in the principle of veracity (truth telling) in the process of disclosing information to patients about their medical diagnosis and prognosis. Yet, informed consent may be in sharp contrast to established cultural norms. For example, Hmong immigrants often believe that discussing a potential health problem before it occurs increases the likelihood of its occurrence (Boult & Boult, 1995). Families may be unwilling to relinquish control over the patient to health care professionals. For example, families of Middle Eastern descent (e.g., Egyptians and Iranians) may be wary of allowing health care professionals to make decisions that might imply that a patient's condition is bleak; they believe that to do so implies that one has given up faith that God has the power to intervene. Additionally, followers of Islam may not permit disclosure of a poor prognosis such as cancer. They believe that this disclosure diminishes the self because it indicates a lack of faith in Allah (Lipson & Hafizi, 1998; Meleis & Meleis, 1998).

In a study of Chinese, Hispanic, African, and Euro Americans, autonomy was not the primary principle that framed health care decisions (Koenig, 1994). Rather, the moral imperative became the obligation of the family to protect the patient's quality of life by not disclosing information. In contrast, in a study of consent agreement, oncologists believed a frank and honest discussion with the patient about their diagnosis and prognosis helped forge a partnership between the patient and the physician (Good, 1991). The physicians emphasized a biomedical understanding of the disease and treatment anchored in Western concepts of legal and ethical ideas of patients' rights.

Blackhall and colleagues (1995) reported important cultural differences in patients' attitudes and preferences toward advance directives. They explored advance care planning among Euro, African, Mexican, and Korean Americans. The Euro and African Americans preferred an autonomous approach to decision making, consistent with mainstream U.S. norms and biomedical practices. In contrast, the Korean and Mexican Americans adopted a family-based decision-making model. Additionally, African

Americans were less likely to complete advance directives than were Euro Americans. Although Tulsky, Cassileth, and Bennett (1997) identified no relationship between frequency of having a DNR (do not resuscitate) order and ethnicity of hospitalized AIDs patients, they did find that African Americans were more likely than Anglos or Latinos to have the orders written later, that is after they were in the hospital for a week or more. Possible reasons for delayed DNR orders in African Americans include a sense of hopelessness, less decision-making control, lower quality care, distrust of the Anglo medical establishment, and poor communication with the physician.

Information regarding end-of-life decisions is not evenly distributed across populations. Physicians may fail to inform some people from non-English speaking or minority ethnic groups (Caralis et al., 1993; Finucane, Shurmway, Powers, & D'Alessandri, 1988). Additionally, a telephone survey of 1,016 people recently discharged from one of four New York hospitals (Mezey, Leitman, Mitty, Bottrell, & Ramsey, 2000), found that most Hispanic patients had never heard of advanced directives. Finally, in a recent review of the literature on end-of-life decision making in adult ICUs, physicians were found to often make end-of-life decisions with minimal input from nurses, patients, or family members (Baggs & Schmitt, 2000). Baggs and Schmitt (2000) anticipate that this practice will increase because of more closed ICUs, cost savings through earlier timing of DNR orders, and increased use of DNR decisions in ICUs. This will continue to place minority elders and family preferences at odds with current practices.

Other common areas of diversity in decision making include withdrawal of care, heroic measures, and organ donation. The withdrawal of life supports (ventilators) or withdrawal of feeding and hydration may be considered purposeful killing by some groups. A recent review concluded that African Americans often disapprove of passive euthanasia, as well as assisted or unassisted suicide for terminal patients (Mouton, Johnson, & Cole, 1995). Although many groups have traditionally believed their religions prohibited organ donation, this is increasingly less so. For example, followers of Islam may now accept organ donations, if the donor consented in writing; adherents of Judaism may require consultation with a rabbi prior to consenting. On the other hand, many ethnic families are concerned that their relatives will be mutilated and suffer, or that their organs will be sold or used for experimentation (McQuay, 1995).

Treatment decisions are often a balancing of expectations deriving from patients' cultural beliefs and those of biomedicine. Use of blood products represents one such situation. Based on Genesis 9:3-6 and Acts 15:28-29, Jehovah's Witnesses believe the act of taking blood is a sin that prohibits entry into Heaven, results in excommunication from the church, and dissolves their relationship with God (Salipante, 1998). Consequently, standard health care practices for human blood transfusion must be modified. Blood substitutes that are acceptable include Hetastarch, crystalloid solutions, and synthetic colloids. Salipante (1998) provides a summary of preop-

362 Social and Policy Issues

erative blood-conservation strategies including adequate preoperative
hemoglobin, erythropoietin, iron and folic acid supplements before surgery. Intraoperative measures include hemodilution, hypothermia, Desmo-
pressin, and Aprotinin; postoperative strategies include the use of
protamine sulfate, aminocaproic acid, erythropoietin, iron, and folic acid.

Interventions generally recommended for ethical decision making at
the end of life include: more sensitive provision of information (such
as linguistically appropriate brochures); improved collaboration among
providers, patients, and families; early discussion of advanced directives for
some groups, and revisiting the discussion as necessary; flexibility in family
access to elder; promotion of continuity of care; support of open communication from patient, family, and significant others; provision of a nonchaotic
environment for family decision making, help for the elder/family to clarify
the patient/family role in decision making; emotional support; education
of families on options; and encouragement of families to communicate
with health care providers (Baggs & Schmitt, 2000).

FAMILY RESPONSE

Because of family beliefs about causality and treatment for critical illnesses,
a family's behaviors in response to a critically ill elder may include the
bringing in of traditional foods or remedies to the ICU. Some of these
foods and remedies may be helpful, some neutral, and others harmful. For
example, among Asian elderly, ginseng is commonly used to retain vitality;
however, it may also have antihypoglycemic effects that may potentiate or
counteract other medications. Further, many herbal drugs used by Asian
elders have anticholinergic properties that make the elders more susceptible to acute confusion (Douglas & Fujimoto, 1995). Some home remedies
commonly used by African Americans also may have considerable health
risks. For example, sassafras root bark contains a hepatotoxic agent, and
sulfur (used to treat dyspnea) can induce metabolic acidosis (Boyd,
Shimp, & Hackney, 1984). Thus, although folk remedies may be an important part of a family's ideal treatment, their use in critical care warrants
close evaluation.

Ethnic elders may use rituals and symbols to give meaning, hope, and
protection to the critical health experience. Within a cultural context,
rituals facilitate an understanding of the contradictory and complex aspects
of human existence. They provide a means of expression and management
of strong emotions by their prescribed and repetitive nature, which eases
feelings of impotence and anxiety (Myerhoff, 1982), and they provide order
and structure at times of chaos and crisis. For example, Taiwanese ICU
patients expressed the need to ask for protection from ancestors/gods
while in the ICU (Shih, 1997). For the critically ill, medallions, icons, or
amulets may be viewed as essential objects to their survival. Symbolic and

ritualistic objects (e.g., Bible, cross) are present in many Western hospital rooms. Each culture has symbols of faith, comfort, and hope.

Rituals or ceremonies may provide comfort, hope, and sustenance for the ethnic elder during critical illness (Cates, 1996; Huttlinger & Tanner, 1994; Tripp-Reimer & Sorofman, 1998). In Western culture the last rites (Anointing of the Sick) for Catholics is one such ceremony that may be used at the time of death as well as for healing. Other examples of healing ceremonies include a joining of the family members and healers (e.g., medicine man, curandero, shaman) with the ill elder. One example is the burning of sage by Lakota (Sioux). For many Native Americans, sage is an herb with strong healing properties: it purifies an area as well as tribal persons who inhale its smoke. Although traditional healers usually do not practice in ICUs, their inclusion should be facilitated on patient/family request. Common practices include prayers, chanting, incense, corn ceremonies, and singing rituals.

Ethnic groups often desire to perform certain rituals immediately before or after death. Most rituals involve rites related to the critically ill elders, assisting them to transition to a different plane. However, some rituals are more for the living, aiding their expression of grief and beginning the breaking of ties to the deceased. Common Islamic rituals at the time of death include facing the elder toward Mecca and ritual washing of the patient, the family praying at the bed of the elder (including the recitation of the Declaration of Faith), preparation of the body by a person of the same sex, and ground burial. Common Hindu rituals include providing the critically ill elder with water from the River Ganges, holy readings and prayers, preparation of the body by the family, gloved handling of the body by nonfamily, and cremation.

Critical care nurses can facilitate healing ceremonies through an awareness and sensitivity to requests of the patient and family; provision of a safe, respectful, and private environment; and flexibility with unit routines. Strategies for staff to facilitate healing ceremonies include an assessment of the benefits and risks of the ceremony. Chrisman (1986) recommends orienting staff and any affected patients to the ceremony. This includes providing information about the purpose, nature, and significance of the ritualistic activities, as well as the length of the ceremony, number of persons involved, space needed, potential noise, and smells that may emerge.

ETHNOGERIATRIC NURSING PRACTICE IN CRITICAL CARE

This section of the chapter focuses on specific practice concepts for culturally competent ethnogeriatric critical care. Communication strategies are discussed, recommendations for problem-focused cultural assessments are highlighted, and culturally appropriate interventions are discussed.

Communication

The ability to establish and maintain rapport is essential for assessment and care of ethnic elders and their families. Rapport is affected by patient and family expectations regarding the nursing role as well as common communication patterns. Expectations affect how patients/families respond to ICU nurses. Some groups' views of nurses are rather rigid; nurses may only be expected to carry out physicians' orders rather than making independent health care judgments. In part, these views may stem from the patient/family's knowledge of nursing in their country of origin. In many Asian hospitals, family members commonly provide all support tasks such as bathing, feeding, and comfort measures for hospitalized persons, whereas the nurses provide strictly medical care such as injections.

Additionally, the degree of intimacy influences the interaction among ethnic elders, family members, and health care professionals. This intimacy may range from a preference for very formal interaction to a need for a close personal relationship with the health professional. For example, Southeast Asians often expect the health professional to be an authoritarian or directive figure. The professional is often viewed as a social "superior" and this may produce the potential for problematic communication. The emphasis on social harmony may prevent the Southeast Asian client from fully expressing concerns or feelings. It may also give the health care professional the impression that the client agrees with or understands a discussion when in fact his or her nodding or smiling may only reflect a desire for interpersonal harmony (Tripp-Reimer, 1984; Uba, 1992). In contrast, Mediterranean and Middle Eastern patients seek a greater degree of intimacy. They may seek to draw health practitioners into their family system, involving them in personal activities and social functions. When relationships are well established, they may also call their health care professional during nonwork hours (Lipson & Meleis, 1983).

Health care professionals may overlook an important information source if they are unaware of the meaning of a client's nonverbal behavior. Volume, speed, and directness of conversation are influenced by cultural values. Many groups value indirectness and subtly in speech. Other important features include facial expression, handshaking, silence, eye contact, and proxemics. For example, Clark (1983) describes an elderly Soviet woman who interpreted nurses' smiles as gestures of insolence and lack of seriousness. On the other hand, smiling and handshaking may be integral parts of sincere interactions among Hispanic clients.

The meaning of silence may also vary considerably. For some groups silence is extremely uncomfortable, and they attempt to fill in every gap in the conversation. In contrast, many Native Americans often consider silence essential to understanding: they believe a person needs to fully consider what another has said before giving a response. When traditional Chinese and Japanese are silent it does not necessarily indicate that they have completed talking; it may mean they wish the nurse to consider the content of what they have said before continuing. Asian cultures often view silence as a sign of respect for elders. Many ethnic groups, such as Native Americans and Appalachians, may view direct eye contact as impolite or aggressive and may avert their eyes during an interview. Health professionals may misunderstand this nonverbal behavior. Intensity or volume of speech may also lead to disharmony between patient/family and nurse. Asians or Native American clients may view health practitioners as loud and boisterous.

There are several other important considerations in promoting rapport between individuals from different cultures. In the majority of health care settings, and in particular in the ICU, nurses are perceived as having a position of power relative to the patient; therefore, nurses must understand their mandate to initiate dialogue. This dialogue should be initiated in the preferred communication style of the cultural group. When possible, the patient's primary language should be used.

A common language helps to communicate both content and empathy. When the patient's primary language is not the same as the nurse's, two main options are available. The first is the use of an interpreter. Suggestions of interpreter alternatives are provided in Table 21.1. Interpretation is a complex process that involves a person speaking in one language and another person speaking in a different language with an interpreter deciphering two linguistic codes with separate cultural and sociopolitical characteristics and producing an equivalent message (Enslein, Tripp-Reimer, Kelley, Choi, in press). According to Title VI of the Civil Rights Act of 1964 and the 1998 Guidance Memorandum, interpretation services are to be provided at no cost or additional burden to the persons who are receiving services from any federally assisted program. With this mandate it is essential that the critical care nurse use interpreters if available, and work with the health care agency to make them available if they are not.

Problem-Focused Cultural Assessment

In providing care to families dealing with a critical illness, cultural assessment is an essential area of clinical practice. Within the health care literature, a number of guidelines for the content and process of cultural assessment have been established. A complete cultural assessment may include eliciting information regarding patterns of communication, family structure and relations, religion, values, health beliefs and behaviors. These guidelines however, suffer from a lack of clinical applicability because of time constraints, especially in the critical care environment. Furthermore, it is rare that an exhaustive cultural assessment will be necessary in most clinical situations. Cultural assessment should be tailored to the presenting care issue and associated intervention areas (see Table 21.2). This assessment is conducted with an awareness that cultural affiliation provides a

TABLE 21.1 Interpreter Alternatives

Interpreter alternatives	Description	Strengths	Limitations
Professional interpreters on staff	• Agency employs and trains interpreters who are available for interpreting languages that are most frequently represented in the particular patient population.	• Available during operating hours. • Consistent personnel foster rapport and trust with clients and health care providers.	• Not a feasible, cost-effective alternative for small agencies. • Not all languages covered.
On-call interpreters	• Agency maintains a list of interpreters of various languages who are willing to interpret as need arises. • May be paid or volunteer.	• Covers a broader variety of languages.	• May have questionable interpretation abilities unless the agency has a method of testing each person. • May be trained or untrained. • Untrained interpreters make more errors: omissions of pertinent information, additions of information that the client did not say, substitutions of information, condensed summaries that omit details, and breeches of confidentiality. • Dependent upon the availability of the interpreter at the time one is needed.

TABLE 21.1 *(continued)*

Interpreter alternatives	Description	Strengths	Limitations
Bilingual staff	• Health care staff (nurses) or support staff (e.g., dietary aides or security personnel) are temporarily utilized as the need arises to interpret for patients with whom they would otherwise have no contact.	• Availability	• Inconsistent availability • May experience conflict of duties between the roles for which they were hired and the ad hoc interpreter duties. May create resentment in staff member or co-workers. • May be unfamiliar with specialized vocabulary. • Usually untrained. • Untrained interpreters make more errors: omissions of pertinent information, additions of information that the client did not say, substitutions of information, condensed summaries that omit details, and breeches of confidentiality. • Inconsistent ability
Family members or friends	• Family or friends who accompany the patient to the agency are used as interpreters	• Availability	• Untrained, thus likely to make errors (see above). • Usually unfamiliar with specialized vocabulary.

(continued)

TABLE 21.1   *(continued)*

Interpreter alternatives	Description	Strengths	Limitations
			• May interfere with family dynamics, confidentiality, or revelation of sensitive information. • Use of children for interpretation is never appropriate except in emergency situations until other alternatives can be arranged.
Telephone interpreter services	• Language Line Service (formerly AT&T Language Line Service; 1-800-752-0093) provides over-the-phone interpretation for agency or individual use. Agencies needing at least 20 minutes of interpretation per month would establish Subscribed Interpretation that involves a $200 set-up fee, and at least $50 charges per month for usage. Interpretation rates range from $2.20 to $4.50 per minute based upon the language and time of day (Language Line Service, 1999).	• Covers over 140 languages • Available 24 hours/day, 7 days/week. • Interpreters are native speakers with training in interpretation and basic health care terminology. • Rapid access. • Training kit for users includes a video and quick reference guides.	• Speaker phone needed for easiest use. • Requires prior arrangement by agency to establish an account. • Interpreters may or may not be trained in mental health applications.

TABLE 21.1 *(continued)*

Interpreter alternatives	Description	Strengths	Limitations
On-line translation services	• Internet Web sites that translate typed statements into other languages. An example is Babylon.com	• Immediate 24 hours/day availability.	• Requires a computer with internet access. • Requires that the client be able to read, and to type responses. • Diaz-Duque (1999) has found them to be ineffective. Simple statements translate well; however the more complicated or ambiguous the statement, the more likely that the translation will be incorrect or incomprehensible.
Interpretation software	• Interlingua computer software is a developing technology that will interpret conversation as it occurs. The developers at Carnegie Mellon University explain that the programs are context dependent and must be developed for specific types of situations (McCollum, 1999). May be a future alternative.	• Private	• Immediate access • Not currently available for health care applications. • Requires computer with audio input and output, and internet access.

©Janet Enslein 1999.

TABLE 21.2   Problem Focused Cultural Assessment

Assessment	Issues	Assessment example* Data from intake interview with patient, her eldest son, daughter-in-law, and daughter.
General assessment Overview of patient and family cultural characteristics and issues	• Ethnicity • Length of time in the United States • Degree of affiliation with ethnic group • Religion • Expected/Preferred level of participation • Pattern of decision-making (individual, family, contact person) • Preferred communication style(s)	• 76 y/o Korean American woman • Immigrated in 1972 under Immigration Act of 1965. • Speaks limited English. Lives in urban Korean enclave with eldest son and daughter-in-law. • Buddhist • Daughter-in-law is the primary hands on care provider whenever she has health problems. • Son is primary decision-maker • Formal greeting (Mrs.). Prefers that you address son with any questions. Indirect eye contact. Son and daughter-in-law also request written information.
Problem-specific assessment Information with reference to the specific health problem (e.g. pain, disclosure of terminal illness, death preparation)	• Meaning of the critical health problem • Explanation as to cause(s) of the critical health problem (individual and family member(s)). • Impact of the critical health problem on the family system	• Uncontrolled angina secondary to severe myocardial infarction explained as *Ah-poom nida* (severe pain) caused by imbalance (too much worry) and bad luck.

TABLE 21.2 *(continued)*

Assessment	Issues	Assessment example* Data from intake interview with patient, her eldest son, daughter-in-law, and daughter.
		• Family values of cohesion, interdependence, and harmony upset with elder's uncontrolled pain. The patient used to care for her grandchildren when her daughter-in-law was at work. Now, because of her illness, the family is looking for someone to take care of the grandchildren. Furthermore, the daughter-in-law cannot go to work because she is expected to stay with her mother-in-law. • Family members at bedside.
Intervention-specific evaluation assessment Information with reference to management of the specific health problem(s)	• What things did they or others do to manage/treat the health problem in the past (e.g. acute pain treatments, management of dyspnea, healing rituals, death preparations)? • How do they expect the problem to be treated in the ICU (desire for biomedical and/or traditional treatments, rituals and symptom management)?	• Does not drink cold or iced fluids to prevent imbalance and pain. • Uses *hanyak* (herbal medicine) and a *hanui* (medicine doctor) who has provided acupuncture for her pain. • With pain often cries, moans and will flail about. Does not respond to the pain scale for expressing pain. Will talk of "great suffering."

(continued)

TABLE 21.2 *(continued)*

Assessment	Issues	Assessment example* Data from intake inter-view with patient, her el-dest son, daughter-in-law, and daughter.
		• Expects medicine will be given to relieve the pain (preferably PO and IV). • Expects to remain in bed and that a family member (preferably the daughter-in-law) will remain nearby to provide for needs.
Intervention-specific evaluation assessment Information regard-ing patient (family) and provider ex-pected outcomes (ef-fects) of treatment for the specific criti-cal care problem.	• Clarification of ex-pected outcomes and evaluation criteria • Strategies to re-negoti-ate intervention spe-cific	• Son states that he ex-pects his mother will be without pain, this means that she is able to rest, eat and sleep comfortably. • The son is the pri-mary decision-maker, however, he will of-ten consult with his siblings and other family members. Con-sequently, extra time may be needed for him to make deci-sions.

*Adapted from Reardon (1996). *Koreans.* In J. Lipson, S. Dibble, and P. Minarik, *Culture & nursing care: A pocket guide* (pp. 191–202). San Francisco, CA: UCSF Nursing Press.

background or clues for assessment, but each ethnic elder and his or her family must be approached as individuals whose cultural affiliation is influenced by rate of acculturation, as well as personal adherence to the cultural system. There are excellent handbooks that can be placed in the ICU reference area that provide short cultural overviews to assist nurses in gaining rapid general knowledge about specific ethnic groups. Two excel-lent resources are Lipson, Dibble, and Minarik (1996), *Culture and Nursing Care: A Pocket Guide* and Purnell and Paulanka (1998), *Transcultural Health Care: A Culturally Competent Approach.*

A cultural assessment is a systematic appraisal of beliefs, values, and practices conducted in order to determine the context of client needs to best tailor nursing interventions. In the first stage of cultural assessment, the nurse performs a general assessment to obtain an overview of the characteristics of the client and identifies areas that potentially require more in-depth assessment. Topics included at this level include ethnicity, degree of affiliation with ethnic group, religion, patterns of decision making, and preferred communication styles (Tripp-Reimer, Brink, & Saunders, 1984).

Subsequently, the nurse elicits cultural information that is problem or situation specific. That is, the nurse obtains information with reference to the pertinent clinical domain (e.g., heart failure, diabetes, or end-of-life care). At this level, the nurse, the patient's and family's beliefs about the problem, previous as well as anticipated treatment, and prognosis are explored.

The next phase of the initial assessment is directed at eliciting detailed cultural factors that may influence intervention strategies. For example, consider that an elder is undergoing surgery, information on decision-making patterns, consent, acceptable treatment options (e.g., use of blood products), and organ donation may be warranted. On the other hand, if postdischarge cardiac rehabilitation and dietary education are the planned intervention, then detailed information would be collected regarding the elder's access to transportation, safe environments for walking, current and preferred diet, specifics regarding food preparation (including who does the preparation and when meals are eaten), and the meaning of food in the life of the elder.

Evaluation is the next phase of a focused cultural assessment. The views of patient and family are integral to evaluating the planned interventions. Evaluation is best carried out through clarification of outcome criteria that are congruent with patient, family, and provider health expectations. With ongoing changes in critical care, negotiation of intervention and treatment goals are essential.

SUMMARY

Cultural competence builds on the concepts of cultural awareness, knowledge, and sensitivity with the goal of providing culturally appropriate interventions. With the rapid increase in the proportion of ethnic elders in the United States, cultural competencies are increasingly important in critical care settings. Patient and family beliefs about a particular illness, appropriate therapies, death, and the role of families may provide points of conflict with ICU staff or opportunities to provide tailored family-focused care. This chapter has provided a brief introduction and examples of ways in which the cultural dimension may affect the ICU experience. It has also provided suggestions for enhancing intercultural communication and conducting focused cultural assessments in critical care environments. These strategies should aid in partnering health care providers and ethno-geriatric patients and their families.

REFERENCES

Baggs, J. G., & Schmitt, M. H. (2000). End-of-life decisions in adult intensive care: Current research base and directions for the future. *Nursing Outlook, 48,* 158–164.

Blackhall, L. J., Murphy, S. T., Frank, G., Michel, V., & Azen, S. (1995). Ethnicity and attitudes toward patient autonomy. *Journal of the American Medical Association, 274,* 820–825.

Boult, L., & Boult, C. (1995). Underuse of physician services by older Asian-Americans. *Journal of the American Geriatrics Society, 43,* 408–411.

Boyd, E. L., Shimp, L. A., & Hackney, M. J. (1984). *Home remedies and the Black elderly: A reference manual for health care providers.* Ann Arbor, MI: University of Michigan Press.

Brangman, S. A. (1995). African-American elders: Implications for health care providers. *Clinics in Geriatric Medicine, 111,* 15–24.

Brod, M., & Heurtin-Roberts, S. (1992). Cross-cultural medicine a decade later. Older Russian èmigrès and medical care. *Western Journal of Medicine, 157,* 333–336.

Burlingame, V. S. (1999). *Ethnogerocounseling: Counseling ethnic elders and their families.* New York: Springer Publishing Co.

Caralis, P. V., Davis, B., Wright, K., & Marcial, E. (1993). The influence of ethnicity and race on attitudes toward advance directives, life-prolonging treatments, and euthanasia. *Journal of Clinical Ethics, 4,* 155–165.

Cates, P. (1996, August). Secret ceremony. What was happening in room 319? *Nursing96,* 72.

Cheung, F. K., & Snowden, L. R. (1990). Community mental health and ethnic minority populations. *Community Mental Health Journal, 20,* 277–291.

Chrisman, N. (1986). Transcultural care. In D. Zschoche (Ed.), *Mosby's comprehensive review of critical care* (pp. 58–69). St. Louis, MO: Mosby.

Clark, M. (1983). Cultural context of medical practice. *Western Journal of Medicine, 139,* 806–810.

Diaz-Duque, O. F. (1999, December). Interpreters in health care settings: Cultural and language issues. Paper presented at the University of Iowa Hospital School, Iowa City, IA.

Douglas, K. C., & Fujimoto, D. (1995). Asian Pacific elders: Implications for health care providers. *Clinics in Geriatric Medicine, 111,* 69–82.

Enslein, J., Tripp-Reimer, T., Kelley, L., & Choi, E. (in press). *Evidence based protocols.* Iowa City, IA: University of Iowa Gerontological Nursing Interventions Center.

Finucane, T. E., Shurmway, J. M., Powers, R. L., & D'Alessandri, R. M. (1988). Planning with elderly outpatients for contingencies of severe illness: A survey and clinical trial. *Journal of General Internal Medicine, 3,* 322–325.

Good, M. D. (1991). The practice of biomedicine and the discourse on hope: A preliminary investigation into the culture of American oncology. In B. Pfleiderer & G. Bibeau (Eds.), *Anthropologies of medicine: A colloquium on West European and North American perspectives* (pp. 121–136). Heidelberg, Germany: Vieweg, Bertelsmann.

Goodwin, J. S., Black, S. A., & Satish, S. (1999). Aging versus disease: The opinions of older Black, Hispanic, and Non-Hispanic White Americans about the causes and treatment of common medical conditions. *Journal of the American Geriatrics Society, 47*, 973–979.

Greenwald, H. P. (1991). Interethnic differences in pain perception. *Pain, 44*, 157–163.

Haley, W., Han, B., & Henderson, J. (1998). Aging and ethnicity: Issues for clinical practice. *Journal of Clinical Psychology in Medical Settings, 5*, 393–409.

Huttlinger, K., & Tanner, D. (1994). The Peyote way: Implications for culture care theory. *Transcultural Nursing Society, 5* (2), 5–11.

Keller, M., Leventhal, H., Prohaska, T., & Leventhal, E. (1989). Beliefs about aging and illness in a community sample. *Research in Nursing and Health, 12*, 247–255.

Klein, S. (Ed.). (1995). *A national agenda for geriatric education: White papers* (Vol. 1). Rockville, MD: U.S. Department of Health & Human Services Public Health Service, Health Resources & Services Administration Bureau of Health Professions.

Koenig, B. A. (1994). Cultural diversity in decision-making about care at the end of life. In *Dying, decision-making, and appropriate care* (pp. 1–18). Washington, DC: Institute of Medicine, National Academy of Science.

Koopman, C., Eisenthal, S., & Stoeckle, J. D. (1984). Ethnicity in the reported pain, emotional distress and requests of medical outpatients. *Social Science and Medicine, 18*, 487–490.

Kosko, D. A., & Flaskerud, J. H. (1986). Mexican American, nurse practitioner, and lay control group beliefs about cause and treatment of chest pain. *Nursing Research, 36*, 226–231.

Lipson, J., Dibble, S., & Minarik, P. (Eds.). (1996). *Culture & nursing care: A pocket guide.* San Francisco, CA: UCSF Nursing Press.

Lipson, J., & Meleis, A. (1983). Issues in health care of Middle Eastern patients. *Western Journal of Medicine, 139*, 854–861.

Lipson, J. G., & Hafizi, H. (1998). Iranians. In L. D. Purnell & B. J. Paulanka (Eds.), *Transcultural health care: A culturally competent approach* (pp. 323–351). Philadelphia: F. A. Davis.

Lipton, J., & Marbach, J. (1984). Ethnicity and the pain response. *Social Science and Medicine, 19*, 1279–1298.

Lopez, J., & Hendrickson, S. (1990). Family visits and different cultures. *Axon, 12* (3), 59–62.

Mardiros, M. (1984). A view toward hospitalization: The Mexican American experience. *Journal of Advanced Nursing, 9*, 469–478.

McCollum, K. (1999). A computer program provides spontaneous translation in multiple languages. *Chronicle of Higher Education, 45* (49), A28.

McQuay, J. E. (1995). Appendix. Cross-cultural customs and beliefs related to health crises, death, and organ donation/transplantation: A guide to assist health care professionals understand different responses and provide cross-cultural assistance. *Critical Care Nursing Clinics of North America, 7*, 581–594.

Meleis, A. I., & Meleis, M. (1998). Egyptian-Americans. In L. D. Purnell & B. J. Paulanka (Eds.), *Transcultural health care: A culturally competent approach* (pp. 217–243). Philadelphia: F. A. Davis.

Mezey, M., Leitman, R., Mitty, E., Bottrell, M., & Ransey, G. (2000). Why hospital patients do and do not execute an advance directive. *Nursing Outlook, 48*, 165–171.

Moon, A., & Williams, O. (1993). Perceptions of elder abuse and help-seeking patterns among African-American, Caucasian American, and Korean-American elderly women. *Gerontologist, 33,* 386–395.

Mouton, D. P., Johnson, M. S., & Cole, D. R. (1995). Ethical considerations with African-American elders. *Clinics in Geriatric Medicine, 11* (1), 113–129.

Myerhoff, B. (1982). Rites of passage: Process and paradox. In V. Turner (Ed.), *Celebration: Studies in festivity and ritual* (pp. 108–135). Washington, DC: Smithsonian Institute Press.

Neill, K. (1993). Ethnic pain styles in acute myocardial infarction. *Western Journal of Nursing Research, 15,* 531–547.

Perkins, H. S., Supik, J. D., & Hazuda, H. P. (1993). Autopsy decisions: The possibility of conflicting cultural attitudes. *Journal of Clinical Ethics, 4,* 145–154.

Putnam, R. D. (2000). *Bowling alone. The collapse and revival of American community.* New York: Simon & Schuster.

Reizian, A., & Meleis, A. (1986). Arab-Americans' perceptions of and responses to pain. *Critical Care Nurse, 6* (6), 30–37.

Ross, H. (2000, August). Studies explore patient, physician perspectives on treating pain effectively. *Closing the Gap,* 7–8.

Rukholm, E., Bailey, P., & Coutu-Wakulczyk, G. (1991). Family needs and anxiety in ICU: Cultural differences in Northeastern Ontario. *Canadian Journal of Nursing Research, 23* (3), 67–81.

Salipante, D. (1998). Refusal of blood by a critically ill patient: A healthcare challenge. *Critical Care Nurse, 18* (2), 68–76.

Saravanabhavan, R. C., & Marshall, C. A. (1994). The older native American Indian with disabilities: Implications for providers of health care and human services. *Journal of Multicultural Counseling and Development, 22,* 182–194.

Shih, F. (1997). Perception of self in the intensive care unit after cardiac surgery among adult Taiwanese and American-Chinese patients. *International Journal of Nursing Studies, 34* (1), 17–26.

Sotomayor, M. (1990). *In triple jeopardy: Aged Hispanic women.* Washington, DC: National Hispanic Council on Aging.

Strogatz, D. (1990). Use of medical care for chest pain: Differences between Blacks and Whites. *American Journal of Public Health, 80,* 290–294.

Sung, T. (1990). A new look at filial piety: Ideals and practices of family-centered parent care in Korea. *Gerontologist, 30,* 610–617.

Tripp-Reimer, T. (1984). Cultural assessment. In J. Bellack & P. Bamford (Eds.), *Nursing assessment: A multidimensional approach* (pp. 226–246). Monterey, CA: Wadsworth Health Sciences.

Tripp-Reimer, T. (1999). Culturally competent care. In M. Wykle & A. B. Ford (Eds.), *Serving minority elders in the 21st century* (pp. 235–247). New York: Springer Publishing Co.

Tripp-Reimer, T., Brink, P., & Saunders, J. (1984). Cultural assessment: Content and process. *Nursing Outlook, 32,* 78–82.

Tripp-Reimer, T., & Sorofman, B. (1998). Greek-Americans. In L. D. Purnell & B. J. Paulanka (Eds.), *Transcultural health care: A culturally competent approach* (pp. 301–322). Philadelphia: F. A. Davis Company.

Tulsky, J., Cassileth, B., & Bennett, C. (1997). The effect of ethnicity on ICU use and DNR orders in hospitalized AIDS patients. *Journal of Clinical Ethics, 8,* 150–157.

Uba, L. (1992). Cultural barriers to health care for Southeast Asian Refugees. *Public Health Reports, 107,* 544–548.

United States Department of Health and Human Services. (1993). *Toward equality of well being: Strategies for improving minority health* (DHHS Pub. # 93-50217). Washington, DC: U.S. Government Printing Office.

Villarruel, A. (1995). Mexican-American cultural meanings, expressions, self-care and dependent-care actions associated with experiences of pain. *Research in Nursing & Health, 18*, 427–436.

Zborowski, M. (1952). Cultural components in response to pain. *Journal of Social Issues, 8* (4), 16–30.

Zborowski, M. (1969). *People in pain.* San Francisco: Jossey-Bass.

Zola, I. K. (1966). Culture and symptoms: An analysis of patients' presenting complaints. *American Sociological Review, 31*, 615–630.

22

Legal Issues

Gloria C. Ramsey

Professional communities around the globe are struggling with legal and bioethical dilemmas brought about by the advances in medicine and technology. From the beginning of life to the end of life, the advances in technology and medicine influence the way health care professionals provide care and the expectation of patients and families. As a result of these advances, issues concerning end-of-life decision making have become increasingly more significant for health care professionals—particularly nurses. Questions concerning self-determination and decision making related to termination of life-sustaining treatment, care of the dying, decision-making capacity, and allocation of scarce resources have sparked much debate while bringing nurses into daily contact with potential ethical and legal dilemmas.

Geriatric nursing care is eminently more important because Americans are living longer, and nurses see the "best" case and "worst" case of the use and abuse of our technology. Technology has resulted in our ability to substantially prolong the lives of seriously ill elderly persons. For example, cardiopulmonary resuscitation (CPR), mechanical respiration, and tube and intravenous feedings offer substantial opportunities to extend the lives of elderly persons. Thus, for the geriatric critical care nurse, questions arise, such as: Do patients have a "right to die." How should patients be involved in the decision-making process regarding their own care? What is the role of the nurse in making these decisions? Who is best able to make decisions for the patients if they are unable to speak for themselves? When, if ever, should life-sustaining treatments be withheld or withdrawn? When, if ever, should caregivers' ethical and moral beliefs override the beliefs and values of the patient? Can and should caregivers be able to make treatment decisions? Should issues of cost and allocation of resources affect treatment decisions?

Because nurses are legally responsible and accountable for the health care patients and families receive, nurses must know the relevant laws affecting the elderly and address the current controversies to ensure that individual rights are protected. In this chapter, legal implications of end-of-life care and implications for geriatric nurses are discussed.

IS LAW THE SAME AS ETHICS?

Law and ethics are similar in that they have developed in the same historical, social, cultural, and philosophical soil (Davis, Aroskar, Liaschenko, & Drought, 1997). Black's *Law Dictionary* defines law as "that which is laid down, ordained, or established; a body of rules of action or conduct prescribed by controlling authority and having binding legal forces; and that which must be obeyed and followed by citizens subject to sanctions or legal consequences" (1990, pp. 884–885). The law may be better defined as the sum total of rules and regulations by which a society is governed. Ethics, as discussed in an earlier chapter, are informal or formal rules of behavior that guide individuals or groups of people.

In other words, legal rights are grounded in the law and ethical rights are grounded in ethical principles and values. The law establishes rules that define a person's rights and obligations and the appropriate penalty for those who violate it. The law describes how government will enforce the rules and penalties. Legal obligations are not new to geriatric critical care nurses. There are many laws that affect the practice of nursing, and nurses must be able to differentiate ethical issues from those that are strictly legal or clinical.

THE LAW AND ADVANCED CARE PLANNING: PURPOSE AND TYPES OF ADVANCE DIRECTIVES

At the onset, let it be said that decisions about advance care planning, and especially about forgoing treatment, call for careful thinking and communication. Decisions about care at the end of life ought to be made in accordance with an individual's wishes, preferences, beliefs, and values. The decision is not about what you would do, but what the individual's wishes are. No one should be subject to medical care against his or her wishes. Accordingly, it is to support this view that the law related to end-of-life care was established.

Nurses must know that each state has its own law regarding the use of advance directives (see Appendix A). Nurses should know the formalities for executing an advance directive, which type is recognized in the state they practice, and what limitations there are, if any, for honoring an advance directive.

Purpose

Meisel (1995) argues that advance directives have three major purposes. First, advance directives are a mechanism by which individuals can exercise control over their bodies. This document will allow individuals to direct the kind of medical care they want or do not want in the event that they do not have the decisional capacity when a decision needs to be made. Advance directives generally are discussed in the context of the right to forgo life-sustaining treatments; however, they also may be used to direct the administration of treatment. Advance directives are intended to effect a person's own choice and self-determination even when the individual no longer possesses this capacity (Meisel, 1995).

Second, advance directives provide guidance, especially to health care professionals, regarding how to proceed with decision making about life-sustaining treatment in the face of diminished capacity. When patients lack decision-making capacity, a great deal of confusion can arise in the clinical setting as to how health care decisions are to be made, who has the authority to make them, and what the treatment decisions should be. Advance directives empower health care professionals to proceed with a clinical decision making and not rely on the court for intervention.

Third, advance directives provide immunity from civil and criminal liability, under certain circumstances. All advance directive statutes contain provisions that grant immunity to health care professionals when they act in good faith and in accordance with state statutes respecting advance directives (Meisel, 1995). Because more and more judicial opinions evolve out of the advance directive legislation, this provision is most important.

Types of Advance Directives

When discussing advance directives, know that there are two types: the living will and the durable power of attorney for health care.

Living Wills

A living will is a directive that documents specific instructions to health care providers about particular kinds of health care treatment an individual would or would not want to prolong life. Generally, living wills are used to declare wishes to refuse, limit, or withhold life-sustaining treatment under certain circumstances should the individual become incapacitated and is unable to communicate. An individual may execute a living will to instruct health care professionals not to administer any "extraordinary treatment," "heroic treatment," "artificial treatment," or "life support" in the event of terminal illness. Furthermore, living wills also can be used to give instructions about what kind of treatment an individual wants to have administered (Meisel, 1995). Although most states have detailed living will statutes, living wills are not recognized by statute in New York, Massachusetts, and Michigan (Meisel, 2000).

Durable Power of Attorney for Health Care

A Durable Power of Attorney for Health Care (DPAHC) is a document that permits an individual to designate another person to make health care decisions for them should they lose decision-making capacity. The person who is appointed by the patient to make decisions is called a health care proxy, health care agent, attorney-in-fact, or surrogate. The term "durable power of attorney" should be used to refer to the document used to appoint this person. The language used varies from state to state, and nurses must become familiar with their own state's language.

One major distinction that nurses should know about between a DPAHC and a living will is that the DPAHC may be used for all health care decisions and not limited to withholding or withdrawing life-sustaining treatment. A DPAHC does not require that an individual know in advance all the decisions that may arise. A health-care proxy can interpret and carry out the patient's wishes as medical circumstances change and can make treatment decisions when need be.

One important fact for nurses to be mindful of is that advance directives are effective only when it is determined that the individual is incompetent or lacks decision making. As long as the patient retains decision-making capacity, his or her decisions should govern. When the patient is deemed to lack decision-making capacity, the health care proxy is authorized to make treatment decisions on behalf of the patient and in accordance with the patient's stated wishes. The health care proxy is bound to make the kinds of decisions the patient would make had he or she the capacity to do so. In situations in which the patient has never been competent, or there is no clear and convincing evidence of what the person would have wanted, the health care proxy is to make decisions in the "best interest" of the patient.

Combination Directives

A number of states have a single advance directive statute that combines elements of a living will and a DPAHC into a single document. A combination document arguably avoids many of the pitfalls of each document alone. If the instructions are too general, the health care proxy has the authority to determine whether instructions should be applied under the specific circumstances. If the instructions are too specific and do not address the particular situation at hand, the health care proxy has the discretion to apply them or not. Nurses should advise patients that they should have a discussion with their health care proxy, informing them that they have been named and what role they wish the health care proxy to assume. Communication is the most effective way to ensure that the patient's wishes are known and that the health care proxy is aware of the appointment.

Oral Advance Directives

Although a written advance directive is preferable, courts view oral advance directives favorably, especially living wills. Even when state statutes recognize written advance directives, oral directives have been found to be legally operative in a number of jurisdictions. The more specific the oral advance directive, the more likely it is to be enforced and have clinical and legal significance.

Family Consent Laws

Many people are under the impression that their family members will be allowed to make the proper decisions for them should the need arise and therefore, see no need to formally execute an advance directive (Furrow, Greaney, Johnson, Soltzfus, & Schwartz, 1995). Traditionally, health-care professionals and the courts have also relied on families to make health care decisions for family members, without any legal authority. In 1983, the President's Commission concluded that, given this practice, family decision making had gained and should be accorded legal acceptance. The Commission pointed out five reasons why deference to family members is appropriate when done in consultation with the physician and other health care professionals:

1. The family is generally most concerned about the good of the patient.
2. The family usually is the most knowledgeable about the patient's goals, preferences, and values.
3. The family deserves recognition as an important social unit that, within limits, ought to be treated as a responsible decision maker in matters that intimately affect its members.
4. Especially in a society in which many other traditional forms of community have eroded, participation in a family often is an important dimension of personal fulfillment.
5. Because a protected sphere of privacy and autonomy is required for the flourishing of this interpersonal union, institutions and the state should be reluctant to intrude, particularly regarding matters that are personal and on which there is a wide range of opinion in society.

Family consent statutes vary from state to state. Some have been added to state living will statutes to provide an alternative mechanism for making life-sustaining treatment decisions for individuals who do not have an advance directive; others are free-standing statutes that apply to either life-sustaining treatment or health-care decisions generally.

THE PATIENT SELF-DETERMINATION ACT

Another law—the first federal law to focus on advance directives and the right of adults to refuse life-sustaining treatment—is the Patient Self-Determination Act (PSDA) of 1991. The PSDA, effective as of December 1, 1991, was motivated by concerns that in the absence of clear directives regarding views on life-sustaining treatment, patients do not have their views respected when they become incapacitated. Thus, it was the intent of Congress vis-à-vis this law to require that facilities participating in the Medicare and Medicaid program must provide written information to individuals about their right to participate in medical decision making and to formulate advance directives (ANA, 1991). The key provisions of the legislation require facilities to provide

1. *written information* to each adult individual concerning "an individual's rights under State law (whether statutory or as recognized by the courts of the State) to make decisions concerning such medical care, including the right to accept or refuse medical or surgical treatment and the right to formulate advance directives."
2. *written policies* of the provider or organization respecting the implementation of such advance directives
3. *inquiry* as to whether a person has an advance directive
4. *documentation* in the patient's medical records whether the individual has executed an advance directive
5. *nondiscrimination,* that is, not to condition the provision of care or otherwise discriminate against an individual based on whether the individual has executed an advance directive
6. *compliance* with requirements of state laws respecting advance directives at facilities of the provider or organization
7. *education* for staff on issues concerning advance directives and provision for community education regarding advance directives

The PSDA does not provide guidance to resolve conflicts among family members and the patient, nor does it address the difficult clinical and ethical questions related to decisionally incapacitated patients who have never executed an advance directive. The PSDA neither creates nor affects requirements with respect to informed consent to medical care or determination of mental capacity.

DO NOT RESUSCITATE DIRECTIVES

Do not resuscitate (DNR) orders are not per se a type of advance directive. Yet, this legislation is important in end-of-life care. DNR is defined as not using CPR. Whether or not to initiate CPR requires careful attention to ethical, legal, professional, and institutional policies.

Health care professionals are never required legally to do procedures that are clearly futile. In fact, nurses and other health care professionals might be sued for performing CPR without consent when the current medical literature indicates that such procedures are futile or the treatment will not be effective.

In 1988, New York became the first state to enact DNR legislation, and it required that consent to CPR be presumed. If physicians do not want to resuscitate patients, they must obtain the patient's consent and proceed with writing the order (Swidler, 1989). Obtaining a DNR order is critical if the patient wishes to avoid this type of treatment.

What nurses need to know about DNR directives is that patients have a right to refuse CPR and may request DNR orders after they have been informed of the risks and benefits involved (ANA, 1992). Open communication is important to ensure that the decision is acceptable to all parties involved. If the physician is unable to write a DNR directive or comply with the patient's request, the physician has a duty to notify the patient or family and assist the patient to obtain another physician. Nurses ought to be aware when such dilemmas are present and act on behalf of patients. In addition, nurses need to know which patients have a DNR directive, the institutional policy and law governing the use of directives (Appendix B), the patient's wishes regarding interventions to be withheld, and their own values toward the decision to withhold treatment. The medical record should clearly indicate the terms of the directive and whether the terms accurately reflect the patients' current stated preferences. "Slow codes" or "partial codes" or any actions that lead the patient's family to believe a full intensive code is being done when it is not are unethical and could give rise to legal implications (Meisel, 1995).

ADVANCE DIRECTIVES IN RELATIONSHIP
TO NURSING PRACTICE

End-of-life care is certainly in the minds of nurses today and is an issue for geriatric critical care nurses. Nurses should not hesitate to participate in ethical and legal discussions related to end-of-life decision making and to better understand current controversies in end-of-life care, such as pain and symptom management, withholding and withdrawing life-sustaining therapies, and barriers to practice.

Overall, surveys report that the general public supports advance directives (Emanuel, 1995; Gordon & Dunn, 1992); however, there is still a low number of patients who actually complete them. The literature suggests that more patients would complete advance directives if they had more information and assistance in completing them (Emanuel, Barry, & Stoeckle, 1991; Mezey, Leitman, Mitty, Bottrell, & Ramsey, 2000) and if physicians initiate the topic (Emanuel, 1995). Patients want the physician with whom they have a relationship to initiate and discuss end-of-life care and living wills (Emanuel et al., 1991). Even patients at higher risk of becoming decisionally incapable were not more likely to complete advance directives. Completion, however, is more concentrated among white patients with higher education and income levels.

To that end, a number of educational interventions have been implemented to address these issues. There is evidence to suggest that health care providers can make a difference in whether patients discuss end-of-life care with their family or friends or complete advance directives. Although many patients discuss advance care planning with their families, other patients find it difficult to initiate such discussions (Elpern, Yellen, & Burton, 1993). Health care professionals and nurses in particular can open up discussion between families and patients by providing a format for such discussions or use advance directives to minimize conflicts between patients and their families.

On the other hand, patients indicate that they complete advance directives to ease the financial and emotional burden on their families and to support decision making (Mezey, Ramsey, Mitty, & Rappaport, 1997). Patients indicate that an advance directive is unnecessary because they believe that family members would "know what to do" when the time came. Studies show that patients who feel that others will make appropriate decisions were more likely to have adult children than those who did not (Elder, Schneider, Zweig, Peters, & Ely, 1992). Nurses and other health care providers should be aware of these sentiments and, when appropriate, involve family members in these discussions. Nurses and other providers need to consider that older persons' values about health and the importance thereto may be different than younger persons' values. Older persons might refuse to formulate an advance directive out of concern for the family and the conflicts that such a document might generate (Stetler, Elliott, & Bruno, 1992).

Another issue that influences comfort or discomfort of patients or families in discussing advance directives concerns the question of autonomy and how one defines it. Health-care providers need to approach advanced directives with cultural sensitivity and cultural competence. Fears that an advance directive permits providers to withhold care or that it will lead to lesser quality of care may be at the root of the rejection of advance directives for some patients. People may be concerned that once an advance directive is completed and it contains a statement to withhold treatment, providers will devote less attention to their care and may withhold more treatment than was desired (Caralis, Davis, Wright, & Marcial, 1993).

Socioeconomic and cultural factors substantially influence decisions to complete an advance directive. Studies are confirming that people with less education or lower income or who are African American or Hispanic are less likely to formulate advance directives (High, 1993; Mezey, Leitman,

Mitty, Bottrell, & Ramsey, 2000; Robinson, DeHaven, & Koch, 1993). Several explanations are plausible. Individuals with these sociodemographic characteristics are less likely to have regular access and availability to health care. For these persons, limiting any medical care would seem unnecessary because they already have too little, not too much. They are also less likely to have exposure to the concept of advance directives (Mezey, 1997). Furthermore, most physicians are White; people who have experienced discrimination throughout their lives may particularly distrust the intent of health care providers and may question their motives. Non-White patients are less likely than white patients are to discuss end-of-life decisions with a white physician. Moreover, certain cultural factors in non-White communities may prohibit discussions of death and dying and find that the cultural differences are barriers to meaningful discussions.

Moreover, providers are particularly hesitant to approach patients about directives when the issue of stopping or withdrawing treatment is imminent (Solomon et al., 1993). Many providers erroneously perceive that there is a legal difference between forgoing and discontinuing treatment. Physicians and nurses, for example, are unsure about a patient's legal right to discontinue nutrition and hydration (Olson, 1993). Under such circumstances, providers need to be concerned about the extent to which patients (and health care proxies) are correctly informed about treatment alternatives and consequences and know the relevant laws.

In long-term care, discussing advance directives poses particular issues. In some cases, nursing home residents may not have any family or friends with whom to discuss such issues, or a relative may live at some distance and rarely visit. Health care providers can sensitize residents to the need for advance directives under such circumstances. Should the resident decide to execute a DPAHC, providers need to be vigilant that the health care proxy will be available, willing, and able to act in the resident's best interest. Residents with fluctuating decision-making capacity may vary in their ability to fully or even partially participate in decisions about their care. If that is the case, providers need to carefully and critically work at not abrogating resident's rights while shielding those who are decisionally incapable from making inappropriate decisions.

INFORMED CONSENT

Every human being of adult years and sound mind has a right to determine what shall be done with his or her own body (*Schloendorff v. Society of New York Hospital* [1914]). Accordingly, the fundamental goals of informed consent are patient autonomy and self-determination (*in re Farrell* [1987]). This goal is effected by allowing patients to make their own decisions about their health care based on their values for as long as they are able.

A second goal of informed consent is to empower patients to exercise their right to autonomy rationally and intelligently (Meisel, 1995). There is no guarantee that providing patients with relevant information about treatment will result in intelligent decisions, nor does it guarantee that they will use the information provided; however, without such a requirement the likelihood of rational decision making is diminished (Meisel, 1995). The patient's right to consent presumes the fact that the patient has sufficient information to make a reasonable decision.

Consent to treatment is only valid when the patient has the capacity to consent (Meisel, 1995). "Competence" and "capacity" are not the same, yet they are frequently considered to be the same. Competency to make health care decisions is a legal term that is determined only by a court. The law presumes that all adults are competent and have decision-making capacity (Applebaum & Grisso, 1988) to make health decisions, and the assumption is ordinarily correct (Meisel, 1995). To be considered competent an individual must be able to comprehend the nature of the particular action in question and be able to understand its significance. One need not be adjudicated incompetent to lack the capacity to consent to medical treatment and one who is adjudicated incompetent does not necessarily lack the capacity to consent (Meisel, 1995).

Capacity, on the other hand, is determined not by the courts but rather by clinicians who assess functional capabilities to determine whether or not it is lacking. Incapacity is not determined solely by a medical or psychiatric diagnosis, rather it rests on the judgments that an informed lay person might make (Mezey, Mitty, & Ramsey, 1997).

The basic elements of a valid consent, the determination that a patient has sufficient decisional capacity to consent or refuse treatment, are based on the observation of a specific set of abilities: (1) the patient appreciates or understands that he or she has the right to make a choice; (2) the patient understands the medical situation, prognosis, risks, benefits, and consequences of treatment (or not); (3) the patient can communicate the decision; and (4) the patient's decision is stable and consistent over a period of time (Roth, Meisel, & Lidz, 1977).

Not all health decisions require the same level of decision-making capacity in order to make a decision. Decision-making capacity is not an "on–off switch" (Mezey, Mitty, & Ramsey, 1997); you do not either have it or not. Rather, during the past 20 years, as a part of the "right to die" movement, bioethicists and lawyers have suggested that capacity be viewed as "task specific" rather than in general terms (Mezey, Ramsey, Mitty, & Rappaport, 1997). An individual may be able to perform some tasks adequately, may have the ability to make some decisions, but is unable to perform all tasks or make all decisions. The notion of "decision-specific capacity" assumes that an individual has or lacks capacity for a particular decision at a particular time and under a particular set of circumstances (Mezey et al., 1997; Mezey, Teresi, et al., 2000). Most people have sufficient cognitive capability to make some, but not all, decisions (Miller, 1995).

Nurses can make a valuable contribution in ensuring that the informed consent process is accurately met (Davis, 1989). Yet, nurses have little training in assessing decision-making capacity (Mezey, Ramsey, Mitty, & Rappaport, 1997). Nurses must become proficient in assessing decisional capacity and become active participants in discussions with other members of the health care team when determining decisional capacity. Those with the most knowledge of the patient should be asked to contribute meaningful and relevant information about the person. When nurses and other health care professionals learn how to objectively assess capacity, two types of errors will be avoided: mistakenly preventing persons who ought to be considered capacitated from directing the course of their treatment and failing to protect incapacitated persons from the harmful effects of their decisions (President's Commission, 1982). Nurses at all educational levels should make efforts to meet their legal and ethical obligations so that patients will retain their rights to make decisions for as long as they are able.

EDUCATION OF NURSES AND OTHER HEALTH CARE PROFESSIONALS REGARDING ADVANCE DIRECTIVES

Education can change nurse's comfort with and willingness to approach patients about advance directives. When they are well informed and comfortable with their own feelings, they are more likely to initiate discussion about advance directives. Physicians who are educated about directives are more comfortable with such discussions and have more discussions with their patients, and their patients complete more advance directives than do patients of physicians who are not educated about directives (Greenberg, Doblin, Shapiro, Linn, & Wenger, 1993; Robinson et al., 1993).

Education requires more than a description of the law and the steps to be taken in formulating directives. Nurses and other health care providers need to learn how to discuss advance care planning with patients and families, assess decisional capacity to execute a directive, identify methods to help patients analyze the benefits and burdens of decisions, and resolve conflicts among staff with different values and beliefs about end-of-life treatment. Education should also include the dissemination and discussion of treatment guidelines, attention to the psychology of decision making, and a dialogue between those who develop ethical recommendations and those who must carry them out at the bedside (Solomon et al., 1993).

Finally, it is important that providers review with patients how and with whom they should communicate that a directive has been formulated. People need to be encouraged to discuss their values and health-care preferences with their health-care proxy (if one is appointed), their family, and a personal physician, if they have one. A study of recently discharged hospital patients with advance directives documented that less than 15% were asked about an existing advance directive during their hospitalization, 60% of patients did not disclose to the hospital staff that they had a directive, and only 35% informed their physician about their advance directives (Mezey et al., 1997). Although failure to communicate this information might be attributed to the patient's presumption that the directive would not be relevant for the hospital stay, selective disclosure may reflect a patient's misunderstanding or fear, or both, about their use.

SUMMARY

Advance directives, DNR orders, and court and legislative actions are all important mechanisms for nurses to consider when seeking ways to resolve the legal and ethical dilemmas that exist when caring for patients at the end of life. Nurses must have opportunities to critically think and articulate their views and positions on dilemmas that they face as individuals and professionals. Ethics committees, ethics rounds, grand rounds, ethics colloquium, courses in basic nursing education, continuing education offerings, and conferences all provide forums for nurses, students, faculty, and clinicians to enhance their ethical and legal awareness. The American Nurses Association Center for Ethics and Human Rights is one rich resource for nurses who seek consultation and ethics information. There are a number of resources available to support the nurse who seeks to empower patients and families (Appendix C). Nurses are the eyes, ears and mouth for those for whom we provide care. Our ethical responsibility as set forth in the ANA Code of Ethics (ANA, 1985) and our legal responsibilities discussed earlier make nurses accountable. If we lose our accountability, we clearly lose of profession. "RN" does not mean Risk Not. We must be risk takers while we advocate and educate our patients and families. Gaining ethical and legal competence will ensure that we fulfill our commitment as members of the profession.

REFERENCES

American Nurses Association. (1985). *Code for nurses with interpretative statements.* Washington, DC: American Nurses Association.

American Nurses Association. (1991). *Position statement on nursing and the Patient Self Determination Act.* Washington, DC: American Nurses Association.

American Nurses Association. (1992). Position statement on nursing care and do-not-resuscitate orders. Washington, DC: American Nurses Association.

Applebaum, P. S., & Grisso, T. (1988). Assessing patient's capacities to consent to treatment. *New England Journal of Medicine, 319,* 1635–1638.

Black, H. C. (1990). *Law dictionary* (6th ed.). St. Paul: West Publishing.

Caralis, P. V., Davis, B., Wright, K., & Marcial, E. (1993). The influence of ethnicity and race on attitudes toward advance directives, life-prolonging treatments, and euthanasia. *Journal of Clinical Ethics, 4* (2), 155.

Davis, A., Aroskar, M., Liaschenko, J., & Drought, T. (1997). *Ethical dilemmas & nursing practice* (4th ed.). Stamford, CT: Appleton & Lange.

Davis, A. J. (1989). Clinical nurses; ethical decision making in situations of informed consent. *Advances in Nursing Science, 11* (3), 63–69.

Elder, N. C., Schneider, F. D., Zweig, S. C., Peters, P. G., & Ely, J. W. (1992). Community attitudes and knowledge about advance care directives. *Journal of the American Board of Family Practice, 5,* 565–572.

Elpern, E. H., Yellen, S. B., & Burton, L. A. (1993). A preliminary investigation of opinions and behaviors regarding advance directives for medical care. *American Journal of Critical Care, 2,* 161–167.

Emanuel, L. L. (1995). Advance directives: Do they work? *Journal of the American College of Cardiology, 25,* 35–38.

Emanuel, L. L., Barry, W., & Stoeckle, J. D. (1991). Advanced directives for medical care—A case for greater use. *New England Journal of Medicine, 324,* 889–895.

Farrell, In re, 529 A.2d 404 (N. J. 1987), Aff'g 514 A.2d 1342 (N. J. Super. Ct. Ch. Div. 1986).

Furrow, B., Greaney, T., Johnson, S., Soltzfus, J. T., & Schwartz, R. (1995). *Health Law, 2,* 369.

Gordon, G. H., & Dunn, P. (1992). Advance directives and the Patient Self-Determination Act. *Hospital Practice, 27* (4A), 39–40, 42.

Greenberg, J. M., Doblin, B. H., Shapiro, D. W., Linn, L. S., & Wenger, N. S. (1993). Effect of an educational program on medical student's conversations with patients about advance directives. *Journal of General Internal Medicine, 8,* 683–685.

Haas, J. S., et al. (1993). Discussions of preferences for life sustaining care by persons with AIDS. *Archives of Internal Medicine, 153,* 1241–1248.

High, D. M. (1993). Advance directives and the elderly: A study of intervention strategies to increase use. *Gerontologist, 33,* 342–349.

Meisel, A. (1995). *The right to die* (Vol. 2). New York: Wiley Law.

Meisel, A. (2000). *The right to die* (Vols. 1 & 2). New York: Aspen Law & Business.

Mezey, M., Leitman, R., Mitty, E., Bottrell, M., & Ramsey, G. (2000). Why hospital patients do and do not execute an advance directive. *Nursing Outlook, 48,* 165–171.

Mezey, M., Mitty, E., & Ramsey, G. (1997). Assessment of decision-making capacity: Nurse's role. *Journal of Gerontological Nursing, 23* (3), 28–35.

Mezey, M., Ramsey, G., Mitty, E., & Rappaport, M. (1997). Implementation of the Patient Self-Determination Act (PSDA) in nursing homes in New York City. *Journal of the American Geriatrics Society, 45,* 43–49.

Mezey, M., Teresi, J., Ramsey, G., Mitty, E., & Bobrowitz, T. (2000). Decision-making capacity to execute a health care proxy: Development and testing of guidelines. *Journal of the American Geriatrics Society, 48,* 179–187.

Miller, T. (1995). Advance directives: Moving from theory to practice. In P. R. Katz, R. L. Kane, & M. Mezey (Eds.), *Quality care in geriatric settings* (pp. 68–87). New York: Springer.

Olson, E. (1993). Ethical issues in the nursing home. *Mount Sinai Journal of Medicine, 60,* 555–559.

President's Commission for the Study of Ethical Problems in Medicine and Biomedical and Behavioral Research. (1983, March). Deciding to forego life-sustaining treatment (pp. 55–68). Washington, DC: United States Government Printing Office.

Patient Self-Determination Act of 1991, Pub. L. No. 101-508, '4206, 4751 [hereinafter OBRA], 104 Stat. 1388-115 to 117, 1388-204 to 206 (codified at 42 U.S.C.A. '1395cc(f) (1) & id. '1396a(a) (West Supp. 1994).

Robinson, M. K., DeHaven, M. J., & Koch, K. A. (1993). Effects of the patient self-determination act on patient knowledge and behavior. *Journal of Family Practice, 37,* 363–368.

Roth, Y. L., Meisel, A., & Lidz, C. W. (1977). Tests of competency to consent to treatment. *American Journal of Psychiatry, 134,* 279–284.

Schloendorff v. Society of New York Hospice., 105 N. E. 92 (N. Y. 1914).

Solomon, M. Z., O'Donnell, L., Jennings, B., Guilfoy, V., Wolf, S. M., Nolan, K., Jackson, R., Koch-Weser, D., & Donnelley, S. (1993). Decisions near the end of life: Professional views on life-sustaining treatments. *American Journal of Public Health, 83* (1), 4–23.

Stetler, K. L., Elliott, B. A., & Bruno, C. A. (1992). Living will completion in older adults. *Archives of Internal Medicine, 125,* 954–959.

Swidler, R. (1989). The presumption of consent in New York State's do-not-resuscitate law. *New York State Journal of Medicine, 89,* 69–72.

APPENDIX A: ADVANCE DIRECTIVE LEGISLATION (DURABLE POWER OF ATTORNEY FOR HEALTH CARE AND LIVING WILL)

ALABAMA	Alabama Stat. §22-8A-2 to -10 (1997)
ALASKA	Alaska Stat. §13.26.338 to .353
ARIZONA	Ariz. Rev. Stat. Ann. §36-3201 to -3262 (1994)
ARKANSAS	Ark. Code Ann. §20-17-201 to -218
CALIFORNIA	Cal. Probate Code §4600 to -4779
COLORADO	Colo. Rev. Stat.§15-14-503 to -509
CONNECTICUT	Conn. Gen. Stat. §1-43 and §19a-570 to -579 (1993)
DELAWARE	16 Del C. §2501 to 2518
DISTRICT OF COLUMBIA	D.C. Code Ann. §21-2201 to -2213
	Phone: 1-800-MED-ETHX Fax: (202) 687-6770
	E-mail: Medethx@gunet.gerogetown.edu
	Phone: (202) 687-8099 Fax: (202) 687-8089
	National Reference Center for Bioethics Literature
	(at Kennedy Institute of Ethics)
	Web site: http://guweb.georgetown.edu/nrcbl/
FLORIDA	Fla. Stat. §765.101 to -.401
GEORGIA	O.C.G.A. §31-36-1 to -13 (1990)
HAWAII	Hawaii Rev. Stat. 551D, 327E
IDAHO	Idaho Code §§39-4501 to -4509
ILLINOIS	755 ILCS 45/1-1 through 4-12
INDIANA	Ind. Code Ann. §30-5-1 to 30-5-10 and Ind. Code Ann. §16-36-1-1 to -14
IOWA	Iowa Code Ann. §44B.1 to .12 (West Supp. 1991)
KANSAS	Kan. Stat. Ann. §§58-625 to -632 (Supp. 1994)
KENTUCKY	Ky. Rev. Stat. §§311.621 to .643 (Supp 1994)
LOUISIANA	La. Rev. Stat. Ann 40:1299.58.1 to .10 (West 1997)
MAINE	Me. Rev. Stat. Ann. tit. 18A, §5-801 to §5-817 (West 1995)
MARYLAND	Md. Code Ann. [Health-Gen.]. §§5-601 to -608
MASSACHU-SETTS	Mass. Gen. Laws Ann. Ch. 201D (West Supp. 1991)
MICHIGAN	Mich. Comp. Laws Ann. §700.496(West 1991)
MINNESOTA	Minn. Stat. §§145C.01 to .15 (1993)
MISSISSIPPI	Miss. Code Ann. §41-41-201 to -229
MISSOURI	Mo. Ann. Stat. §404.700 to .735 and §800–870 (West 1991)
MONTANA	Mont. Code Ann. §50-9-101 to -111, and -201 to -206 (1991)
NEBRASKA	Neb. Rev. Stat. §§30-3401 to -3434 (1993)
NEVADA	Nev. Rev. Stat. §§449.800 to .860 (Supp. 1989)

NEW HAMPSHIRE	N.H. Rev. Stat. Ann. §§137-J:1 to -J:16 (1993)
NEW JERSEY	N.J. Stat. Ann. §26:2H-53 to -78 (West 1993)
NEW MEXICO	N.M. Stat. Ann. §24-7A-1 to -16 (1997)
NEW YORK	N.Y. Pub. Health Law §2980 to 2994
NORTH CAROLINA	N.C. Gen. Stat. §32A-15 to -26 (1993) Also N.C. Gen. Stat. §122C-71 to -77
NORTH DAKOTA	N.D. Cent. Code §§23-06.5-01 to -18 (1993)
OHIO	Ohio Rev. Code §§1337.11 to .17 (Anderson Supp. 1991)
OKLAHOMA	Okla. Stat. Ann. tit. 63, §3101.1 to -.16 (West 1993) [See Okla. Sess. Law Serv. Ch. 251 (H.B. 1353) enacted 11995 for mental health advance directive]
OREGON	Or. Rev. Stat. §§127.505 to .640 (1993) [See Or. Rev. Stat. 127.700 to .735 (1993) for mental health advance directive.]
PENNSYLVANIA	Pa. Stat. Ann. tit. 20, §§5401 to 5416 (1993)
RHODE ISLAND	R.I. Gen. Laws §23-4.10-1 to -12 (Supp. 1993)
SOUTH CAROLINA	S.C. Code §62-5-501 and 62-5-504
SOUTH DAKOTA	S.D. Codified Laws Ann. §§34-12C-1 to -8, and §§59-7-2.1 to -2.8 (Supp. 1992)
TENNESSEE	Tenn. Code Ann. §§34-6-201 to -214 (Supp. 1991)
TEXAS	Tex. [Civil Practice & Remedies] Code Ann. §135.001 to -.018
UTAH	Utah Code Ann. §75-2-1101 to -1118 (Supp. 1993)
VERMONT	Vt. Stat. Ann. tit. 14, ª3451 to 3467 (1989)
VIRGINIA	Va. Code §54.1-2981 to -2993 (Supp. 1992)
WASHINGTON	Wash. Rev. Code Ann. §§11.94.010 to .900 (Supp. 1990)
WEST VIRGINIA	W. VA. Code §16-30A-1 to -20
WISCONSIN	Wis. Stat. Ann. §155.01 to .80 and 243.07(6m)
WYOMING	Wyo. Stat. Ann. §§3-5-201 to -213

APPENDIX B: DO NOT RESUSCITATE LEGISLATION
(DNR ORDERS)

ALASKA	Alaska Stat. §18.12.035-.100
ARIZONA	Ariz. Rev. Stat. Ann. §36-3251
ARKANSAS	Ark. Code Ann. §20-13-901 to -908
CALIFORNIA	Cal. Probate Code §4753; Cal. Health & Safety Code §1569.74
COLORADO	Colo. Rev. Stat.§15-18.6-101 to -108
CONNECTICUT	Conn. Gen. Stat. Ann. §19a-580d
FLORIDA	Fla. Stat. §401.45(3)
GEORGIA	Ga. Code Ann §§.31-39-1 to -9
HAWAII	Haw. Rev. Stat. 321-229.5
IDAHO	Idaho Code §§39-151 to -165
ILLINOIS	Ill. Ann. Stat. Ch. 210, §45/2-104.2
INDIANA	Ind. Code Ann. §16-36-5
KANSAS	Kan. Stat. Ann. §§65-4941 to -4948
LOUISIANA	S.B. 209, 1999 Reg. Sess. (La.1999), codified at La. Rev. Stat. Ann §40:1299.58.2, 58.3, & 58.7-10
MARYLAND	Md. Code Ann. Health-Gen. §§5-608
MICHIGAN	Mich. Comp. Laws Ann. §§333.1051-.1067
MONTANA	Mont. Code Ann. §§50-10-9-101 to -107
NEVADA	Nev. Rev. Stat. Ann. §§450B.400 -.590, as amended by A.B. 73, 70th Regs. Sess. (Nev. 1999)
NEW JERSEY	N.J. Stat. Ann. §26:2H-68
NEW MEXICO	N.M. Stat. Ann. §§24-10B-4(J)
NEW YORK	N.Y. Pub. Health Law §§2960–2979
OHIO	Ohio Rev. Code Ann. §§2133.02
OKLAHOMA	Okla. Stat. Tit.63, §§3131.1-.14, as amended by H.B. 1381, 47th Leg., 1st Sess. (Okla.1999)
PENNSYLVANIA	Pa. Cons. Stat. Ann. tit. 20, §5413.
RHODE ISLAND	R.I. Gen. Laws §23-4.10; R.I. Gen. Laws §23-4.11-14
SOUTH CAROLINA	S.C. Code Ann. §§44-78-10 to 65
TENNESSEE	Tenn. Code Ann. §68-11-224; Tenn. Code Ann. §68-140-601 to -604
TEXAS	Tex. Health & Safety Codes §§674.001-.024 1999; Tex.S. B. 1260
UTAH	Utah Code Ann. §75-2-1105.5
VIRGINIA	Va. Code Ann. §§54.1-2982,-2987.1,-2901,63.1-174.3, as amended by 1999 Va. Acts 814 (Supp. 1992)
WASHINGTON	Wash. Rev. Code Ann. §43.70.480.
WEST VIRGINIA	W. VA. Code §§16-30C-1 to -16
WISCONSIN	Wis. Stat. Ann. §154.17-,29
WYOMING	Wyo. Stat. §§35-22-201 to 213

APPENDIX C: BIOETHICS RESOURCES

1. American Hospice Foundation
    1130 Connecticut Ave, NW suite 700
    Washington, DC 20036-4101
    Phone: (202) 223-0204
    Fax: (202) 223-0208
    E-mail: ahf@msn.com

    Publications include
      Grief at Work
      Grief at School
      Grief and Faith

2. Academy of Hospice Nurses
    Susan Ridel, President
    3320 Bradford Road
    Cleveland Heights, OH 44118
    Phone: (561) 265-1293
    Fax: (561) 265-1293

3. American Nurses Association (ANA)
    ANA Center for Ethics and Human Rights
    600 Maryland Ave., SW, suite 100 West
    Washington, DC 20024-2571
    Phone: (202) 651-7055
    Fax: (202) 651-7001

    Publications include
      Code for nurses with interpretive statements
      Communique (quarterly newsletter)
      Position statements on assisted suicide and active euthanasia, do-not-
        resuscitate, Comfort and relief, Patient Self-Determination Act
      Selected bibliographies on ethical issues such as end-of-life decisions,
        foregoing artificial nutrition and hydration, nursing ethics
        committees, and assisted suicide and euthanasia

4. The American Society of Bioethics and Humanities
    4700 West Lake Ave.
    Glenview, IL 60025
    Phone: (847) 375-4745
    Fax: (847) 375-4777

    Publications Include:
      International Journal of Nursing Ethics

5. Choice In Dying
    475 Riverside Drive Rm. 1852

New York, NY 10115
Phone: (212) 870-2003
Fax: (212) 870-2040

Choice In Dying
National Office
1035 30th St., NW
Washington, DC 20007
Phone: (202) 338-9790
(800) 989-WILL
Fax: (202) 338-0242
Web site: http://www.choices.org

Publications Include:
Questions and Answers: Advance Directives and End-of-Life Decisions
Questions and Answers: You and Your Choices; Advance Medical Directives Physician Assisted Suicide
Questions and Answers: You and Your Choices
Questions and Answers: Dying at Home
Questions and Answers: Medical Treatments and Your Advance Directives
Questions and Answers: Artificial Nutrition and Hydration and End-Of-Life Decision Making
Questions and Answers: Cardiopulmonary Resuscitation
Questions and Answers: Do-Not-Resuscitate Orders, and End-of-Life Decision
Questions and Answers: What Every Professional Should Know
Brochures: Talking About Your Choices
Videos: Whose Death is it, Anyway? (PBS special)

6.   The Hastings Center
     Route 9D
     Garrison, NY 10524-5555
     Phone: (914) 424-4040
     Fax: (914) 424-4545

     Publications Include:
     Hastings Center Report

7.   Hospice and Palliative Nurses Association
     Medical Center East, suite 375
     211 North Whitfield St.
     Pittsburgh, PA 15206-3031
     Phone: (412) 361-2470
     Fax: (412) 3612425

     Publications Include:

Standard of Hospice Nursing
Terminal Restlessness
Symptom Management
Algorithms for Palliative Care

8. The Kennedy Institute of Ethics
    Box 571212
    Georgetown University
    Washington, DC 20057-1212

Policy Issues

Ethel Mitty

The advocacy role of nursing is implicit in the social contract of the nursing profession with society and in our professional code of ethics. As such, we are committed to act assertively on behalf of a client's safety, well-being, and empowerment. An advocate defends or promotes the rights of others and strives to change systems to meet those needs. Nursing's ability to provide high-quality nursing care cannot be based solely on appropriate education of its practitioners, continuing development of competencies, and setting-specific evidence-based practice. Continuing nursing effectiveness requires health care policies and programs that facilitate what nursing does best for our culturally and socioeconomically diverse populace. To make this happen, nurses caring for the critically ill elderly must understand policy making and the actions it requires of us.

This chapter begins by defining policy making, describes the process, and identifies significant health-delivery issues that have an impact on care of the elderly. The middle section provides a historical view of health policies and programs, their intent, achievements, and failures. Actions and attitudes associated with policy development and promulgation—the advocacy role of nursing as an expression of nursing accountability—constitutes the last section of the chapter.

HEALTH POLICY DYNAMICS

The *policy process* directs attention to public problems and acts on them. Public policy emerges from the policy process. Politics is the use of power to facilitate or inhibit policy enactment. A policy is a political decision to implement a program that will achieve societal goals (Cochran & Malone, 1995) and represents the influence and power that government has on the lives of its citizens (Peters, 1986). Health policy is a decision that primarily affects those who deliver and receive health care, that is, health care professionals, institutions, and the patient (or client, consumer). Diers (1985) noted the difference between policy and politics: policy deals with the "shoulds" and "oughts"; it sets goals and directions for achieving them.

A health policy is but one of many public policies, such as education, defense, transportation, environment, and safety, that affect the common weal. The demand for health care *services* to accommodate the "idea" of health must be weighed and prioritized against other needs that could powerfully affect health status, such as sanitation and nutrition. In the American system of government, there is no single policy maker but, rather, involvement of and influence by the three branches of federal government—executive, legislative, and judicial; the three levels of government—federal, state, and local; the media; the public; and interest groups. It can be argued, furthermore, that there is no "public interest" but rather multiple publics and stakeholders each with their own interests.

Two opposing views dominate thinking about American health care: that it is primarily a private health care system or that it is government directed by virtue of being government funded. To a certain extent, both perspectives are accurate. Most health care systems in the United States, other than the government owned and operated VA system, are owned and managed by for-profit and not-for-profit organizations and providers. On the other hand, almost half of all health care expenditures in the United States are government funded and although this is a smaller proportion in comparison with other industrialized nations, government involvement in health care is significant. The physician fee-for-service model is, in fact, heavily supported by the Medicare and Medicaid funding streams. In addition, many of the departments and agencies of the federal government are a major source of funds for medical research.

Public policy can be defined by its level of impact (Peters, 1986). A "policy choice" is a decision made by an elected representative, including the President, a program administrator, civil servant or pressure group to use public power to achieve a certain end. A "policy output" can be a program or action to put the policy choice into motion. At this level, the government or its agent is spending money (taxpayer dollars and other revenues) to hire people, develop technology, purchase sites or equipment, or enforce regulations that affect the lives of all or some of the citizenry. The third level is, in a sense, the most obvious—"policy impact"—the effect of policy choices and outputs. Inasmuch as policy development is a messy process involving many people and parties, a desired intended effect may be distorted or lost as the idea becomes translated into action. Thus, it is important that nurses understand the dynamic and political context of policy making so that networks and alliances can be forged with other groups whose interests and goals are similar.

Clearly, the health of individuals, groups of people, and large populations are affected by health policy choices and outputs. However, it is important to realize, also, that health policy influences the type, intensity, location, and remuneration for nursing practice. The *Nursing Agenda for Health Care Reform* (1991) established nursing as the profession that was most invested in working toward health. Health goals were not just medical but included prevention and health promotion goals. Basic concepts of the *Agenda* were enhanced access to health care service through the delivery of primary health care in community settings, consumer responsibility for personal health and self-care, and cost-effective therapeutic options delivered in the most appropriate settings.

Instruments and the Environment of Public Policy

Law and regulation, services, funding, and "moral suasion" are instruments of government that influence social, economic, and health behavior and produce change in the lives of the populace (Peters, 1986). The road taken will vary with the likelihood that the method is politically acceptable, the degree to which it is a break with or continuance of tradition, and its probable effectiveness. Law and regulation are uniquely a government prerogative and generally require back-up enforcement, monitoring, and sanctions for failure to comply or honor the intent of the law or the inherent obligations of the citizenry. Interestingly, however, law also creates or defines citizens' fundamental rights, such as access to health care. Disagreement over whether the right to health care is an equal right to a basic minimum of care or a right to equal care influences the nature and demand for health care reforms.

Government services can be directly or indirectly provided. Indeed, there is significant concern about the role of federal and state government as a direct provider, such as government ownership and management of prisons and psychiatric hospitals. In some cases, the government contracts with and financially subsidizes a quasi-governmental body that will provide services, such as Amtrak (Peters, 1986). The government can "deem authority" to an organization, such as the Independent Peer Review Organizations (IPRO) and Joint Commission for the Accreditation of Healthcare Organizations (JCAHO), to monitor operations in which the government has financial or regulatory interest. Funding in the form of money transfers to citizens, as with the Social Security program, is intended to facilitate the individual citizen's access to policy goals—basic necessities of life. Critics of the Social Security program and of categorical grants—monies for specific purposes—argue that decision making concentrated at the federal level does not represent local needs or goals. Block grants for broad categories, for example, primary care community health centers, are awarded to states with few strings. Money spent based on local discretion and needs assessment appears to be more satisfactory but raises concerns that citizens with similar needs in different states will have their needs differentially met. Thus, issues of access and quality are raised once again.

Moral suasion, the nation's history, and the political and socioeconomic environment can influence policy development and the creativity and strength brought to policy enactment. It is critically important to understand the ideological context of public policy; ideologies are selective and competitive and seek to dismiss what another ideology holds as unrebuttable fact or assumption. If the citizenry distrusts the government, questions its motives, or is otherwise disheartened by the actions or legitimacy of its elected representatives, then exhortation on behalf of the public interest are unlikely to raise support for a public program, especially if it imposes burdens in the form of taxes or other disincentives. Historically, citizens of this country want limited government in their economic, social and private lives while demanding government action to protect the marketplace economy, improve education, and ensure access to and quality of health care. Americans demand the right to participate in government but see it in terms of local control. Low voter turnout for national, state, and local elections is troubling and appears to refute the notion of a politicized citizenry.

Federalism and Public Policy

More than 200 years ago, the constitutional notion of federalism was a means to prevent domination of one point of view or faction over all others. From the latter part of the 19th century and through most of the 20th century, conservatives used the term to justify less national or federal and more state and local control; liberals used the term to support federal government programming, funding and regulation. The terms "new federalism" or "devolution" connotes the changing relationship between federal, state, and local government as they sort out their roles and responsibilities and is based on the theory that state and local governments can do better than the federal government in providing services to their citizens (Watson & Gold, 1997). Policy responsibility is removed from the federal government and passed to state and local government through a variety of mechanisms that increase states' flexibility in compliance with federal regulations. As such, the nation "has fifty separately directed laboratories in which to experiment with the design of public policies" (Sapolsky, Aisenberg, & Monroe, 1987, p. 135).

States need assistance in meeting four key policy areas: encouraging Medicaid clients to enroll in managed care, expanding insurance coverage for children, making insurance more affordable for small business owners, and containing long-term care costs. The federal government continues to guarantee some level of welfare and medical support to, in particular, children, the elderly, disabled, and chronically ill who meet defined criteria of need. Absent this nationally directed coverage and given state and local incentives to control costs, there is fear that the demise of national entitlements will tear holes in the safety net. Several states have initiated programs that combine elements of local control, education, welfare, health and social service partnership boards overseeing the allocation and administration of block grants and waivered programs. The present system of creating and administrating public policy, that is, programs, is best characterized as interdependence and overlapping authority characterized by complex reimbursement mechanisms, regulations, expectations, and responsibilities. The Urban Institute is conducting a large multiyear study of devolution based on the premise that the states are leading the way in redesigning the nation's safety-net policy; thus, it is important to know and understand what each state is doing (Sparer, 1998).

Setting the Agenda

The policy process is complex because of the very nature of the problem(s) under consideration and the competing and confusing world where the problem lives and is described. An issue is "placed on the agenda" of public interest because of the perception that something is wrong and it can be improved by public (policy) activity. Some problems go through an "issue attention cycle;" they generate enormous public concern, congressional hearings, some type of response from the government, and then disappear—not necessarily because the problem has been adequately addressed but because of cost and funding realities and the difficulties of policy enactment (Peters, 1986). Examples of such issues are national health insurance, noise abatement, and pollution control. It is suggested that every problem should be presented with a tentative solution before presenting it for the agenda; if the issue is seen as unfixable by public action, it is unlikely to gain the attention of policy or decision makers.

The policy cycle moves through four stages: policy formulation, adoption, implementation, and evaluation. This is hardly a linear process, however; in most cases, several stages are occurring at the same time, but one stage will be more prominent than another will. In addition, nongovernmental stakeholders are involved by design or through lobbying, networking, and political action throughout the process.

HEALTH POLICIES AND PROGRAMS

Across the country, politicians and the public of every political (or apolitical) inclination feel that the problems of the health care system are those of access, quality, and cost. The United States spends more on health care than on defense. Since 1965, the year the Medicare and Medicaid programs were instituted, health care expenditures have grown from 6.2% of the Gross Domestic Product (GDP) to 14% in 1995 or one of every seven dollars from public and private sources, annually (Cochran, Mayer, Carr, & Cayer,

1999). Forty-five percent of total health care costs are reimbursed from government sources; 22%, private pay; 34%, insurance (Cochran et al., 1999). The mix of private, public, and insurance financing in the United States is generally not the model in other industrialized countries, where physician reimbursement is capitated, the physician is a salaried employee of a provider organization, or fee schedules are negotiated between the government and providers. Staff model health maintenance organizations (HMOs) and captivated managed care delivery systems have made significant inroads since the 1990s in this country, in some cases adapting aspects of other country's health care systems to the United States delivery system.

Issues in medical ethics (e.g., genetic testing, reproductive technology, euthanasia and physician-assisted suicide, and abortion), iatrogenic practice errors that cost millions of dollars annually and have high morbidity and unacceptable mortality rates, and the exponential increase in medical technology and the pharmaceutical emporium that promises endless life are claiming judicial attention in heretofore unknown domains. As noted by Cochran and colleagues (1999), many conditions once managed by the nation's moral, religious, and criminal justice systems, such as alcoholism, family violence, elder and child abuse, and workplace anxiety, are now classified as illnesses warranting attention by health care professionals.

The demand for a national health care insurance system continues. National health care insurance can be classified into two types (Cochran et al., 1999). In countries with a national health service, the government owns and operates the health care institutions; health care professionals (including physicians) are employees of the government. The most well-known prototype is the system of socialized medicine in Great Britain, in which there is very little private practice. Universal health insurance, typified by the systems in Germany, Sweden, France, and Italy, is government-mandated insurance coverage through the employer or other private policies; the government insures those citizens unable to obtain private insurance. Government control and operation of the provider system can vary; the system is not socialized medicine. In both systems, wealthy clients can seek private care. In the United States, the elderly and those nonelderly who are poor or "medically indigent" are guaranteed medical insurance by the government or through tax subsidies (Cochran et al., 1999).

The services covered in other nations is broader and more intensive than they are in the United States and include home health care, nursing home care, medications, eyeglasses, dental services, and social worker home visits. Although coinsurance and deductibles are generally high, patients have fewer out-of-pocket costs than hospitalized patients do in the United States (Cochran et al., 1999). Comparing the costs of care with other countries, health care services in the United States cost more and provide fewer services. Multinational studies of health care systems have not found a direct relationship between higher costs and better health outcomes.

Life expectancy for the elderly is highest in the United States among all nations, but we are only equal to or lag behind other countries in infant mortality. A paradox of American health care is that it is cure rather than care oriented; acute medical care has priority over chronic conditions. Disease prevention, health promotion and education, and alternatives to institutional long-term care receive minimal attention and funding. Many health system analysts believe that if access is increased, we will be unable to contain costs at present spending levels or quality will suffer; conversely, if costs are restrained, then quality or access will diminish.

Access, Cost, and Quality Issues

Health care economists generally feel, based on extensive analyses of national and international data, that there is no relationship between the percent of the GDP spent on health care and life expectancy, given a reasonable level of industrialization. In spite of more than 60 years of health services research, there is no consensus on the number of people who do not receive adequate health care or whether access is getting better or worse (Berk & Schur, 1998). The issue appears to be more methodological than conceptual. Interestingly, estimates of unmet need are generally lower when survey response rates are higher and are explained by the presumption that if an individual is interested in a subject, he or she will respond to questions about it (Berk & Schur, 1998). Conversely, low response rates might be reflecting only those who had access problems; the remaining pool of potential respondents found the subject of no interest to them. Inequity in access to health care is primarily attributed to resource distribution imbalance (Cochran et al., 1999). In short, those with greatest need for health care services do not reside in areas with the greatest distribution of resources, such as hospitals, physicians, nursing homes, clinics, wellness centers, dentists, mental health professionals, and so on. There are more physicians per 1000 population in urban and suburban areas compared with rural areas. The distribution of medical care appears to be more on the basis of ability to pay rather than on need.

The number of people who lack of health insurance, currently estimated at approximately 43 million Americans, 10 million of whom are children, is stable despite transient differences in exactly who is affected; that is, an employed insured worker today can be out of work tomorrow; tomorrow, a formerly unemployed and uninsured worker secures a job and insurance coverage. According to Cantor, Long, and Marquis (1998), the U.S. Census Bureau reports that individuals with a high school education or less are twice as likely to lack health care insurance as those with a college degree. Inadequate access, compounded by not having health insurance, forces many patients to present themselves for treatment at an emergency department, by which time the illness may be far advanced and more difficult and costly to manage. Uninsured individuals residing in states with a higher percentage of uninsured citizens are more likely to be in poorer health than is an insured individual in a state with fewer uninsured citizens (Cantor,

Long, & Marquis, 1998). Health status and functional limitations are important determinants in the decision by some elderly with Medicare coverage to purchase additional private health care insurance (Wilcox-Gok & Rubin, 1994).

Fear of losing insurance coverage is associated with the phenomenon known as "job lock"—staying at a job that might be unsatisfying for any number of reasons rather than risk not having coverage with a new employer. Industry downsizing that caused many white collar and middle class workers to lose their jobs and health insurance and an increase in the number of part-time positions driven, in part, by employers wanting to reduce their health coverage costs for full-time workers, further complicates the health care access issue. Almost one half of U.S. companies indicated that they contributed half or less to their workers' insurance premiums (Johnson & Bender, 1996). The Health Insurance Portability and Accountability Act of 1996 seeks to increase the number of people who have, and maintain their access to, health insurance. Insurance coverage for preexisting conditions, pooled risk for the hard-to-insure, front- and back-end coverage, community versus experience rating, and mandated coverage are additional aspects of health care insurance being observed and tested.

The enormous increase in health care costs during the 1960s to 1980s was due, for the most part, to the fact that there was no incentive to keep fees and costs down because providers would be reimbursed by insurers or public programs. Higher costs were "passed through" as higher costs to employers or to private policy holders in the form of increased premiums. Other third party payers, Medicare and Medicaid, fostered greater use of services by virtue of expanding the population of covered beneficiaries and the services covered.

Research, development, and operating costs of medical technology are expensive and have replaced diagnostic and invasive procedures in some, but not all, cases. In some instances, new procedures are added to the plethora of available interventions. Competition between providers to have prestige services, duplicating a service that may not be needed in the geographic area but that may be attractive for network selection, is subsidized, in effect, by patients and their insurers. Other causes of high health care costs are the federal tax policy that holds employer contributions tax exempt and individual medical expenses above a certain percent tax deductible. Employees are encouraged to use deductible medical expenses and take additional income as a health insurance benefit.

Health care expenditures are currently slightly over 1 trillion dollars annually, up from 700 billion dollars in 1990. Per capita expenditures are approximately $4000 per annum. The public-sector share in bearing the costs of reimbursement is approximately 47%, an overall increase of 5% since 1989. The annual increase in public-sector spending is slightly over 9% and is, in fact, slowing down each year. Debate continues as to whether the dip in total health care expenditures in the early 1990s was real or a bookkeeping artifact related to the distribution of costs and expenditures. Those who felt that health care costs actually did go down attribute it to the growing number of uninsured citizens going without health care; the early effects of capitated health services delivery contracts negotiated between employers, providers (hospitals, physicians), and managed care organizations; the Balanced Budget Act of 1997, and federal efforts to combat fraud and abuse. However, the average annual growth in private sector costs is now creeping upward; at 12% during 1975–1989, private sector costs dipped to as low as 4.8% in 1997 and were 6.9% in 1998. In addition, there is upward pressure on insurance premiums and higher out-of-pocket costs for prescription medications, particularly among the elderly.

Overall, health care spending was 13.5% of the GDP in 1998, the smallest claim of health spending on national resources in 5 years. Analysts suggest that this is probably due to employer pressure on employees to select lower cost managed care plans, low general and medical-specific inflation, voluntary price caps imposed by some providers out of concern about health care reform cost containment, and excess capacity of some providers, such as hospitals, that forced them to seek managed care contracts with subsequent downward pressure on prices.

The quality of health care delivered is not the same as quality of health achieved. Patients and providers do not necessarily have the same notion of quality. For example, quality can be construed as being pain and symptom free, a successful surgery, return to work, the relationship with the provider, absence of nosocomial infection, no medication errors, and so on. In a sense, the question is, how much quality do you get for the dollar spent? Cost-effective analysis (CEA) looks at whether the same level or type of outcome can be achieved with different cost inputs, as for example, staffing models. However, CEA makes implicit value assumptions about quality about which the public may not agree.

Rationing and the Compression of Morbidity

A nurse at the bedside, in the clinic, on a home visit, and in executive management makes decisions about the allocation of finite resources. At the level of policy choice and output, resource allocation decisions can be construed as what it is reasonable for the old to demand of the young, or conversely, what the young are obligated to provide the elderly. The allocation of scarce resources is, perhaps, more a moral than a medical or scientific decision. All health care systems ration care and rationalize their decisions. Rationing to control costs and resource use draws on notions of the meaning of health, the value of life, quality of life, imminence of death, and futility.

Setting limits on the medical goals for the elderly is based on the premise that medical interventions should not be used to simply extend the life of the elderly but should be used for "achievement of a natural and fitting life span and thereafter for the relief of suffering" (Callahan, 1987, p. 53) and the prevention of premature aging. The mere suggestion that a segment of society should receive less medical care is reprehensible to most citizens. Furthermore, the proposal does not even begin to address what is a natural life span, quality of life, functionality, or cognition. Given the skepticism that many young employed citizens of this country have about the solvency of the Social Security system when they reach retirement age, it is unclear how willingly they will accept additional payroll taxation for benefits that are unlikely to be available to them. Intergenerational conflict about resource allocation is not characteristic of American society, although on a smaller scale, aging communities have voted down school and library budgets.

Age-related proposals for health care rationing presuppose scientific knowledge about the natural life span and that most elderly will live comfortably and healthily until some precipitating event ends their lives quickly. Furthermore, there is no assurance that money saved by rationing health care to one group would be spent wisely or effectively on services for another group (Daniels, 1986). The drive for cost containment should not cloud the fact that social health policy decisions will differentially affect the haves and the have-nots, and has racial and cultural implications.

The financing structure of Medicare and Medicaid encourages the shift to Medicare coverage and hospitalization, whether admitted from a nursing home or the community. Frequently cited data purport to indicate that a significant number of hospitalized elderly consume a disproportionate amount of Medicare dollars in their last year of life. Yet, subsequent analyses find that the number of Medicare beneficiaries receiving intensive life-sustaining technology is very small and would represent, had such care been withheld, a very small savings to the Medicare program. Watson, Bubolz, Lynn, and Teno (1998) simulated reduced hospitalization rates based on current use. They reported that savings from fewer hospitalizations were sufficient to purchase almost 50 home visits by nurses and still have funds remaining that could be used to purchase services for community-based residents with the greatest need. The growth in home and community-based waiver programs (Medicaid) and the increase in Medicare skilled home care benefits encouraged the phenomenal growth in home care expenditures: 28 billion dollars in 1995. Some HMOs developed innovative ways to care for those with chronic illnesses that the fee-for-service system was unable to construct or provide but might emulate (Fox, Etheridge, & Jones, 1998). At the same time, however, we need to be cautious about medicalizing home care to the point where both the client and the caregiver become victims of an albeit well-intentioned system.

The compression of morbidity paradigm posits reduction of overall morbidity and health care costs by virtue of shortening the time period between onset of old-age disability and the age of death. The theory suggests that delay in the onset of disability can be brought about by aggressive efforts toward disease prevention, health promotion, and reduction in health risks

(Fries et al., 1994; Vita, Terry, Hibert, & Fries, 1998). Data are still out as to how application of this theory would appear in practice and what exactly preventive practice would look like. Evidence about the degree of preventive care in managed and nonmanaged care practice remains equivocal.

NURSING ADVOCACY AND PUBLIC POLICY

Nursing is in a unique position to make valuable contributions to the health policy debate, decisions, and strategies for moving a program forward to goal achievement. In addition to the data generated by our drive for evidence-based practice, we can be the bearers of patients' words and feelings, words spoken directly to us. This is information power, a power that other health care professionals do not have because they are not with the patient 24 hours a day. Just as patient's words and conditions influence our actions to achieve their care goals, our words and actions are a base of power to influence health care policy goals.

The President's Commission (1983) on access to health care articulated principles that remain as cogent now as then and can inform and guide the nursing profession's approach to health care policy. The Commission concluded that American society is ethically obligated to provide equitable access to health care based on a special understanding of health care in "relieving suffering, preventing premature death, restoring functioning, and increasing opportunity" (p. 4). In addition, the Commission felt that equitable access to an adequate level of health care should be possible without imposition of excessive burdens. Adequate care was construed as a "floor" below which no one should fall, "not a ceiling above which no one could rise" (p. 4). Ultimate responsibility for ensuring that society met its obligation resides with the government, even if the process is a combination of public and private arrangements. In the Commission's view, cost-containment measures that increased existing inequalities or were barriers to the achievement of equity were morally unacceptable (Williams, 1986).

Practical decision-making in the political arena "seeks the right decision for *this* issue in *this* political climate at *this* time" (Stevens, 1985, p. 19). American history tells us that we should not expect dramatic breakthroughs and major changes in health care delivery; we tend to proceed by evolution, not revolution. Systems seek homeostasis and will tolerate small changes rather than resist them, as it would a major innovation. Political systems that rely on democratic processes tend to seek and accept only those changes that are acceptable to the majority of its citizens. There is historic tension between the "experts" and the "common man," but the nurse advocate is in the unique position of occupying both roles; we are providers as well as patients in the pursuit of our own health status goals.

Power is the ability to influence others to achieve goals; it includes coaching, mentoring, teaching, and facilitating. Five key power bases are coercive, reward, legitimate, referent, and expert power (French & Raven, 1957). Coercive power is based on fear, the ability to punish or withhold what is desired, whereas reward power is the ability to grant what is valued, such as, money, material, information, and connections. Legitimate power is positional; power is ascribed to the holder of an accepted position or status in an organization or group. Referent and expert power are personal, achieved powers. Expert power means that an individual has the knowledge and skills that are needed by others. Referent power generally means personality characteristics that others would like to emulate. Two additional power bases emerged with the explosion of information and communication technologies. Information power, as noted previously, is the possession of selected information desired by others. Network or connection power is the association with or access to people perceived as powerful or who can help achieve goals. Nurses have been politically active for years; yet, the notion that we have power and have used it is an uncomfortable image for some nurses.

Participation in Public Policy

Drawing on the work of Kalisch and Kalisch (1982), Yoder-Wise (1999) described four levels of political activism. "Apathetics" belong to no professional association nor do they serve on any committee at the workplace; if they are on a committee, they are unproductive. "Spectators" belong to one or more associations, rarely if ever go to a meeting or serve on a committee, and only occasionally read an article about trends or issues in nursing and discuss it with a colleague. "Transitionals" are actively involved in an association, attend meetings, are knowledgeable about and discuss nursing issues with colleagues, and assume leadership roles at work and in their professional organizations. The highest level of activist, the "gladiator," has a leadership role in state and national professional associations. A nurse at the transitional or gladiator level characterizes the mature professional concerned about health care delivery beyond the confines of the setting.

Cohen and colleagues (1996) conceptualized a framework of the political development of the nursing profession that is useful for looking back at our accomplishments and forward to our strategies for goal achievement. Four stages are described on four parameters: the activity associated with the stage, language used, coalition building, and "nurses as policy shapers" (p. 260). A professional organization, group, or individual can be in more than one stage of political development at the same time; there can be movement back and forth between stages, and activities inherent in one stage can or should be carried into a later stage. In looking at the four stages—"buy-in," "self-interest," "political sophistication," and "leading the way"—what begins as a reactive focus on nursing issues widens into a focus on health issues and then to social policy issues that include health care among them. Language development moves from learning political language and presentation that is understood by non-nurses in the policy debate to articulate reconceptualization of the policy concern. Tentative participation in nurse-based coalitions matures to participation in broader health groups, such as a national multidisciplinary task force, to creating coalitions with non-nursing organizations that share nursing's health policy concerns. As policy shapers, nursing professionals begin to be sought for key health policy positions because nursing expertise and knowledge can initiate health policy ideas.

Different groups have power or dominion over different policy ideas. Establishing an agenda for health care is quintessentially political; "control of the agenda gives substantial control over ultimate policy choices" (Peters, 1986, p. 42). The fourth stage described by Cohen et al. (1996), "leading the way," is grounded in the firm belief that nursing values such as health promotion, self-directed care, holism, and cultural competency need to be at the policy table precisely because no other interest group represents citizens' health care beliefs and wishes.

Health-policy activism on an individual, group, and organizational basis is achieved by developing written and oral communication skills, networking, coalition building, collegiality and collaboration with other health professions, and building a constituent base from the local citizenry. Nursing leadership development and health-policy studies should be part of the required undergraduate nursing curriculum and a core component of graduate nursing education, regardless of nursing specialty. Ongoing policy research on the interrelationship between policy, nursing practice, and patient outcomes is vital to nursing's ability to influence the agenda for health care delivery. In addition, we must use and press for (if not conduct ourselves) health services research for information on what works and when, where, and at what cost in order to inform our vision and goals for the organization and financing of health care.

CONCLUSION

In those countries with universal access to health care, mortality continues to be linked to socioeconomic status (SES); higher income is associated with greater longevity. Health services research in the United States indicates that the difference in health outcomes between rich and poor is far greater than race or ethnic differences; the disparity in mortality between rich and poor is based on SES. Not having at least a high school education is associated with greater morbidity and mortality than for those with a high school education or some college. This tells us two things: economic and social policies should consider the health consequences of enactment, and health status involves more than the delivery of health care. History notes the significant decline in mortality among those age 65 to 85 in the years following passage of the Social Security Amendment in the 1940s, guaranteeing a basic income to those older than 65.

Healthy People 2010 (HP2010) is a guide to better health that was developed and supported by "partners" from state and federal government, business and industry, communities, and more than 350 national health professional organizations, including nursing. Among the goals of this 10-year national program are to increase the quality and years of healthy life, reduce avoidable morbidities, and lessen disparities due to race and culture in health care access. Leading health indicators of HP2010 include physical activity, overweight and obesity, tobacco use, substance abuse, responsible sexual behavior, mental health, injury and violence, environmental quality, immunization, and access to health care. The goals of HP2010 are congruent with those of the nursing profession and are the basis of educational efforts by federal, state, and other health plans to reach out to our diverse citizenry and make a difference in disease prevention and health promotion. The potential and power of nurses to contribute to the development of a more humane and responsive health care system—recognizing that health status is more than the delivery of health care, per se—is our ethical obligation to society as surely as we are obligated to advocate for and "be with" our patients.

REFERENCES

American Nurses Association. (1991). *Nursing agenda for health care reform.* Kansas City, MO: American Nurses Association.

Berk, M. L., & Schur, C. (1998). Measuring access to care: Improving information for policymakers. *Health Affairs, 17* (1), 180–186.

Callahan, D. (1987). *Setting limits. Medical goals in an aging society.* New York: Simon & Shuster.

Cantor, J. C., Long, S. H., & Marquis, M. S. (1998). Challenges of state health reform: Variation in ten states. *Health Affairs, 17* (1), 191–200.

Cochran, C. E., Mayer, L. C., Carr, T. R., & Cayer, N. J. (1999). *American public policy. An introduction* (6th ed.). New York: Worth Publishers.

Cochran, C. L., & Malone, E. F. (1995). *Public policy: Perspectives and choices.* New York: McGraw-Hill.

Cohen, S. S., Mason, D. J., Kovner, C., Leavitt, J. K., Pulcini, J., & Sochalski, J. (1996). Stages of nursing's political development: Where we've been and where we ought to go. *Nursing Outlook, 44,* 259–266.

Daniels, N. (1986). Why saying no to patients in the United States is so hard: Cost containment, justice and provider autonomy. *New England Journal of Medicine, 314,* 1380–1383.

Diers, D. (1985). Policy and politics. In D. Mason & S. Talbott (Eds.), *Political action handbook for nurses.* Menlo Park, CA: Addison-Wesley.

Fox, P. D., Etheridge, L., & Jones, S. B. (1998). Addressing needs of chronically ill persons under Medicare. *Health Affairs, 17,* 144–151.

French, J., & Raven, B. (1957). The bases of social power. In D. Cartwright (Ed.), *Studies in social power.* Ann Arbor: University of Michigan, Institute for Social Research.

Fries, J. F., Koop, C. E., Sokolov, J., Beadle, C. E., & Wright, D. (1998). Beyond health promotion: Reducing health care costs by reducing need and demand for medical care. *Health Affairs, 17,* 70–84.

Johnson, H., & Bender, D. S. (1996). *The System. The American way of politics at the breaking point.* New York: Little, Brown.

Kalisch, B. J., & Kalisch, P. A. (1982). *Politics of nursing.* Philadelphia: J. B. Lippincott.

Peters, B. G. (1986). *American public policy: Promise and performance* (2nd ed.). New York: Chatham House.

President's Commission for the Study of Ethical Problems in Medicine and Biomedical and Behavioral Research. (1983). *Securing access to health care: The ethical implications of differences in the availability of health services* (Vol 1). Government Printing Office, No. 040-000-00472-6. Washington, DC: Government Printing Office.

Sapolsky, M., Aisenberg, J., & Monroe, J. A. (1987). The call to Rome and other obstacles to state-level innovation. *Public Administration Review, 47,* 135.

Sparer, M. (1998). Devolution of power: An interim report card. *Health Affairs, 17* (3), 7–16.

Stevens, B. (1985). Nursing, politics, and policy formulation. In R. Wieczorek (Ed.), *Power, politics and policy in nursing.* New York: Springer.

Vita, A. J., Terry, R. B., Hibert, H. B., & Fries, J. F. (1998). Aging, health risks, and cumulative disability. *New England Journal of Medicine, 338,* 1035–1041.

Watson, J. H., Bubolz, T. A., Lynn, J., & Teno, J. (1998). Can we afford comprehensive, supportive care for the very old? *Journal of the American Geriatrics Society, 46,* 829–832.

Watson, K., & Gold, S. D. (1997). The other side of devolution: Shifting relationships between state and local governments [On-line]. *The Urban Institute* Available: http://newfederalism.urban.org

Williams, C. A. (1986). Policy issues. In T. T. Fulmer & M. Walker (Eds.), *Critical care nursing of the elderly patient.* New York: Springer.

Wilcox-Gok, V., & Rubin, J. (1994). Health insurance coverage among the elderly. *Social Science and Medicine, 38,* 1521–1529.

Yoder-Wise, P. S. (1999). *Leading and managing in nursing.* St. Louis: Mosby.

Index